The Neuropsychiatry of Headache

The Neuropsychiatry of Headache

Edited by

Mark W. Green, MD

Professor of Neurology, Anesthesiology, and Rehabilitation Medicine, and Director of Headache and Pain Medicine,
Mount Sinai School of Medicine, New York, USA

Philip R. Muskin, MD

Professor of Clinical Psychiatry, Columbia University College of Physicians and Surgeons, Chief of Service: Consultation-Liaison Psychiatry, New York-Presbyterian Hospital,
Columbia University Medical Center, Faculty: Columbia University Psychoanalytic Center for Research and Training, New York, USA

CAMBRIDGE
UNIVERSITY PRESS

CAMBRIDGE UNIVERSITY PRESS
Cambridge, New York, Melbourne, Madrid, Cape Town,
Singapore, São Paulo, Delhi, Mexico City

Cambridge University Press
The Edinburgh Building, Cambridge CB2 8RU, UK

Published in the United States of America by Cambridge University Press, New York

www.cambridge.org
Information on this title: www.cambridge.org/9781107026209

First published 2013

Printed and bound in the United Kingdom by the MPG Books Group

A catalogue record for this publication is available from the British Library

Library of Congress Cataloguing in Publication data
The neuropsychiatry of headache / edited by Mark W. Green, Philip R. Muskin.
p. ; cm.
Includes bibliographical references and index.
ISBN 978-1-107-02620-9 (Hardback)
I. Green, Mark W. II. Muskin, Philip R.
[DNLM: 1. Headache. 2. Comorbidity. 3. Headache Disorders. WL 342]
616.8′491–dc23
2012037118

ISBN 978-1-107-02620-9 Hardback

Contents

Color plates are situated between pp. 72 and 73.

Contributors

Carolyn B. Britton MD
Columbia University,
Neurological Institute,
New York, USA

Dawn C. Buse, PhD
Montefiore Medical Center,
Bronx NY and Albert Einstein College of Medicine,
Bronx, NYC, USA

Rabin Chandran, MD
Associate Professor of Family Medicine
Warren Alpert Medical School of Brown University
and Memorial Hospital of RI,
Pawtucket, USA

Eric D. Collins
Department of Psychiatry,
New York-Presbyterian Medical Center,
New York, USA

Robert P. Cowan, MD FAAN
Department of Neurology,
Stanford University Medical Center,
Stanford, CA, USA

Mark W. Green, MD
Professor of Neurology, Anesthesiology, and Rehabilitation Medicine, and Director of Headache and Pain Medicine, Mount Sinai School of Medicine
New York, NY, USA

Elizabeth Haase, MD
Department of Psychiatry Columbia University
New York, NY, USA

Margaret E. M. Haglund, MD
Columbia University/New York State Psychiatric Institute Department of Psychiatry, NY, USA

Filza Hussain, MBBS
Psychosomatic Fellow,
Columbia University,
New York, USA

Robert G. Kaniecki, MD
Department of Neurology,
University of Pittsburgh,
Pittsburgh, PA, USA

Mallika Lavakumar, MD
Fellow in Psychosomatic Medicine,
Columbia University Medical Center,
New York, USA

Samuel Lieblich, MBBS
Registrar in Psychiatry University of Melbourne
Royal Melbourne Hospital
Melbourne
VIC, Australia

Richard B. Lipton, MD
Montefiore Medical Center,
Bronx NY and Albert Einstein College of Medicine,
Bronx, NYC, USA

Sander Markx, MD, PhD
Department of Psychiatry,
Columbia University Medical Center,
New York, USA

Kathleen Mullin, MD
Department of Neurology, Mount Sinai School of Medicine,
New York, NY, USA

Philip R. Muskin, MD
Professor of Clinical Psychiatry,
Columbia University College of
Physicians and Surgeons,
Chief of Service: Consultation-Liaison Psychiatry,
New York-Presbyterian Hospital,
Columbia University Medical Center,
Faculty: Columbia University
Psychoanalytic Center for
Research and Training,
New York, USA

Justin M. Nash, PhD
Associate Professor of Family Medicine and Psychiatry and Human Behavior, Warren Alpert Medical School of Brown University and Memorial Hospital of RI,
Pawtucket, USA.

Maurice Preter, MD
Assistant Professor of Clinical Psychiatry, Columbia University College of Physicians and Surgeons and Adj. Associate Professor of Neurology,
State University of New York,
Downstate Medical Center,
New York, USA

Lucy Rathier, PhD
Clinical Assistant Professor of Psychiatry and Human Behavior,
Warren Alpert Medical School of Brown University and The Miriam Hospital,
Providence,
USA

Peter A. Shapiro, M.D.
Professor of Clinical Psychiatry, Columbia University,
New York, USA

C. Mark Sollars, MS
Montefiore Medical Center,
Bronx NY, USA

Nomita Sonty, Ph.D, M.Phil
Division of Pain Medicine,
Department of Anesthesiology,
Columbia University,
NY, USA

Preface

Headaches run the gamut from an annoying experience to a symptom of a life altering disorder. While "Not tonight dear, I have a headache," may exist in the common parlance, this statement points to the complex interaction between biology and psychology in the experience of a headache. Psychiatric syndromes are commonly comorbid with headaches. Therefore, any practitioner treating one disorder is likely to encounter the other. There is a well-documented bidirectional influence on the treatment of these disorders; however, it is not always a positive influence. Understanding the complexities of how the conditions and their management influence each disorder is key to a successful treatment outcome of the patient's suffering.

This book is directed towards practicing neurologists, psychiatrists, psychologists, and others involved in the care of headache sufferers. We have brought specialists together from a wide variety of disciplines in order to address the dramatic complexity of the headache sufferer.

We would like to thank the chapter authors who have contributed important information relevant to the care of these individuals. They have given generously of their time, their knowledge, and their clinical expertise to guide practitioners in understanding and treating this diverse patient population.

Mark W. Green, MD and
Philip R. Muskin, MD

Chapter 1

Epidemiology of the psychiatric comorbidities of headache

Kathleen Mullin, Dawn C. Buse, C. Mark Sollars, and Richard B. Lipton

"Comorbidity" refers to the occurrence of two conditions in the same individual at a frequency greater than would be expected by chance. [1] Migraine is comorbid with a number of medical, neurologic, and psychiatric disorders. Examples of medical comorbidities include asthma, [2] coronary heart disease, [3] and chronic pain disorders. [4–7] Neurologic comorbidities include stroke and epilepsy, [8] and psychiatric comorbidities include anxiety, depression, panic disorder, and bipolar disorder. [9,10,]

Comorbidities are best studied in representative samples because the prevalence of disease and the association among disorders is sometimes altered in clinic-based samples. This phenomenon, known as Berkson bias, can lead to under-estimates or over-estimates of the rates of co-occurrence for various disorders. Berkson bias arises when patterns of symptoms influence patterns of care seeking for a range of medical disorders. For example, someone with migraine and depression may be more likely to seek medical care with complaints of head pain and sadness than someone who experiences only one of these disorders. Clinic-based studies of comorbidities are useful for generating hypotheses about comorbidities and for characterizing patient groups. They cannot be relied upon to determine if two conditions are actually occurring together with frequency greater than chance.

Both clinic and population studies suggest that migraine is comorbid with a number of psychiatric disorders including depression, [11,12] anxiety [11,13,14] posttraumatic stress disorder, [15] chronic pain, [6] fibromyalgia, [16] and other medical disorders such as asthma. [2] In addition, rates of a number of comorbid conditions increase with the frequency of migraine attacks, and are higher for episodic migraine (EM) than for chronic migraine (CM). In the American Prevalence and Prevention (AMPP) study, persons with CM ($n = 655$) are about twice as likely than persons with EM (11,249) to have depression, anxiety, and various chronic pain disorders. [2] Respiratory disorders including asthma, bronchitis, and COPD, and cardiac risk factors including hypertension, diabetes, high cholesterol, and obesity are significantly more likely to be reported by those with CM.

The broad range of comorbidities associated with headache, and the increasing risk of comorbidity with headache frequency, have important implications for healthcare professionals. Research indicates comorbidities negatively impact headache-related disability and health-related quality-of-life, further justifying an enhanced understanding of co-existing conditions to inform clinical practice.

This chapter focuses on the psychiatric comorbidities of migraine and other headache disorders. The nature of epidemiologic research, the importance in differentiating between population and clinic-based studies, the clinical relevance of comorbidity, and the potential mechanisms that link migraine to its psychiatric comorbidities are discussed. Several key studies are examined as to what they reveal about psychiatric comorbidities and headache disorders.

Epidemiology

Epidemiology is the study of the distribution and determinants of health-related states or events in human populations and its application to the prevention and control of health problems. [17,18] Broadly, epidemiologists focus on populations and the collective health of a community, whereas clinicians focus on the health of individual patients assessed one at a time. The

The Neuropsychiatry of Headache, ed. Mark W. Green and Philip R. Muskin. Published by Cambridge University Press.

population focus makes it easier to study risk factors and protective factors for illness. The developmental perspective includes understanding the natural history of a condition within a population, over time, as well as over the lifespan of an individual. The developmental perspective takes into account the rate of onset or incidence of a condition and the average duration of a condition as well as its natural progression.

Epidemiology not only involves the study of the distribution of health-related states or events in human populations; epidemiologists also provide data for directing public health action. [19] Results of epidemiologic studies can provide public health officials with information about who is at greatest risk for disease, where the disease is most common, when the disease occurs most frequently, and what public health programs might be most effective. This information can then lead to more efficient resource allocation and programs designed to educate, prevent, and control disease spread. The results of epidemiologic studies provide a wealth of information that goes beyond the individual patient at a particular point in time to provide a more comprehensive understanding of disease processes.

Epidemiologists use a variety of study designs to identify the distribution, determinants, and natural history of disorders in populations. Cross-sectional studies are often performed to document disease prevalence, or the number of people afflicted with a given disease at a single point in time. [20] Although these studies provide insight into communities at risk, they do not illuminate etiology. Cross-sectional studies are useful for documenting comorbidity, but leave many questions unanswered. Case-controlled studies identify persons with the disorder (cases) and persons without (controls) and attempt to elucidate exposures that precede the onset of the disease. These exposures can include environmental or genetic factors or the occurrence of a comorbid disorder. This study design is particularly useful in studying rare diseases and serves as a good first step in trying to identify a cause/effect relationship. If the identified cases have headaches, the case control design can determine if a comorbid condition is associated with an increased rate of migraine onset but not the converse. The principal limitation of the case control design is recall bias.

Prospective or cohort studies measure host and environmental factors at a time zero and then follow subjects over time to elucidate factors which predict onset of disease. Temporal relationships can be established and confounders can be more easily controlled. However, prospective studies are more costly and, due to a long follow-up period, more sensitive to subject attrition. [18] If the cohort includes persons with and without migraine, the rate of disease onset in persons with migraine can be determined. To establish a bidirectional relationship, both persons with migraine and the comorbidity need to be sampled in order to determine the rate of onset of each disorder in those who have the other disorder.

Once a relationship is demonstrated, experimental research (i.e., randomized clinical and preventative trials) may be useful. For the study of comorbidity itself, randomized trials are not possible. One can assess the influence of the comorbidity on prognosis and determine if treating migraine improves the outcomes for the comorbid disorder, and if treating the comorbid disorder improves migraine outcomes. The experimental design allows investigators to measure the effect of a manipulated independent variable on outcome measures. For study accuracy, attention must be paid to standardization, replicability, and control. [21] Most clinical trials have a control group, which does not receive the experimental treatment, randomization in which the subjects are assigned to control or treatment group without bias, and blinding of the examiners to the status of each participant as experimental or control subject.

Methodological issues may limit studies. It is imperative, when investigating a possible diagnostic relationship, that consistent diagnostic criteria be established and utilized reliably. Unfortunately, a great portion of the studies done to investigate migraine comorbidities were performed prior to the establishment of the International Headache Society Criteria, which limits their validity. Studies must be adequately powered and bias must be limited. The ideal study for investigating a potential comorbid relationship is a bidirectional, population-based study of incidence, where a population that has only migraine is followed over time to assess whether or not they develop a second diagnosis. Concurrently, a sample with a diagnosis of interest is followed over time to see if they develop migraine.

Psychiatric comorbidities in headache

Several large-scale population-based studies have confirmed clinicians' longstanding suspicions: depressive and anxiety disorders are more prevalent in patients with headache. [22] Thus far, clear associations have been established between migraine and Major Depression, anxiety disorders, posttraumatic stress disorder (PTSD), substance abuse, bipolar disorder, suicide attempts, and childhood maltreatment and abuse. [23] Much research involving migraine and mood disorders, including numerous prospective, large-scale, population-based studies, have focused on depression. Population-based studies examining the prevalence of depression in migraine patients report ranges from 3.8% to 57.0% compared with the general population lifetimes', rates of 16%. [13, 24–27]

Additionally, anxiety disorders have been found to be significantly associated with migraine in both clinical and community-based studies. When anxiety disorders are further broken down into Generalized Anxiety Disorder and Panic Disorder, both conditions are found independently to have a higher prevalence in patients that suffer from migraines. A population-based study done by Breslau *et al.* in 1991 finds that anxiety disorder is almost twice as likely to be diagnosed in migraineurs than in the general population (> 50% vs. 27% of the general population). [22] A three-fold increase in migraine prevalence in patients with bipolar spectrum disorders has been demonstrated. [28]

Tension-type headache frequently is complicated by comorbid psychiatric conditions as well. Rates of depression and anxiety disorders are significantly higher in this group than in the general population. [29] Other comorbid conditions may include personality disorders and bipolar disorder. However, the rates of these disorders among tension headache patients have not been as well studied. [30]

Chronic daily headache, defined as headache experienced 15 or more days a month, [31] has been associated with higher levels of anxiety and depressive disorders as well. [26] A clinic-based study performed by Juang *et al.* demonstrates that major depression and panic disorders are highly prevalent in patients with tension-type headache and migraine and that these associations are greater when the headaches are transformed to chronic. [13,32]

Patients with migraine and tension-type headache exhibit psychiatric illnesses at a disproportionately higher rate than individuals with no history of recurrent headache. [33,34] These comorbid relationships have been identified in epidemiological research as well as in clinical studies of treatment-seeking patients. [35] Other chapters of this book will outline further distinct psychiatric diagnoses and their relationship to the varying headache types in further detail.

Understanding the mechanisms of comorbidity

Several theories explain why two conditions appear to be associated. [36] Sometimes, the association may be a consequence of methodologic artifact such as Berkson bias as discussed above. If symptom features overlap, diagnostic confusion may lead to spurious associations. Sometimes there may be a unidirectional causal link, implying that the presence of one condition predisposes to another. [37] Shared environmental or genetic risk factors may account for the comorbidity. An underlying brain state may arise as a consequence of genetic or environmental factors and predisposes to the comorbid disorders. [36] (See Fig. 1.1.) For example, migraine and epilepsy have been found to be comorbid and both conditions can involve a transient altered level of consciousness. Additionally, transient ischemic attacks and migraine with aura both involve reversible focal neurologic deficits and these conditions have also been found to be comorbid.

Unidirectional causal models suggest that an index disease increases the risk of the comorbid disorder. The relationship between disorders, such as migraine and depression, may be unidirectional or bidirectional. As noted above, for migraine and depression, the association is bidirectional. Breslau and colleagues [38] assess the headache and depression status of 1007 young adults via interview using 1988 International Headache Society (IHS) criteria and NIMHS-DIS, respectively. Three and a half years later, 979 participants are re-interviewed. Persons with migraine (vs. those without) stand a greater risk for major depression (relative risk [RR], 3.2; 95% CI, 2.3–4.6). In addition, persons with major depression (vs. those without) stand a greater risk for migraine (RR, 3.1; (95% CI, 2.0–5.0). [38]

Breslau and colleagues [39] investigate the incidence of new-onset migraine as a function of baseline depression (and vice versa) during a 2-year follow-up period. At baseline, subjects are screened for depression and migraine and fall into one of the following headache groups: Migraine (n = 496), Severe headache (n = 151), or No history of severe headache (n = 539). The lifetime prevalence of depression at baseline is 42.1%, 35.8%, and 16.0% for the Migraine group, Severe headache group, and No history of severe headache group, respectively. In addition, analyses show that the incidence of new-onset depression is 10.5%, 5.1%, and 2.0% in the Migraine, Severe headache, and No history of severe headache groups, respectively. Further supporting the

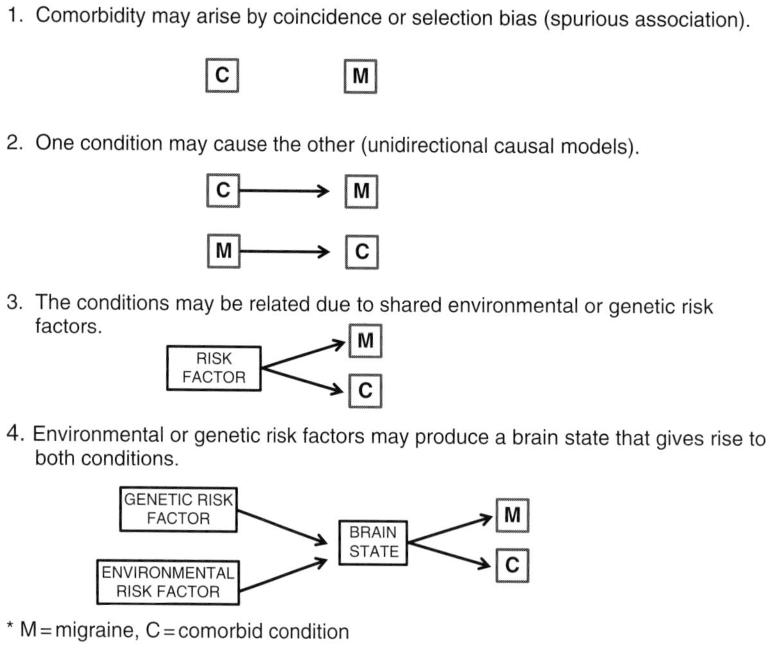

Fig. 1.1. Potential sources of comorbidity.

bidirectional causal model of comorbidity, the incidence of new-onset migraine is 9.3% in control subjects with a history of depression and 2.9% in controls without. No significant associations are found in either direction between other types of severe headache and major depression.

Shared environmental or genetic risk factors represent another possible explanation for the phenomenon of comorbidity. Merikangas and colleagues find a greater incidence of migraine in the relatives of probands with migraine (21%) vs. the relatives of persons without migraine (10%). In parallel, investigators find a greater incidence of depression in relatives of probands with depression (22%) vs. the relatives of persons without depression (10%). Given that little cross-transmission of migraine and depression between probands and relatives is found, these comorbidities may be due to non-genetic factors that aggregate within families. Therefore, investigators suggest that depression might be a pathological condition resulting from migraine or the diathesis, which results in both depression and migraine. [40]

In a separate longitudinal study, Merikangas and colleagues demonstrate a familial association between migraine and affective/anxiety disorders, although the rates of anxiety and depression are elevated only in conjunction with migraine (OR, 2.3; 95% CI, 1.29–4.0), indicating a syndromic relationship between migraine and affective/anxiety disorders. [28] Environmental and genetic risk factors may produce a latent brain state that precipitates co-existing conditions; that is, conditions share a pathophysiologic mechanism. For example, cortical excitability is seen in both migraine and epilepsy. Regarding migraine and mood disorders specifically, Burstein *et al.* propose that several brain areas, including the hypothalamic, limbic, and cortical regions, are activated during migraine. [41] Pain signals are conveyed through trigeminovascular projections to areas of the brain that are competent to produce migraine symptoms as well as depression. Consistent with this hypothesis, some researchers speculate that serotonergic and dopaminergic dysfunction underlies the comorbidity of depression and migraine. [42,43,44] Because altered levels of serotonin are often observed during migraine attacks, migraines are frequently treated with selective serotonin agonists (i.e., triptans). Experimental evidence suggests that persons with anxiety and persons with migraine have a polymorphism in the 5-HT transporter gene. [45] The established relationship between depression/anxiety and serotonergic dysfunction warrants speculation that the source of migraine and mood/anxiety disorder comorbidity is aberrant serotonin signaling. Moreover, migraine is often accompanied by dopaminergic symptoms such as nausea and vomiting. Experimental data reveal higher levels of dopamine receptors on peripheral lymphocytes of persons with migraine relative to controls, indicating a hypodopaminergic state in migraineurs. The link between dopamine deficiency and depression is equally well established. Thus, reduced dopamine levels may contribute to the comorbidity of depression and migraine.

Both migraine and depression may be mediated by the cascade of neuronal events associated with central sensitization and its clinical marker, allodynia. [46] Cutaneous allodynia (CA) is indicative of central sensitization, a state in which abnormally excited neurons cause a reduced pain threshold and hypersensitivity to noxious and innocuous stimuli alike. Lending additional support to the latent brain state model of comorbidity is the discovery that migraineurs with major depression (vs. those without depression) experience worse cutaneous allodynia (CA). Bigal and colleagues analyze data from 16 573 study participants with "severe headache" who completed the Allodynia Symptom Checklist (ASC-12) and the PHQ-9 for depression. The incidence of CA (as determined by ASC score ≥ 3) is 68.3% in persons with CM, compared with 63.2% in persons with EM ($P< 0.01$). Severe CA, (ASC score ≥ 9), was highest among persons with CM (28.5%) compared to those with EM (20.4%). In all persons with headache, regardless of type, the CA severity is highest among respondents who are depressed, with CM respondents having the highest ASC-12 sum scores. In adjusted analyses, depression has an incremental influence on the prevalence of CA. Compared to persons with no depression, persons with mild depression have a prevalence ratio (PR) of 1.22 (95% CI, 1.10–1.35). Persons with moderate depression and moderately severe depression are also more likely to have CA compared to those without depression (PR, 1.4; 95% CI, 1.23–1.58 and PR, 1.51; 95% CI, 1.34–1.96, respectively). The PR for CA is highest in those with severe depression (PR, 1.62; 95% CI, 1.34–1.96). [47]

The psychiatric comorbidities of headache are clinically important

Understanding the psychiatric comorbidities of headache is important for many reasons. [36,48] These comorbidities, particularly depression and anxiety, are extremely common in persons with migraine and have implications for diagnosis, treatment and our understanding of disease mechanisms. When conditions are comorbid, the usual principle of diagnostic parsimony (find a single unifying diagnosis that accounts for the patient's signs and symptoms) does not apply. Once a diagnosis of migraine has been established, it becomes more likely that psychiatric comorbidities are present, warranting a heightened index of suspicion.

The existence of comorbidities also has implications for treatment, creating opportunities and imposing limitations. Treatment choices should be informed by comorbid conditions. For example, treatment with a tricyclic antidepressant may benefit both disorders in a patient with migraine and depression, though undertreatment of depression is possible. Conversely, a known comorbid condition may impose therapeutic limitations. For example, depression is viewed as a relative contraindication for the use of beta-blockers in migraine.

Efforts to understand these relationships are informed by the directionality of association. In 1994, Breslau and colleagues demonstrate that there is a bidirectional relationship between depression and migraine, with each condition increasing the incidence of the other. [38] These bidirectional relationships challenge simple unidirectional causal models. For example, migraine is unlikely to be just a somatic manifestation of depression because migraine onset may precede depression onset. Conversely, depression is unlikely to be a consequence of recurrent episodes of unpredictable pain, a form of learned helplessness, because depression may precede migraine onset. The complexity is illustrated by a small, open-label pilot study showing that a treatment that reduces headache frequency without acting on the central nervous system (onabotulinum toxin A), also relieved depressive and anxious symptomology. [49] These findings further emphasize the need to recognize an underlying psychiatric condition prior to developing a treatment plan. Once comorbidity and its directionality are established, further investigations can clarify the shared pathophysiology of the disorders.

Comorbidities may also influence the clinical course and prognosis of migraine, potentially leading to increased migraine-related disability and impact, diminished health-related quality of life, and poor treatment outcomes. Psychiatric comorbidities can influence the frequency and severity of migraine, and impact disease prognosis, treatment, and clinical outcomes. [50,51] Some psychiatric comorbidities, including depression and anxiety, have been associated with increasing migraine attack frequency, or progression from episodic to chronic migraine. [12,14] Migraine can be conceptualized as a chronic disorder with episodic manifestations. [52] The clinical course is variable. Patients with migraine may remit spontaneously for unknown reasons, they may continue to have intermittent attacks for many decades, or they may develop a clinically progressive disorder characterized by attacks of increasing frequency at times leading to headaches on more days than not. Episodic migraine (EM) is defined as meeting ICHD-2 criteria for migraine with an average of 14 or fewer headache days per month. Chronic migraine (CM) is defined as headache on 15 or more days per month for at least 3 months. The process of developing CM from EM, sometimes termed "transformation" or "progression," occurs in approximately 2.5% of persons with EM annually. [53] Transformation is associated with various modifiable (e.g., medication overuse, BMI) and unmodifiable (e.g., traumatic brain injury) risk factors. Depression and anxiety may be modifiable risk factors for migraine progression. [12,14] Chronic migraine is associated with more substantial disability than episodic migraine in multiple ways. [54] Additionally, psychiatric conditions often affect the coping mechanisms of migraine patients, thereby increasing headache-related disability, reducing quality of life, and often making them more difficult to treat. [55] Jette *et al.* demonstrates in a population-based study that migraine in association with various mental health disorders results in poorer health-related outcomes compared with migraine or with a psychiatric condition alone. [56]

The occurrence of comorbidities may provide clues to mechanisms underlying disease based on environmental or genetic risk factors common to migraine and its coexisting conditions. Further investigations may clarify these mechanisms. For example, it is likely that the co-occurrence of depression and anxiety with migraine may reflect neurochemical alterations common to these disorders.

Conclusion

Headaches are comorbid with many psychiatric disorders including depression and anxiety. Rates of psychiatric comorbidity are even higher among persons with more frequent headache (i.e., CM). Although this elevated rate is confirmed in both population and clinic studies, it remains important to discriminate between these samples as they differ in significant ways. In addition, evidence indicates that co-existing conditions are associated with worse treatment outcomes, increased headache-related disability, and reduced health-related-quality-of-life, further underscoring the need to study and understand comorbidity.

The diagnosis, prognosis, and treatment of migraine are confounded by comorbid psychiatric disorders. The high rates of psychiatric comorbidity with migraine highlights the importance for healthcare professionals (HCPs) to maintain diagnostic vigilance and provide appropriate treatment or referrals when necessary. When comorbid psychiatric disorders are present, it is important to take all disorders into account in formulating a treatment plan and remain mindful of the negative impact that psychiatric disorders can place on treatment outcomes, adherence, and general quality of life. [57–59] Buse, Andrasik, and Sollars [60] and Maizels, Smitherman, and Penzien [61] review and provide suggestions in screening for psychiatric comorbidity among persons with headache.

Many theories exist to explain the associations. These include models of causal link, shared environmental and genetic factors, and latent brain state. Nonetheless, many questions remain unanswered. Additional research is needed to increase our understanding of these relationships and subsequently, to enhance our knowledge of the pathophysiology, directionality, and treatment of both headaches as well as their comorbid psychiatric conditions.

References

[1] Feinstein A. The pre-therapeutic classification of co-morbidity in chronic disease. *J Chronic Dis* 1970; **23**: 455–68.

[2] Aamodt AH, Stovner LJ, Langhammer A, Hagen K, Zwart JA. Is headache related to asthma, hay fever, and chronic bronchitis? The Head-HUNT Study. *Headache* 2007; **47**: 204–12.

[3] Cook NR, Bensenor IM, Lotufo PA, *et al.* Migraine and coronary heart disease in women and men. *Headache* 2002; **42**: 715–27.

[4] El Metwally A, Salminen JJ, Auvinen A, Kautiainen H, Marja Mikkelsson M. Prognosis of non-specific musculoskeletal pain in preadolescents: a prospective 4-year follow-up study till adolescence. *Pain* 2004; **110**: 550–9.

[5] Hestbaek L, Leboeuf-Yde C, Kyvik KO, *et al.* Comorbidity with low back pain: a cross-sectional population-based survey of 12- to 22-year-olds. *Spine* 2004; **29**: 1483–91.

[6] Hagen K, Einarsen C, Zwart JA, Svebak S, Bovim G. The co-occurrence of headache and musculoskeletal symptoms amongst 51,050 adults in Norway. *Eur J Neurol* 2002; **9**: 527–33.

[7] Von Korff M, Crane P, Lane M, *et al.* Chronic spinal pain and physical-mental comorbidity in the United States: results from the national comorbidity survey replication. *Pain* 2005; **113**: 331–9.

[8] Ottman R, Lipton RB. Comorbidity of migraine and epilepsy. *Neurology* 1994; **44**: 2105–10.

[9] Breslau N, Davis GC. Migraine, physical health and psychiatric disorder: a prospective epidemiologic study in young adults. *J Psychiatry Res* 1993; **27**: 211–21.

[10] Lanteri-Minet M, Radat F, Chautard M-H, Lucas C. Anxiety and depression associated with migraine: influence on migraine subjects' disability and quality of life, and acute migraine management. *Pain* 2005; **118**: 319–26.

[11] Zwart JA, Dyb G, Hagen K, *et al.* Depression and anxiety disorders associated with headache frequency. The Nord-Trondelag Health Study. *Eur J Neurol* 2003; **10**: 147–52.

[12] Ashina S, Buse DC, Manack AN, *et al.* Depression: a risk factor for migraine chronification: results from the American Migraine Prevalence and Prevention (AMPP) Study. *Neurology* 2010; 74(Suppl 2): A113. Presented at the 62nd Annual Meeting of the American Academy of Neurology, Toronto, Canada, April 12–17, 2010.

[13] Juang KD, Wang SJ, Fuh JL, Lu SR, Su TP. Comorbidity of depressive and anxiety disorders in chronic daily headache and its subtypes. *Headache* 2000; **40**: 818–23.

[14] Ashina S, Buse DC, Maizels M, *et al.* Self-reported anxiety as a risk factor for migraine chronification. results from The American Migraine Prevalence and Prevention (AMPP) study. *Headache* 2010; **50**(Suppl 1): S4. Presented at the 52nd Annual Scientific Meeting of the American Headache Society, Los Angeles, California, June 24–27, 2010.

[15] Peterlin BL, Tietjen G, Meng S, Lidicker J, Bigal M. Post-traumatic stress disorder in episodic and chronic migraine. *Headache* 2008; **48**: 517–22.

[16] Peres MF, Young WB, Kaup AO, Zukerman E, Silberstein SD. Fibromyalgia is common in patients with transformed migraine. *Neurology* 2001; **57**: 1326–8.

[17] Stedman's Medical Dictionary for the Health Professions and Nursing, 5th edn., New York: Lippincott: Williams & Wilkins, 2005.

[18] Gerstman BB. *Epidemiology Kept Simple: An Introduction to Classic and Modern Epidemiology.* Hoboken, John Wiley & Sons, 1998.

[19] Gordis L. *Epidemiology.* Philadelphia, WB Saunders Company, 1996.

[20] Merrill RM. *Introduction to Epidemiology*. Jones & Bartlett Learning, 2010.

[21] Rothman K, Greenland S. *Modern Epidemiology.* Hagerstown, MD, Lippincott-Raven; 1998.

[22] Merinkangas KR, Angst J, Isler H. Migraine and psychopathology. Results of Zurich cohort study of young adults. *Arch Gen Psychiatry* 1990; **47**: 849–53.

[23] American Psychiatric Association. *Diagnostic and Statistical Manual of Mental Disorders.* 4th edn. Washington, DC: American Psychiatric Press; 2000.

[24] Marazziti D, Toni C, Pedri S, *et al.* Headache, panic disorder and depression: comorbidity or a spectrum? *Neuropsychobiology* 1995; **31**: 125–9.

[25] Mitsikostas DD, Thomas AM. Comorbidity of headache and depressive disorders. *Cephalalgia* 1999; **19**: 211–17.

[26] Verri AP, Cechini AP, Galli C, Granella F, Sandrini G, Nappi G. Psychiatric comorbidity in chronic daily headache. *Cephalalgia* 1998; **18** Suppl 21: 45–9.

[27] Oedegaard K, Neckelmann D, Mykleton A, *et al.* Migraine with and without aura: association with depression and anxiety disorder in a population-based study. The HUNT Study. *Cephalalgia* 2005; **26**: 1–6.

[28] Merinkangas KR, Merinkangas JR, Angst J. Headache syndromes and psychiatric disorders: association and familial transmission. *J Psychiatry Res* 1993; **27**: 197–210.

[29] Heckman BD, Holroyd KA. Tension-type headache and psychiatric comorbidity. *Curr Pain Headache Rep* 2006; **10**: 439–47.

[30] Williams DE, Raczynski JM, Domino J, Davig HP. Psychophysiological and MMPI personality assessment of headaches: an integrative approach. *Headache* 1993; **3**: 149–54.

[31] Silberstein S, Lipton R, Dodick, D. *Wolff's Headache and Other Head Pain.* New York: Oxford University Press; 2008.

[32] Penacoba PC, Fernandez-de-las-Penas CF, Gonzalez-Gutierrez JL, Miangolarra-Page JC, Pareja JA. Interaction between anxiety, depression, quality of life and clinical parameters in chronic tension-type headache. *Eur J Pain* 2008; **12**: 886–94.

[33] Lipchik GL, Penzien DB. Psychiatric comorbidities in patients with headaches. *Semin Pain Med* 2004; **2**: 93–105.

[34] Lake AE, Rains JC, Penzien DB, Lipchik GL. Headache and psychiatric comorbidity: historical Context, clinical implications, and research relevance. *Headache* 2005; **45**: 493–506.

[35] Puca F, Genco S, Prudenzano MP, *et al.* Psychiatric comorbidity and psychosocial stress in patients with tension type headache from headache centers in Italy. The Italian Collaborative Group for the Study of Psychopathological Factors in Primary Headaches. *Cephalalgia* 1999; **19**: 159–64.

[36] Lipton RB, Silberstein SD. Why study the comorbidity of migraine? *Neurology* 1994; **44**: S4–S5.

[37] Merikangas KR, Stevens DE. Comorbidity of migraine and psychiatric disorders. *Neurol Clin* 1997; **15**: 115–23.

[38] Breslau N, Davis GC, Schultz LR, Peterson EL. Joint 1994 Wolff Award Presentation. Migraine and major depression: a longitudinal study. *Headache* 1994; **34**: 387–93.

[39] Breslau N, Lipton RB, Stewart WF, Schultz LR, Welch KM. Comorbidity of migraine and depression: investigating potential etiology and prognosis. *Neurology* 2003; **60**: 1308–12.

[40] Merikangas KR, Risch NJ, Merikangas JR, Weissman MM, Kidd KK. Migraine and depression: association and familial transmission. *J Psychiatry Res* 1988; **22**: 119–29.

[41] Burstein R, Jakubowski M. Neural substrate of depression during migraine. *Neurol Sci* 2009; 30 Suppl 1: S27–31.

[42] Barbanti P, Fabbrini G, Ricci A, *et al.* Migraine patients show an increased density of dopamine D3 and D4 receptors on lymphocytes. *Cephalalgia* 2000; **20**: 15–19.

[43] Ferrari MD, Saxena PR. On serotonin and migraine: a clinical and pharmacological review. *Cephalalgia* 1993; **13**: 151–65.

[44] Hamel E. Serotonin and migraine: biology and clinical implications. *Cephalalgia* 2007; **27**: 1293–300.

[45] Smitherman TA, Penzien DB, Maizels M. Anxiety disorders and migraine intractability and progression. *Curr Pain Headache Rep* 2008; **12**: 224–9.

[46] Finocchi C, Villani V, Casucci G. Therapeutic strategies in migraine patients with mood and anxiety disorders: clinical evidence. *Neurol Sci* 2010; **31** Suppl 1: S95–98.

[47] Bigal ME, Ashina S, Burstein R, Reed ML, Buse DC, Serrano D, *et al.* Prevalence and characteristics of allodynia in headache sufferers: a population study. *Neurology* 2008; **70**: 1525–33.

[48] Scher AI, Bigal ME, Lipton RB. Comorbidity of migraine. *Curr Opin Neurol.* 2005; **18**: 305–10.

[49] Boudreau GP, Grosberg BM, McAllister PJ, Sheftell FD, Lipton RB, Buse DC. Open-label, multicenter study of the efficacy and outcome of onabotulinumtoxin – a treatment in patients with chronic migraine and comorbid depressive disorders. 2nd European Headache and Migraine Trust International Congress – EHMTIC, 241, 2010.

[50] Heckman BD, Holroyd, KA, Himawan L, *et al.* Do psychiatric comorbidities influence headache treatment outcomes? results of a naturalistic longitudinal treatment study. *Pain* 2009; **146**: 56–64.

[51] Holroyd KA, Drew JB, Cottrell CK, Romanek KM, Heh V. Impaired functioning and quality of life in severe migraine: the role of catastrophizing and associated symptoms. *Cephalalgia* 2007; **27**: 1156–65.

[52] Haut SR, Bigal ME, Lipton RB. Chronic disorders with episodic manifestations: focus on epilepsy and migraine. *Lancet Neurol* 2006; **5**: 148–57.

[53] Lipton RB. Tracing transformation: chronic migraine classification, progression, and epidemiology. *Neurology* 2009; **72**: S3–7.

[54] Buse DC, Manack A, Serrano D, Turkel C, Lipton RB. Sociodemographic and comorbidity profiles of chronic migraine and episodic migraine sufferers. *J Neurol Neurosurg Psychiatry* 2010; **81**: 428–32.

[55] Lipton RB, Hamelsky SW, Kolodner KB, Steiner TJ, Stewart WF. Migraine, quality of life, and depression: a population-based case-control study. *Neurology* 2000; **55**: 629–35.

[56] Jette N, Patten S, Williams J, Becker W, Wiebe S. Comorbidity of migraine and psychiatric disorders – a national population-based study. *Headache* 2008; **48**: 501–16[0].

[57] Silberstein SD, Dodick D, Freitag F, *et al.* Pharmacological approaches to managing migraine and associated comorbidities – clinical considerations for monotherapy versus polytherapy. *Headache* 2007; **47**: 585–99.

[58] Buse DC, Andrasik F. Behavioral medicine for migraine. *Neurol Clini* 2009; **27**: 321–582.

[59] Buse DC, Rupnow MFT, Lipton RB. Assessing and managing all aspects of migraine: migraine attacks, migraine-related functional impairment, common comorbidities, and quality of life. *Mayo Clin Proc* 2009; **84**: 422–35.

[60] Buse DC, Andrasik F, Sollars CM. Headaches. In: Andrasik F, Goodie J, Peterson A, eds. *Biopsychosocial Assessment in Clinical Health Psychology: A Handbook.* New York: Guilford Press; 2012.

[61] Maizels M, Smitherman TA, Penzien DB. A review of screening tools for psychiatric comorbidity in headache patients. *Headache* 2006; **46**(Suppl 3): S98–109.

Chapter 2

Migraine

Mark W. Green

"Migraine" is a diagnosis used broadly by headache specialists to describe a phenotype, undoubtedly influenced by many genotypes yet to be identified. The main feature in common among these phenotypes is a low threshold for the development of headache among migraineurs. The International Classification of Headache Disorders, 2nd Edition (ICHD-2) [1] definitions for migraine are far more specific.

Background

The term "migraine" is a derivation of Galen's *hemicrania* that described a paroxymal disorder of severe hemicranial pain, vomiting, and photophobia often relieved by darkness and sleep. Hemicrania was corrupted into low Latin as *hemigranea* and *migranea* and eventually became *migraine*. However, the term led many practitioners to assume that migraine had to be associated with unilateral head pain; in fact it is commonly bilateral. When the condition is mild, many with this distribution come to be diagnosed as having *tension headache*.

Diagnosis and clinical features

Although many variations exist, migraine is typically a recurring headache syndrome associated with other neurological symptoms, frequent symptom-free intervals, and is commonly provoked by stereotyped triggers. Adult women are more commonly affected, while childhood migraine has a greater prevalence in boys.

Most migraine is without aura, accounting for 80% of attacks. This means that no focal neurological complaints precede or accompany attacks; however, prodromal symptoms commonly precede migraines, and the physiologic basis for this is poorly understood. Prodromes are not included in the ICHD-2 criteria for migraine diagnosis. These prodromal symptoms include yawning, food cravings (often for chocolate), mood changes including depression or euphoria, various gastrointestinal complaints involving diarrhea, cold hands and feet, and frequent urination. In Blau's review on prodromes in 1980, he wrote that "George Eliot felt 'dangerously well before an attack' and Sir John Forbes had an 'irresistible and horrid drowsiness'; Lady Conway ate her supper with a 'greedy appetite,' and DuBois Reymond's migraines were 'in general preceded by constipation'." [2]

IHS Criteria for Migraine without Aura

- At least five attacks
- Headache attacks lasting 4–72 hours
- Headache with at least two of the following:
  - Unilateral location
  - Pulsating quality
  - Moderate to severe pain
  - Aggravation of avoidance of physical activity
- During headache at least one of the following:
  - Nausea and/or vomiting
  - Photophobia and phonophobia
- Not attributed to another disorder

IHS criteria notwithstanding, migraine headache is not always unilateral and not always pulsatile. Osmophobia, aside from photophobia and phonophobia, is common with migraine but is not a criterion for the diagnosis according to the ICHD-2 guidelines. Although not specific, the worsening of migraine with activity is the most sensitive criterion. The term *photophobia* describes the experience of an uncomfortable sensation of glare when exposed to light and often includes the effect of light enhancing the pain of

The Neuropsychiatry of Headache, ed. Mark W. Green and Philip R. Muskin. Published by Cambridge University Press.

migraine, both of which have a different physiologic basis. [3] These features explain the behavior of a sufferer during a severe attack: lying still in bed in a dark and cool room.

20% of migraineurs have an aura and the ICHD-2 criteria are as follows:

Migraine with Aura

- At least two attacks fulfilling criteria B-D
- Aura consists of one of the following no motor weakness
  - Fully reversible visual symptoms including positive and or negative features
  - Fully reversible sensory symptoms including positive and or negative features
  - Fully reversible dysphasic speech disturbance
- At least two of the following
  - Homonymous visual symptoms and or unilateral sensory symptoms
  - At least one aura symptom develops gradually over 5 minutes and or different symptoms occur in succession over >5 minutes
- Headache fulfills criteria for migraine without aura
- Not attributed to another disease

Intl Classification of Headache Disorders: 2nd edn. *Cephalalgia.* 2004; 24 (Suppl 1): 26–27. The international Classification of Headache Disorders. 2nd ed. Cephalalgia. 2004; 24 (suppl 1): 1–160.

Auras are predominantly visual, and if sensory systems or language become impaired, these phenomena usually follow visual aura. A migraine aura emanating from the occipital lobe is commonly experienced as scintillation, often followed rapidly by a scotoma. Fortifications are also common. The aura may begin in the center of a homonomous field, commonly enlarge and move across the visual field over 20 minutes, migrating to the periphery of one visual field, and then resolving. Recognizing their anatomic location in the cortex, these phenomena can be calculated to move at 2–6 mm/minute. After the aura there is a prolonged period of inhibition. This demonstrates a pattern of positive symptoms followed by negative symptoms, key in recognizing the episode as a migraine aura (Fig. 2.1).

The symptoms of migraine vary widely between attacks. Many practitioners and sufferers report only severe attacks as migraine. Some patients have frequent milder attacks as well, reflective of their lowered threshold for headache.

Attacks are often triggered by internal or external factors or a combination of both. Internal factors include menstruation, stress, and relaxation following stress, and sleep deprivation or oversleeping. External factors can include various foods including alcohol, missing a meal, smoke, change in weather, and certain visual patterns or scents. [4] Migraineurs are often bothered by the use of an opticokinetic drum during a neurological examination. Vertigo and motion sickness are commonly associated with migraine, but motion can also be a trigger of an attack. Carsickness, particularly in children, is common. One study suggested that, in those having migraine with aura, light was a frequent trigger, and in women without aura, menstruation was a frequent trigger. [5] The Greek physician Paulus Aegineta in the sixth century AD wrote "each of these affections is a permanent pain of the head, liable to be increased by noises, cries, a brilliant light, drinking of wine or strong-smelling things which fill the head. Some feel as if the whole head were struck, and some as if one half, in which case the complaint is called hemicrania. When the affection is seated within the skull, the pain extends to the roots of the eyes, and when externally it spreads around the skull." The trigger does not define the headache in that there are no actual *stress headaches, rainy day headaches* or *menstrual headaches.*

Migraine auras commonly precede the headache, but can develop in association with head pain. Some sufferers develop auras without any associated head pain. These episodes are often referred to as "acephalic migraines" and are more common after the age of 40. C. Miller Fisher described them as "late-life migraine accompaniments" but they can occur in younger individuals. [6] If these are periodically associated with head pain, a migrainous diagnosis can be made with increased confidence.

Sensory auras can occur as well as dysphasia or motor weakness. They may appear sequentially; the common order is visual auras first, then sensory auras second. Positive followed by negative features are characteristic. In the visual system, this is usually a scintillation followed by a scotoma. In sensory auras, this generally means tingling followed by numbness.

Pathophysiology

If migraine is a phenotype caused by multiple genotypes, the question arises: what is the final common pathway that defines a migraine?

It is often useful to view a migraine as a low threshold for the development of headache. Mundane triggers,

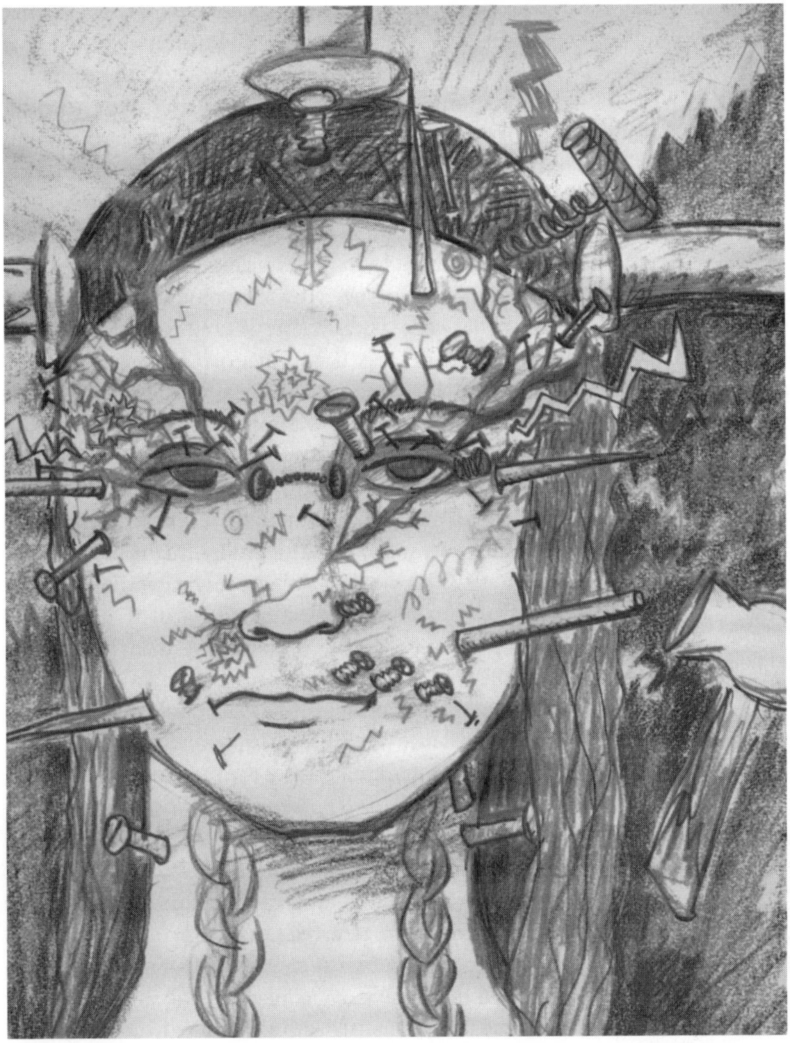

Fig. 2.1. Patient's drawing of their migraine.

which are innocuous to others, can initiate a paroxysm of events that lead to a migraine attack. Most headaches triggered by stress, weather change, modest amounts of alcohol, or menstruation, are migraines. Similar attacks can be induced by extraordinary triggers in most individuals who are not migraineurs.

In 1873, Liveing's publication *A contribution to the Pathology of Nerve Storms* recognized the similarity of migraine and epilepsy. K.S Lashley, a neuropsychologist who suffered from migraine with aura, charted his own fortification spectra. He calculated that his aura marched across his occipital cortex at a rate of 3 mm/minute. He also speculated that there was a leading edge involving an intense excitation of neurons, followed by a dramatic wave of inhibition of activity of the visual cortex.

Leão first described cortical spreading depression (CSD) in 1944. This was accidentally identified during experiments intended to trigger epilepsy. He then proposed that this was the biological basis of a migraine aura. [7] CSD involves a brief wave of activation of neurons and glia, followed by a wave of depression of neuronal activity, slowly propagating from the occipital lobe, although involving the cerebellum, hippocampus and other regions. It is associated with a profound increase in extracellular potassium and various neurotransmitters, with a subsequent increase in intracellular sodium and calcium. These ionic shifts are responsible for the DC potential shift that is recorded when this event is identified. This wave travels at 2–5 mm/minute. The term "cortical spreading depression" is unfortunate and might have better been described as "cortical spreading activation," as it is a positive wave spreading slowly across the cortex followed by a wave of inhibition. This wave of depolarization commonly originates in the occiput. The positive waves appear to correlate with the positive neurological complaints of scintillations and tingling; whereas the negative wave may explain the scotoma and numbness. Functional magnetic resonance imaging and magnetoencephalography have identified events in migraine, which are concordant with what Leão observed, providing further evidence for this theory.

It is this hyperexcitable cortex that may be the common thread between a migraineur and an individual with bipolar depression, anxiety and social phobias, and epilepsy. The hyperexcitability can be due to pathology such as inherited channelopathies, mitochondrial dysfunction involving energy metabolism, or locally or globally reduced levels of brain magnesium. Certainly, many other mechanisms are possible in the myriad genotypic forms of migraine.

This hyperexcitability can be demonstrated clinically. When individuals have a transcranial magnetic stimulator applied to the occipital scalp, all see phosphenes, bright lights similar to common visual migraine auras. Yet migraineurs, with and without aura, develop phosphenes at a much lower threshold than controls. [8] Dr. Hubert Airy observed the fortification spectra of migraine in the nineteenth century, stating that these resembled a "fortified town with bastions all around it," and "spectrum" suggested an apparition or specter. This hallucination involves enlarging serrated edges of a hallucinated C. If high contrast, angulated, flashing lines are presented to anyone, the primary visual cortex is activated. Migraineurs, when presented the same stimulus, develop activations of regions well beyond the primary visual cortex. [9] This process may be activating linear-detector neurons in the primary visual cortex, and will frequently trigger an attack. Migraineurs commonly dislike visualizing certain patterns with high contrast, including strobes and glare. When an opticokinetic drum is used in the examination of a migraineur, they report more illusions and dislike the procedure. Occipital cortical excitability, associated clinically with photophobia, can be detected on PET studies during a migraine and following treatment, even with resolution of the attack, but not interictally. [10]

Many practitioners were taught, or at least influenced by the theory of Dr. Harold Wolff. Wolff claimed that the aura of migraine was largely due to cerebral vasoconstriction and the headaches were due to cerebral vasodilatation. Graham and Wolff demonstrated that the administration of ergotamine reduced the amplitude of pulsations of the temporal artery and often reduced head pain. [11] It was assumed that the extracranial circulation was primarily responsible for headaches. All of this led to the development of vasoconstricting medications for the acute treatment of migraine. It is of interest that ergotamine tartrate, which is a potent arterial vasoconstrictor, was promoted for the acute treatment, whereas dihydroergotamine, a weak arterial vasoconstrictor, was largely ignored. Changes in cerebral blood flow are indeed seen with migraine. The hyperemia of CSD is associated with release of a variety of chemicals including potassium, ATP, and glutamate as well as others. By diffusing into the leptomeninges, CSD can activate cranial meningeal nociceptors, which are first-order trigeminal neurons. [12] The pulsatile quality of pain with a migraine might be due to these sensitized nociceptors detecting normal CSF pulsations, rather than the pulsations emanating from meningeal blood vessels. Another component of migraine pain can be due to dural plasma protein extravasation accompanied by a sterile neurogenic inflammation. [13] The "neurogenic inflammation" of the meninges is mediated through 5-HT1B receptors, and an inflammatory response involving plasma extravasation is mediated through 5-HT1D receptors. This leads to the release of a variety of proinflammatory agents including neurokinin A, calcitonin gene related peptide (CGRP), bradykinin, and prostanoids. This helps explain why a severe attack of migraine is so similar phenomenologically to an attack of meningitis with throbbing head pain, nausea, photophobia and phonophobia, and neck pain. Vasodilation does not appear to account for the pain of migraine. Vasoactive intestinal peptide (VIP), a transmitter involved in parasympathetic transmission, is a powerful cerebral vasodilator, but is not a migraine trigger. The blood flow changes might, to a large extent, reflect the metabolic response to a brain undergoing activation and depression of neuronal activity. It has been shown that blood vessels dilate ahead of CSD and vasoconstriction from CSD is unlikely to be the cause of an aura. [14]

In 1960 Kimball demonstrated that intravenous serotonin could terminate a migraine attack. [15] At the same time, there were unacceptable side effects, similar to those seen with a carcinoid syndrome. Later studies revealed that there are many serotonin receptors and that it was possible to alter brain serotonin more selectively. Triptans are agonists of presynaptic inhibitory 5-HT1B and 5-HT1D receptors, and some show affinity for the 5-HT1F receptor. However, blockers of neurogenic plasma protein extravasation alone, such as neurokinin-1 receptor antagonists, are not effective in the prophylaxis of migraine. Methysergide was said to be a "serotonin antagonist" and was an effective preventive antimigraine agent. Drugs causing serotonin release, such as SSRIs, can trigger headaches, and platelet serotonin levels are known to fall as a migraine attack begins. Until the release of triptans, however, this area of research was not very fruitful in producing effective preventive or acute migraine drugs.

PET imaging on a patient who fortuitously developed a migraine without aura while undergoing the study, showed the development of widespread cerebral changes. [16] It has been questioned whether this individual might have had an aura; but the changes extended far beyond what might have explained any minor visual disturbance, even if present. Other groups have imaged migraines with aura showing effects consistent with CSD. Abnormal brain stem activation with PET is also seen in migraine, in particular the dorsolateral midbrain and pons. [17] These regions are involved in modulating traffic from the cortex.

Although migraine is felt to be a neuronal condition, astrocytes are also involved. Astrocytes regulate the extracellular microenvironment of the brain normalizing levels of glutamate, potassium, and magnesium. These cells communicate via calcium waves. The spread of these waves is identical to the waves of CSD and, and like CSD, can be multifocal. [18] Therefore glia may be actively involved in the initiation and potentiation of CSD and communicate with neurons, each other, and endothelial cells. [19]

The changes in blood flow are complex and poorly understood. Typically there is an initial hyperemia of the brain followed by a prolonged oligemia. [20] Blood vessels in the brain may also be involved, not simply by responding passively to metabolic requirements of the brain during a paroxysm of cortical spreading depression, but possibly by signaling astrocytes and neurons.

It is of interest that migrainous auras typically begin in the occiput, in distinction to auras of epilepsy that commonly originate in the temporal lobe. It appears that some migraines may be derived from abnormalities in astrocytes. The occipital cortex has the lowest neuronal to glial ratio, which might cause a particular vulnerability for this region. Areas of the brain with a higher neuronal density appear to be less vulnerable to CSD.

Migraineurs commonly exhibit a variety of headaches, all of which are considered to be part of the "spectrum of migraine." Some of these differences may be due to epigenetic variations. Other differences are due to variable regions within the trigeminovascular system that become variably involved in the attacks. Migraineurs often discuss how their migraines start like *tension headaches*, then become *migraines*, or vice versa. The primary trigeminal afferents reside in the trigeminal ganglion. These are bipolar neurons, with a branch projecting into the pia and dura innervating blood vessels, and a branch projecting to the trigeminal nucleus caudalis. Cell bodies of the second-order trigeminovascular neurons are present in the upper cervical segments. The reported "tension headache" can be on the basis of pain referred through the trigeminal nucleus caudalis and its afferents, in the same way that angina can present with alternating chest pain, left arm pain, and jaw pain.

Migraines are frequently associated with autonomic symptoms of eye tearing and nasal congestion. This frequently leads to a misdiagnosis of migraines as "sinus headaches": a popular, but unscientifically based diagnosis made in the United States.

It is unclear whether frequent migraine attacks can lead to clinically relevant neurological dysfunction. Migraine appears to be associated with oxidative stress, and deposition in the midbrain is also associated with oxidative stress and correlates with the "burden of migraine." [21]

Other forms of migraine

Basilar migraine is an unusual form of migraine accompanied by impaired brainstem function. The common symptoms include vertigo, dysarthria, and diplopia. A mild or dramatic change in sensorium is frequently seen. All of these symptoms may persist for many minutes, like other migraine auras, and may be followed by a pulsatile occipital headache. Although this occurs at any age, it is difficult to diagnose with certainty in the elderly who are more likely to have posterior circulation ischemic attacks with associated headache. Hemiplegic migraine can occur sporadically or in families. The convincingly genetic forms of migraine are associated with hemiplegic migraine. Hemiparesis occurs at various stages of the attacks, and typically there is a contralateral head pain. The laterality varies with attacks. One gene for familial hemiplegic migraine maps to chromosome 19 in half of the families. Missense mutations are seen within the CANA1A gene, which encodes a P/Q type calcium channel subunit that is only seen within the brain. This leads to an increase in presynaptic calcium with subsequent elevations in glutamine, the most powerful excitatory amino acid, and ultimately precipitates the development of cortical spreading depression. Mutations of ATP1A2 gene encode a catalytic subunit of a sodium–potassium ATPase. This second form of hemiplegic migraine is highly comorbid with epilepsy. This trait is expressed primarily in astrocytes in adults, and likely causes an impairment of their ability to clear glutamate. It also provides evidence of the importance of glia in migraine pathogenesis. Some non-familial forms of hemiplegic migraine have the same genetic basis. A third type of familial hemiplegic migraine is caused by a mutation in the SCN1A gene, leading to a gain in function in the sodium channel which causes sodium influx into the neuron. This is also comorbid with epilepsy.

Ophthalmoplegic migraine is now considered to be a cranial neuralgia, rather than a variant of migraine.

Precipitating factors

The triggers of migraine are mundane; largely relevant because they can trigger attacks in migrainous individuals who possess a low threshold for the development of attacks. Through a variety of mechanisms, they all alter neuronal and possibly glial excitability.

Foods reported to be migraine triggers are vast, and often unscientifically based. Many contain tyramine, a product of fermentation. Wines and beers are often potent triggers, containing alcohol, histamine, tyramine, and sulfites. Red wine is more likely to trigger migraines than white wine as it contains higher levels of phenolic amines and histamine. Chocolate contains phenylethylamine. Citrus fruits contain phenolic amines. Processed meats may contain nitrites. Monosodium glutamate, often in high concentrations in many snack foods, is claimed to trigger migraine. Since glutamate in the brain is known to enhance CSD, this is plausible. Similarly, the artificial sweeter aspartame can trigger attacks, and aspartic acid is also a potent excitatory amino acid in the brain. Caffeine is a constituent of many over-the-counter migraine agents. Chronic overuse of caffeine, more than 200 mg daily, may increase headache frequency over time. Headaches may develop between uses from caffeine withdrawal.

Obesity is associated with an increase in migraine disability and frequency in both children and adults. [22] The connection may be due to proinflammatory mediators seen with obesity, which are capable of triggering migraine pain. Some examples are calcitonin gene-related peptides and cytokines. [23] Obese women can develop significant amounts of extraovarian estrogen synthesis from adipose tissue, which also can increase the risk of migraine, particularly migraine with aura. [24] Weight loss can improve migraines in such patients. Bariatric surgery in those who are morbidly obese can also be effective in improving migraines. [25] A disproportionate number of obese individuals have comorbid hypersomnia sleep apnea syndrome, which might increase the burden of headache. Migraine frequency is reduced in those treated with continuous positive airway pressure [26]; however, not all studies have supported a relationship of migraine and obstructive sleep apnea. [27]

Migraine treatment

There are three major approaches to the treatment of migraines. As migraine is frequently not properly diagnosed, treatments for "the headache" are often inappropriate and ineffective.

Non-medication therapies

The first approach involves non-medication therapies. Evidence-based guidelines support the use of cognitive behavior therapy. [28] Biofeedback typically involves autogenic training to elevate skin temperature and reduce electromyographic response. [29] Acupuncture, hypnosis, physical therapy, chiropractic manipulation, and massage have less evidence supporting their effectiveness in the treatment of migraines. Trigger management is also important when physician and patient understand which triggers are relevant in an individual's headache pattern.

Acute treatment

There are many agents available for the acute treatment of migraine. In the past, acute antimigraine agents were developed to be powerful arterial constrictors. Triptans, as well as ergot alkaloids, and some non-steroidal anti-inflammatory agents block plasma extravasation. They may also reverse vasoconstriction. Unfortunately, the therapeutic gain of existing agents is about 30% at 2 hours and absolute response may not exceed 70%. There is, therefore, significant room for improvement. [30]

Both the time that the headache takes to reach full intensity and the timing of nausea, if it occurs, are important treatment considerations. Migraineurs have been shown to have impaired gastric motility, even between attacks. [31] The presence of nausea likely further delays the absorption of oral agents. Since acute agents are far more effective if administered early in an attack, delays in absorption reduce efficacy and increase the chance that the headache will recur, even if originally improved by medication. Headaches that build very rapidly or with early nausea might require an agent administered parenterally or intranasally.

Many recent trial designs, beginning with the triptan studies, treated attacks only when the pain was moderate to severe. This might have been necessary to gain regulatory approval to treat moderate to severe attacks. In retrospect this paradigm often failed to produce a clear dose–response. Efficacy, in these protocols, was defined as going from moderate to severe headache to mild or no headache (a two-point drop). With early intervention, higher doses are typically more effective than lower doses, increase the chance that the subject will be pain free rather than suffer mild pain, and reduce the chance that the attack will recur within 24 hours. Furthermore, early treatment reduces side effects. [32] Because of the high cost of triptans and lack of availability of these agents, patients tend to delay treatment until the pain is severe. Commonly, more medication is required to terminate the attack, and side effects increase with this strategy. All of these facts are important to bring to patients' attention.

Non-steroidal anti-inflammatory medications, typically at high doses, can abort an attack, particularly if administered early. These agents have the advantage that they are safely used in individuals with vascular disease, unlike triptans and ergots. They also have none of the psychoactive effects or sedation seen with opioids and butalbital-containing drugs.

Triptans and ergots are considered to be "migraine specific." This is not entirely true. Although they do not treat non-cephalgic pains, most headache types are responsive to such agents. Improvement of headache symptoms should never be considered as a diagnostic test of migraine.

Regardless of which agent is chosen for acute therapy, early treatment will improve outcomes by increasing both the chance of complete resolution of the attack and the chance that the attack will not recur in the first 24 hours.

Ergots were the mainstay of acute migraine treatment until the 1990s. The widespread use of ergotamine tartrate reflected the fact that migraine pain was felt to be a result of cerebral vasodilation, and ergotamine is a powerful vasoconstrictor. Dihydroergotamine is a potent 5-HT1A agonist as well as having some affinity for the 5-HT1B and 5-HT1D receptors. Many of the adverse events associated with dihydroergotamine are due to affinities for alpha-adrenergic and dopaminergic receptors. Dihydroergotamine (DHE) binds to the dorsal raphe of the midbrain, a region rich in serotonin receptors. Stimulation of the dorsal raphe can trigger headaches similar to migraines. These neurons terminate on cerebral arteries, and neurons which are involved in visual processing in the geniculate body, retina, superior colliculus and the visual cortex. Dorsal raphe neurons are suppressed during sleep. Sleep, particularly in children, often terminates a migraine attack. Rest without sleep is far less likely to stop an attack. It is possible that the central action explains why ergotamine can be effective late in a migraine attack, as opposed to triptans. Currently, dihydroergotamine is used to treat attacks and also used intravenously to treat medication overuse headaches. [33] When used intravenously, an antiemetic must be given concomitantly and some antiemetics are themselves antimigraine drugs, notably prochlorperazine and chlorpromazine. Methylergonovine has been used with some success as a preventive agent.

Triptans are commonly employed in the acute treatment of migraine. Various mechanisms are proposed to explain their efficacy: the ability to constrict intracranial and extracranial vessels, reducing trigeminal nerve activation and the subsequent release of the vasoactive neuropeptides, and inhibition of trigeminal neurons in the brainstem and upper cervical region. Several of these agents are available: sumatriptan, zolmitriptan, rizatriptan, naratriptan, almotriptan, frovatriptan, and eletriptan. Some differences in formulations exist in different countries. The only injectable triptan is sumatriptan. All are available as tablets. Zolmitriptan and sumatriptan are available as nasal sprays and sumatriptan by subcutaneous injection. All are agonists of 5-HT1B and 5-HT1D receptors, and some of 5-HT1F receptors. The 5-HT1B receptors are largely confined to cranial blood vessels and their activation reverses vasodilation. The 5-HT1D receptors are largely confined to peripheral and central trigeminal sensory neurons and activation of these inhibitory receptors blocks sensory transmission. It also blocks the release of proinflammatory peptides, which would otherwise lead to meningeal inflammation and a sterile perivascular inflammatory response.

Differences between triptans include their pharmacokinetic profiles and available delivery systems. They have a variable penetration through the blood brain barrier, partially explained by differences in lipophilicity, but this feature does not appear to influence efficacy. Active metabolites and high degree of lipophilicity are most likely to contribute to differences in the incidence of central nervous system side effects. Differences in oral bioavailability are corrected through dosing. Since nausea and vomiting are common with attacks, the use of oral agents is limited. Triptans have been shown to reduce not only headache, but also nausea, photophobia and phonophobia. As with ergots, triptans possess vasoconstrictive properties and therefore cannot be used in the presence of cardiovascular, cerebrovascular, or peripheral vascular disease. Although there are differences in the tolerability of the triptans, this does not suggest a safety difference between products. Triptans are contraindicated for use in those with vascular disease. They are also contraindicated in basilar migraine and hemiplegic migraine, but they are safe and approved for use in those with visual and sensory auras, although they do not affect the aura. Some nonsteroidal antiinflammatory agents might work synergistically with triptans to enhance efficacy, widen the window of opportunity to effectively treat, and reduce rates of recurrence.

Combination analgesics with butalbital are often used in the acute therapy of migraine in the United States and elsewhere. However, few studies support butalbital use. The significant dissociation between the biological half-life (about 44 hours) and the duration of action (about 4 hours) may account for some of the reasons it often leads to the development of medication overuse headache. Given such a long half-life, there can be drug accumulation with only modest use. Furthermore, barbiturates were commonly employed in the treatment of anxiety in the past, but often triggered depression, one of the most common psychiatric comorbidities with migraine.

Opioids are commonly unsuccessful in the treatment of migraine pain. They can enhance neurogenic inflammation, possibly through degranulation of meningeal mast cells. Cortical glutamate enhances the development of cortical spreading depression. The glutamate transporter enzyme normally returns the molecule into the neuron, but its action is blocked by opioids.

Preventive treatment

There are few agents with strong evidence of efficacy in the prevention of migraine. The predicted response for these agents is a 50% reduction in headaches in 50% of headaches treated after 3 months of treatment. [35] It is hoped, but yet to be proven, that the use of these medications in appropriate individuals will be disease modifying, preventing progression of the disorder that often occurs. Typically, those with six or more attacks monthly are candidates for prophylaxis. However, an individual might have a co-existing medical condition, for example, cardiovascular or cerebrovascular disease, which contraindicates the use of ergots or triptans. In these individuals it is often difficult to manage severe attacks, and prophylaxis might reduce the number of attacks while rendering acute medications more effective. This would reduce the disability of migraine.

The mechanism of antimigraine preventive agents has been obscure. A promising model suggests that the agents effective in the prophylaxis of migraine all suppress CSD. [35] This simulation might help to facilitate the screening of potential antimigraine agents. As is observed clinically and in this model, several weeks of exposure may be necessary to reduce CSD.

Only five agents have level A evidence for efficacy: amitriptyline, divalproex, topiramate, propranolol, and timolol. Among them, few head-to-head trials exist comparing their relative efficacy. Accordingly, the choice is often based on previous failures and comorbid conditions. In terms of comorbidity, the goal is to help treat the comorbid conditions at the same time as migraine, or at least not adversely affect them.

Timolol and propranolol are the two beta-blockers most used in migraine. Clearly, if an individual has co-existing hypertension, it may be possible to treat both conditions with proper dosages.

It is frequently stated that beta-blockers can cause depression, which may be true, yet the supportive studies are scant. These studies often use the concomitant use of antidepressants from pharmacy records to support the diagnosis of depression. It would be expected that the lipophilic beta-blockers would be most likely to cause depression, but this does not appear to be the case.

Presynaptic PQ channels are involved in the regulation of various neurotransmitters, and type 1 familial hemiplegic migraine is known to be associated with an abnormality in these channels. Some practitioners advocate the use of calcium channel blockers, notably verapamil, which is an L-channel blocker. These channels may play a role in nitric oxide inhibition. Yet few studies exist to support this recommendation. Flunarizine has a scientific basis for the prevention of migraine. This drug is not available in the United States.

Small trials support the use of lisinopril, an angiotensin-converting enzyme inhibitor, in migraine. [36] Angiotensin II type-1 inhibitors candesartan and telmisartan have demonstrated efficacy in preventing migraines. [37] The use of these agents might be a logical approach to the treatment of a hypertension in a migraineur.

Amitriptyline has the best evidence for migraine treatment among the "antidepressants." The selective serotonin reuptake inhibitors have little support for their use in migraine prophylaxis, although there are mixed results with fluoxetine. Emerging data is appearing with the use of selective norepinephrine/serotonin reuptake inhibitors. Monoamine oxidase inhibitors have been used in refractory migraine cases for many years but have not been well studied and are reserved for the most recalcitrant cases.

Among "antiepileptic drugs," topiramate and divalproex have grade A evidence of efficacy. There is a known comorbidity of migraine and epilepsy, but most antiepileptic agents are ineffective or minimally effective in the prevention of migraine.

Topiramate is an antiepileptic drug that blocks voltage-sensitive sodium ion channels as well as enhancing GABA A receptors. It is also a calcium L-channel blocker. It has linear kinetics and has a 21-hour half-life. In dose-ranging trials, the optimal dose, a balance of tolerability and efficacy, is 100 mg. This is significantly less than is usually used in the treatment of epilepsy. Topiramate was originally developed, but never marketed, as a treatment for diabetes. Topiramate is commonly selected for prophylaxis for the fact that, unlike most of the antimigraine agents, administration of the drug can induce weight loss. Since obesity is an independent risk factor for migraine disability, this side effect may be advantageous in this group. At the same time, a cognitive blunting, in particular for word retrieval, can occur. Paresthesias and an increased risk of nephrolithiasis are due to its carbonic anhydrase inhibition. The mechanism of action of topiramate is unknown, but it has been shown to block AMP/kainate glutamate receptors and mechanisms of phosphorylation. Topiramate is also a presynaptic sodium and calcium channel blocker. As a carbonic anhydrase inhibitor, topiramate can cause paresthesias, increase the risk of nephrolithiasis, and alter the taste of carbonated drinks. Reduced appetite, drowsiness, and diarrhea are reported. Topiramate also has efficacy in the treatment of migraine in children with a mean dose of 3.5 mg/kg/per day. [38] Topiramate might have some anxiolytic properties. Preliminary data suggest that coadministering topiramate with a beta-blocker may demonstrate therapeutic synergy. [39]

Zonisamide, an agent generally employed as an adjunctive treatment for partial seizures, is a possible alternative to topiramate, as it is better tolerated, but otherwise similar in side effects. These include weight loss, anxiety, paresthesias, and fatigue. It is possible that it is "weaker" than topiramate, and if corrected for efficacy, would not have that advantage. The two agents have not been directly compared. Although dose-ranging data is scant, doses up to 400 mg are reasonable. [40]

Valproate, an antiepileptic agent, increases GABA levels in brain and enhances GABA-mediated responses. It also blocks the degradation of GABA, therefore increasing levels of GABA in both neurons and glia. It is also a sodium ion channel inhibitor. Valproate has a clinical advantage: it can be used intravenously to "load" and treat an acute migraine, although this use is off label. Should chronic use be contemplated, it appears that, in the setting of a loading dose, the oral formulation has to be started concomitantly before there is drug redistribution. Common adverse events include tremor, weight gain, alopecia, nausea and somnolence. Since valproate is also used in the treatment of bipolar disease and epilepsy, this might be a reasonable agent to select if one of these conditions is comorbid with migraine.

There are data on gabapentin that suggest some efficacy in migraine, but this has not been well studied. High doses of 2400 mg daily may be necessary for migraine. A high degree of somnolence is often reported at this dose. It is of interest that agents like gabapentin, carbamazepine, and phenytoin show significant efficacy for neuropathic pain, unlike migraine pain. Agents such as topiramate and valproate, which are effective in migraine, are minimally effective in the management of neuropathic pain. [41] This may reflect different pathways for generation of these syndromes.

Tizanidine, a centrally acting muscle relaxant, may be effective in episodic tension-type headache, and for episodic and chronic migraine. [42] It is an alpha-2 adrenergic presynaptic agonist that inhibits brainstem and spinal cord epinephrine. Its use is often limited by sedation.

Sigma R receptor agonists, including dextromethorphan and memantine, show some promise in migraine prevention, but appropriate dosing and efficacy has not been established.

Small studies have suggested that the atypical antipsychotic agents olanzapine and quetiapine may be of value in migraine prevention. [43] These agents have a high affinity to dopaminergic D4 receptors and 5-HT2 receptors. Sedation and weight gain are often limiting factors in their use.

Triptans are labeled for the acute treatment of migraine, but may be useful for the preemptive treatment of migraine. Those with the longest half-lives, in particular naratriptan and frovatriptan, are usually selected. Examples would be menstrual migraine and weekend awakenings with headaches associated with oversleeping. If these events predictably herald a severe attack, and this occurs infrequently, the use of one of these agents during the prodrome might prevent the attack. Successful preemptive treatment has been accomplished with naratriptan, but likely could be applied to other triptans. [44]

Migraine can be associated with systemic or focal regions of low magnesium in the brain, all of which would increase the likelihood for developing neuronal hyperexcitability. Replacing systemic magnesium can help reduce migraine attacks, but oral forms may lead to diarrhea if administered too rapidly. Intravenous magnesium may be useful in aborting a migraine attack, but if used orally, this is often replaced over several months duration to avoid diarrhea. [45]

Riboflavin, vitamin B2, was studied for migraine prophylaxis at 400 mg daily for 3 months and was significantly effective. Tolerability was acceptable. [46]

Coenzyme Q10 deficiency may also have some effect of migraine disability. It is typically administered at 300 mg daily and used in the morning to prevent drug induced insomnia. [47]

Feverfew (*Tanacetum parthenium*) is an herb that might have some value in the prevention of migraine and possesses anti-inflammatory properties, including supression of prostaglandin synthesis. [48] Adverse event rates are low, but it has antiplatelet properties so might not be safely co-administered with other anticoagulant agents.

Butterbur (petasites), a leukotriene inhibitor, might be effective. [49] One study reported efficacy and tolerability with 75 mg twice a day after 3–4 months of treatment. This agent is potentially teratogenic, carcinogenic, and hepatotoxic. There are large potency differences between butterbur preparations, further confounding clinical trials and therapeutic uses. Montelukast, also a leukotriene inhibitor used in the treatment of allergies and asthma, showed contradictory results in trials.

Acupuncture may have benefit as a migraine preventive agent according to a recent Cochrane review metanalysis. [50] The studies are difficult to interpret, based on methodological study issues and variability in acupuncture techniques. There are no data to support the use of homeopathy as a migraine therapy.

Onabotulinum toxin A injected in pericranial muscles is approved in the United States for the prevention of chronic migraine (more than 15 days monthly with migraine attacks lasting more than 4 hours). Lower frequency of attacks did not appear to respond to this treatment. The mechanism of action of Onabotulinum toxin A is unknown but it is unlikely to primarily involve scalp muscle relaxation. It is known to inhibit substance P, glutamate, and calcitonin gene related peptide. [51] A possible mechanism may involve sensory neurons identified in the scalps of rodents, which traverse the skull and terminate in the meninges. Those who describe an exploding pressure like headache, in distinction to those who describe an imploding or ocular headache, appear to respond better to this treatment. [52] Advantages of Onabotulinum toxin A include the lack of systemic side effects and its compatibility with systemic agents for migraine.

Side effects

Given the modest efficacy of preventive agents and the high frequency of side effects, it is often difficult to convince migraineurs to use these agents. The choice of agent for prevention significantly affects compliance. Most preventive agents for migraine are associated with weight gain, and this effect, along with memory loss and depression, are the most common reasons for rejecting a particular agent. Those sufferers utilizing a high frequency of acute agents are more likely to accept the adverse events associated with preventive agents. Tremor is the most common reason for rejection of drug in elderly individuals. [53]

The serotonin syndrome

The Food and Drug Administration in the United States issued an alert in 2006 that there would be a life-threatening risk when triptans were used in individuals taking selective serotonin reuptake inhibitors and selective serotonin/norepinephrine inhibitors. Given the high comorbidity of migraine and depression, many such exposures have occurred without incident. [54] This assertion has been questioned by the American Headache Society in their position paper, suggesting only Level U evidence to support that recommendation. [55] Clarification of this issue is important in order for clinicians to make rational treatment decisions in those with migraine comorbid with psychiatric disease.

References

[1] The International Classification of Headache Disorders, 2nd Edition. *Cephalalgia* 2004; **24**; (suppl 1): 9–160.

[2] Blau JN. Migraine prodromes separated from the aura: complete migraine. *BMJ* 1980; **281**: 658–81.

[3] Noseda R, Kainz V, Jakubowski M, Gooley J *et al.* A neural mechanism for exacerbation of headache by light. *Nature Neuroscience* 2010; **13**: 239–45.

[4] Kelman L. The triggers or precipitants of the acute migraine attack. *Cephalalgia* 2007; **27**: 394–402.

[5] Russell MB, Rasmussen BK, Fenger K, Olesen J. Migraine without aura and migraine with aura are distinct clinical entities: a study of four hundred and eighty-four male and female migraineurs from the general population. *Cephalalgia* 1996; **16**: 239–45.

[6] Fisher CM. Late-life migraine accompaniments-further experience. *Stroke* 1986; **17**: 1033–42.

[7] Leão A. Spreading depression of activity in the cerebral cortex. *J Neurophys* 1944; **7**: 359–90.

[8] Aurora SK, Ahmad BK, Welch KMA, Bhardhwaj P, Ramadan NM. Transcranial magnetic stimulation confirms hyper excitability of occipital cortex in migraine. *Neurology* 1998; **50**: 1111–14.

[9] Bowyer SM, Aurora SK, Moran JE, Tepley N, Welch KMA. Magnetoencephalographic fields from patients with spontaneous and induced migraine aura. *Ann Neurol* 2001; **50**: 582–7.

[10] Denuelle M, Boulloche, Payoux P, *et al.* A PET study of photophobia during spontaneous migraine attacks. *Neurology* 2011; **76**: 213–18.

[11] Graham JR, Wolff HG. Mechanism of migraine headache and action of ergotamine tartrate. *Arch Neurol Psychiatry* 1939; **39**: 737–63.

[12] Bolay H, Reuter U, Dunn AK, Huang Z, Boas DA, Moskowitz MA. Intrinsic brain activity triggers trigeminal meningeal afferents in a migraine model. *Nat Med* 2002; **8**: 136–42.

[13] Moskowitz MA. Basic mechanisms in vascular headache. *Neurol Clin* 1990; **8**: 801–15.

[14] Brennan KC, Beltran-Parrazal L, Lopez-Valdes HE, Theriot J, Toga AW, Charles AC. Distinct vascular conduction with cortical spreading depression. *J Neurophysiol* 2007; **97**: 4143–51.

[15] Kimball RW, Friedman AP, Vallejo E. Effect of serotonin in migraine patients. *Neurology* 1960; **10**: 107–11.

[16] Woods RP, Iacoboni M, Mazziotta JC. Bilateral spreading cerebral hypoperfusion during spontaneous migraine headache. *N Engl J Med* 1994; **331**: 1689–92.

[17] Bahra A, Matharu MS, Buchel C, Frackowiak PSJ, Goadsby PJ. Brainstem activation specific to migraine headache. *The Lancet* 2001; **357**: 1016–17.

[18] Charles A. Intercellular calcium waves in glia. *Glia* 1998; **24**: 39–49.

[19] Haydon PG, Carmignoto G. Astrocyte control of synaptic transmission and neurovascular coupling. *Physiol Rev* 2006; **86**: 1009–31.

[20] Lauritzen M, Olesen J. Regional cerebral blood flow during migraine attacks by xenon-133 inhalation and emission tomography. *Brain* 1984; **107**: 447–61.

[21] Welch KMA, Nagesh V, Aurora SK, Gelman N. Periaqueductal gray matter dysfunction in migraine: cause of burden of illness? *Headache* 2001; **41**: 629–37.

[22] Hershey AD, Powers SW, Nelson TD *et al.* American Headache Society Pediatric Adolescent Section. Obesity in the pediatric headache population. *Headache* 2009; **49**: 170–7.

[23] Bigal ME, Lipton RB, Holland PR, Goadsby PJ, Obesity, migraine, and chronic migraine: possible mechanisms of interaction. *Neurology* 2007; **68**: 1851–61.

[24] Horev A, Wirguin I, Lantsberg L, Ifergane G. A high incidence of migraine with aura among morbidly obese women. *Headache* 2005; **45**: 936–8.

[25] Bond DS, Vithiananthan S, Nash JM, Thomas JG, Wing RR. Improvement of migraine headaches in severely obese patients after bariatric surgery. *Neurology* 2011; **76**: 1135–8.

[26] Kallweit U, Hidalgo H, Uhl V, Sándor PS. Continuous positive airway pressure therapy is effective for migraines in sleep apnea syndrome. *Neurology* 2011; **76**: 1189–91.

[27] Kristiansen HA, Kvænrner KJ, Akre H, Øverland V, Russell MB. Migraine and sleep apnea in the general population. *J Headache Pain* 2011; **12**: 55–61.

[28] US headache consortium guidelines in: http://www.americanheadachesociety.org/professional_resources/us_headache_consortium_guidelines/

[29] Nestoriuc Y, Martin A. Efficacy of biofeedback for migraine: A meta analysis. *Pain* 2007; **128**: 111–27.

[30] Ferrari MD, Roon KI, Lipton RB, Goadsby PJ. Oral triptans (serotonin 5-HT (1B/1D agonists) in acute

migraine treatment: a meta-analysis of 53 trials. *Lancet* 2001; **358**: 1668–75.

[31] Aurora S, Kori S, Barrodale P, Nelsen A, McDonald S. Gastric stasis occurs in spontaneous, visually induced and interictal migraine. *Headache* 2007; **47**: 1443–6.

[32] Dowson AJ, Mathew NT, Pascual J. Review of clinical trials using early acute intervention with oral triptans for migraine management. *Int J Clin Pract* 2006; **60**: 698–706.

[33] Silberstein SD, Schulman EA, McFadden M. Repetitive intravenous DHE in the treatment of refractory headache. *Headache* 1990; **30**: 334–9.

[34] Ramadan MN, Silberstein SD, Freitag FG, Gilbert TT, Frishberg GM. Pharmacological management for prevention of migraine. Available at http://www.aan.com/public/practiceguidelines.

[35] Ayata C, Jin H, Kudo C, Dalkara T, Moskowitz M. Suppression of cortical spreading depression in migraine prophylaxis. *Ann Neurol* 2006; **59**: 652–61.

[36] Schrader H, Stovner LJ, Helde C, Sand T, Bovim G. Prophylactic treatment of migraine with angiotensin converting enzyme inhibitor (lisinopril): randomised, placebo controlled, crossover study. *BMJ* 2001; **322**: 19.

[37] Tronvik E, Stovner LJ, Helde G, Sand T, Bovim G. Prophylactic treatment of migraine with an angiotensin II receptor blocker. *JAMA* 2003; **289**: 65–9.

[38] Campistol J, Campos J, Casas C, Herranz JL. Topiramate in the prophylactic treatment of migraine in children. *J Child Neurol* 2005; **20**: 251–3.

[39] Pascual J, Rivas MT, Leira R. Testing the combination beta-blocker plus topiramate in refractory migraine. *Acta Neurol Scand* 2007; **115**: 181–3.

[40] Drake ME, Greathouse NI, Renner JB, Armentbright AD. Open-label zonisamide for refractory migraine. *Clin Neuropharmacol* 2004; **27**: 278–80.

[41] Mathew NT, Rapoport A, Saper J, *et al.* Efficacy of gabapentin in migraine prophylaxis. *Headache* 2001; **41**: 119–28.

[42] Krusz JC, Belanger J, Mills C. Tizanidine: a novel effective agent for the treatment of chronic headaches. *Headache* 2000; **11**: 41–5.

[43] Silberstein SD, Peres M, Hopkins MM, Schechter AL, Young WB, Rozen TD. Olanzapine in the treatment of refractory migraine and chronic daily headache. *Headache* 2002; **42**: 515–18.

[44] Luciani R, Carter D, Mannix L, Hempfill M, Diamond M, Cady R. Prevention of migraine during prodrome with naratriptan. *Cephalalgia* 2000; **20**: 122–6.

[45] Mauskop A, Altura BT, Cracco RQ, Altera BM. Intravenous magnesium sulfate relieves acute migraine in patients with low serum ionized magnesium levels. *Clin Sci* 1995; **89**: 633–6.

[46] Schoenen J, Jacquy J, Lanaerts M. Effectiveness of high-dose riboflavin in migraine prophylaxis. *Neurology* 1998; **50**: 466–70.

[47] Sándor PS, Di Clemente L, Coppola G. Efficacy of coenzyme Q10 in migraine prophylaxis: a randomized controlled trial. *Neurology* 2005; **64**: 713–15.

[48] Pfaffenrath V, Diener HC, Fischer M, Friede M, Henneicke-von Zepelin HH. The efficacy and safety of *Tanacetum parthenium* (feverfew) in migraine prophylaxis – a double-blind, multicentre randomized placebo-controlled dose-response study. *Cephalalgia* 2002; **22**: 523–32.

[49] Lipton B, Gobel H, Wilks K, Mauskop A. Efficacy of petasites (an extract from petasites rhizone) 50 and 75 mg for prophylaxis of migraine: results of a randomized, double-blind, placebo controlled study. (abstract). *Neurology* 2002; **58**: A472.

[50] Linde K, Allais G, Brinkhaus B, Manheimer E, Vickers A, White AR. Acupuncture for migraine prophylaxis. *Cochrane Database Syst Rev* 2009 (**1**):CD001218.

[51] Durham PL, Cady R. Insights into the mechanism of onabotulinumtoxin A in chronic migraine. *Headache* 2011; **51**: 1573–7.

[52] Jakubowski M, McAllister P, Bajwa ZH, *et al.* Exploding vs imploding headache in migraine prophylaxis with Botulinum Toxin A. *Pain* 2006; **125**: 286–95.

[53] Kowacs PA, Piovesan EJ, Tepper SJ. Rejection and acceptance of possible side effects of migraine prophylactic drugs. *Headache* 2009; **49**: 1022–7.

[54] FDA Alert. Combined use of 5-hydroxytriptamine receptor agonists (triptans), selective serotonin reuptake inhibitors SSRIs), or selective serotonin/norepinephrine reuptake inhibitors (SNRIs) may result in life-threatening serotonin syndrome. July 2006.

[55] Evans RW, Tepper SJ, Shapiro RE, Sun-Edelstein C, Tietjen GE. The FDA alert on serotonin syndrome with use of triptans combined with selective serotonin reuptake inhibitors or selective serotonin-norepinephrine reuptake inhibitors: American Headache Society position paper. *Headache* 2010; **50**: 1089–99.

Chapter 3

Tension-type headache

Robert G. Kaniecki

Overview

Tension-type headache is the most common form of headache in the general population. It is characterized by recurrent episodes of headache that are relatively featureless and mild to moderate in intensity. The diagnosis is based solely on the history and examination. Exclusion of secondary headaches or forms of migraine is important in the assessment process. Despite extensive investigation the underlying pathophysiology remains a matter of speculation, with peripheral muscular and central nervous system components both likely involved. Treatment has changed little over the past 20–30 years. Simple analgesics are generally helpful for individual attacks while preventive agents are often frustratingly ineffective.

Classification and description

Tension-type headache (TTH) is an ill-defined and likely heterogeneous syndrome. Subclassified along lines of headache frequency, the ICHD-II (International Classification of Headache Disorders, 2nd edition) recognizes infrequent episodic (averaging < 1 day/month), frequent episodic (averaging 1–14 days/month), and chronic (averaging >14 days/month) subtypes (Table 3.1). [1] The phenotypic features are nonspecific, with diagnostic criteria based more on what it *is not* rather than what it *is*. By definition these headaches exhibit pain that is *not* localized, *not* throbbing, *not* aggravated by activity, and *not* severe. Associated neurological, autonomic, or migrainous features are *not* components of this disorder. By definition there is *no* significant nausea, and *no* vomiting. Photophobia and phonophobia *cannot* both be present. The ICHD-II also allows for further subclassification based on the presence or absence of pericranial muscle tenderness. Finally the diagnosis requires the exclusion of secondary headache possibilities.

In episodic tension-type headache (ETTH) the attacks typically last anywhere from 30 minutes to 7 days, while those with chronic tension-type headache (CTTH) may report discomfort of a relatively continuous nature. The majority of episodes develop during waking hours and progression over the course of the day is commonly reported. Nocturnal development of tension-type headache is uncommon and should provoke potential investigation. The most frequently reported triggers for TTH are mental or physical stressors, leading to the maintenance of the term "tension-type" headache in the most recent classification and explaining prior terms such as "stress" and "muscle contraction" headache. Other commonly described triggers include hunger, dehydration, over-exertion, alterations in sleep patterns, caffeine withdrawal, and female hormonal fluctuations. [2]

Table 3.1. Warning signs for secondary headache disorders

1.	First/worst headache
2.	Abrupt onset headache
3.	Progression or fundamental change in pattern of headache
4.	New headache in those less than 5 years old, greater than 50 years old
5.	New headache with cancer, immunosuppression, or pregnancy
6.	Headache with syncope or seizure
7.	Headache triggered by exertion/valsalva/sex
8.	Neurologic symptoms greater than 1 hour in duration
9.	Abnormal general or neurological examination

The Neuropsychiatry of Headache, ed. Mark W. Green and Philip R. Muskin. Published by Cambridge University Press.

Table 3.2. Diagnostic criteria for tension-type headache International Classification of Headache Disorders, 2nd edition

2.1 Infrequent episodic tension-type headache
A. At least ten episodes occurring on < 1 day/month on average (<12 days/year) and fulfilling criteria B–D listed below
B. Headache lasting from 30 minutes to 7 days
C. Headache has at least two of the following pain characteristics • Bilateral location • Mild or moderate intensity (may inhibit, but does not prohibit activity) • Pressing/tightening (non-pulsating) quality • No aggravation through climbing stairs or similar routine physical activity
D. Both of the following • No nausea or vomiting (anorexia may still occur) • No more than one of photophobia and phonophobia
E. Not attributed to another disorder
2.2 Frequent episodic tension-type headache
As 2.1 except for: At least 10 episodes occurring ≥ 1 but < 15 days/month for at least 3 months (≥ 12 and < 180 days/year) and fulfilling criteria B–D above
2.3 Chronic tension-type headache
As 2.1 except for:
A. Headache occurring on ≥ 15 days/month on average for > 3 months (≥ 180 days/year) and fulfilling criteria B–D above
B. Headache last hours or may be continuous
C. Both of the following • No more than one of photophobia, phonophobia, or mild nausea • Neither moderate nor severe nausea nor vomiting

Diagnosis and investigation

The phenotypic features of tension-type headache are non-specific and may be seen with an assortment of secondary headache conditions, which are linked mechanistically to an identifiable structural or physiological disorder. [3] A fundamental criterion to establish a link between an apparent organic condition and headache is the resolution or amelioration of symptoms following treatment of the underlying disorder. Ranging from benign to catastrophic, these conditions frequently present with phenotypic headaches similar to tension-type headaches. Intracranial mass lesions (tumor, subdural hematoma), disorders of cerebrospinal fluid pressure (benign intracranial hypertension, hydrocephalus), joint dysfunction of the cervical spine or temporal-mandibular joint, and systemic conditions such as giant cell arteritis, obstructive sleep apnea, and hypothyroidism may all be present with apparent tension-type headache. Although symptoms may be shared with primary headaches, the secondary headaches often exhibit one of the "red flags" which would help signify organic underpinnings (Tables 3.2). [4]

Due to this extensive symptom overlap between primary and secondary headaches, one feature crucial to elicit during clinical assessment is the temporal pattern of the headache disorder. Headaches described as "new" or "different," as well as those which progress in frequency or intensity, should raise particular concern. Thorough general and neurological examinations are key components to the clinical evaluation, providing additional clues to the potential presence of organic disease. In those patients where such suspicions are raised by the history or examination, further diagnostic workup might include neuroimaging of the brain or cervical spine, cerebrospinal fluid analysis, or serum testing with erythrocyte sedimentation rate and thyroid function studies. [5]

The difficulty in distinguishing episodic tension-type headache from migraine headache, two of the most common episodic headache types, is widely acknowledged. [6] Individuals with episodic migraine often describe milder attacks that may be suggestive of ETTH. An acute migraine often passes through a mild initial phase that may be initially misinterpreted as a tension-type attack. Both of these elements contribute to a high rate of misdiagnosis. Clinicians are likely to diagnose tension-type headache when bilateral or non-throbbing head pain is present, if the patient reports that the headache is triggered by stress or muscle tension, or when neck pain is present. All of these features are common with migraine. Among respondents in the American Migraine Study II who met ICHD criteria but lacked a physician diagnosis of migraine, 32% report a physician diagnosis of tension-type headache. [7] In one study investigating the efficacy of sumatriptan in the range of headaches experienced by migraineurs, 71% of patients initially diagnosed with ETTH have their diagnosis altered to migraine after a detailed review of diary data. [8] Another study demonstrates that 84% of those in the population with self-diagnosed "stress" or "tension" headaches actually meet criteria for migraine. Such diagnostic confusion is not limited to those with episodic headache conditions. [9] Subjects with chronic migraine often define a lower-grade headache that is phenotypically similar to CTTH, particularly in the presence of a medication-overuse component. Since over 90% of patients consulting clinicians for recurrent episodic headache disorders will ultimately be found to have migraine, and only 3% will have tension-type headache, it is imperative to first exclude migraine as a possibility before arriving at a tension-type headache diagnosis. [10]

Epidemiology of tension-type headache

Tension-type headache is the most common primary or secondary headache, with prevalence varying by population, subtype of tension-type headache studied, age, and gender. One large population-based survey in the United States determines an annual prevalence of 38.3% for ETTH and 2.2% for CTTH. [11] Based on pooled results from five population-based studies, the mean lifetime prevalence of tension-type headache in adults is 46% (range 12%–78%). The 2%–3% population prevalence for CTTH is fairly consistent worldwide[12] Although no clear genetic underpinnings have been identified, approximately 40% will report a family history of some form of headache disorder. First-degree relatives have a two to four-fold increased risk of CTTH compared to the general population. Twin studies show no difference in risk between identical and non-identical twins.

The prevalence varies by sex and age. [13] There is a slight female preponderance for ETTH with a F:M ratio of approximately 5:4, although this ratio increases when the headache disorder becomes chronic. Most develop tension-type headache prior to age 30 with peak prevalence in the decade of ages 40–49 and a subsequent decreased prevalence with age in both sexes. [11] Despite such declines the rates of ETTH remain above 25% in the seventh decade of life for both men and women, while 1.5% of men and 2.7% of women continue to report CTTH beyond age 60. There is also a correlation between prevalence of episodic tension-type headache and higher educational level.

Episodic tension-type headache is as prevalent as migraine in both children and adolescents. According to estimates from several population-based studies the mean prevalence in children is 31% (range 10%–72%). [14] Headaches develop at a mean age of 7, with an average duration of 2 hours. Age is again a risk factor as the rate of TTH has been shown to rise in schoolchildren between the ages of 7 and 15. For children, the duration, frequency, intensity, and medication use associated with attacks of ETTH are typically lower when compared to those with episodic migraine. The prevalence of CTTH is lower in children than in adults and estimates generally place it at <1% of this age group. Tension-type headache in children and adolescents is also related to psychosocial factors, with such individuals more likely to report depression, divorced parents, and fewer peer relationships when compared to migraine and headache-free controls. [15]

Partly due to higher population prevalence, the societal impact of tension-type headache is actually greater than that seen with migraine. [12] A number of studies have documented considerable absenteeism with TTH. One study from the United States demonstrated that both ETTH and CTTH cause significant absenteeism, while another from Europe showed the number of lost workdays from TTH was three times higher than that lost to migraine. The economic and social burdens are higher for those with CTTH than with ETTH as measured by several disability instruments including the Migraine Disability Assessment Scale (MIDAS) and the General Health Questionnaire. The impact is particularly high for those with comorbid complications, such as depression as measured by the Beck Depression Inventory. Frequency, rather than severity, of headache appears to deliver a greater impact on disability and quality of life.

Comorbidity of tension-type headache

Tension-type headache is associated with a number of medical and mental health disorders. [16] Migraine represents one such association, but as stated previously it may be difficult to phenotypically distinguish mild migraine from true tension-type headache in those patients appearing to exhibit attacks representative of both conditions. Population studies estimate the prevalence of TTH in those with migraine at 94%, with 56% experiencing frequent episodic TTH. [17] Temporomandibular disorders (TMD) have been linked to both migraine and tension-type headache in several studies, though the relationship may be confounded by the fact that one symptom of temporomandibular dysfunction is headache. One blinded study finds the prevalence of TMD in a headache clinic population to be 56%, with the highest prevalence in those reporting both migraine and tension-type headache. [18] Headache patients with co-existent TMD had a significantly higher likelihood of depression: 71% vs. 34% in those without TMD. Patients with cervical spine discogenic and spondylitic disorders present with features of tension-type headache, and in such patients it may be difficult to distinguish a primary tension-type headache from a secondary "cervicogenic" cause based on clinical criteria alone. The best means of mechanistic connection with either TMJ dysfunction or cervical spine disease requires significant improvement or eradication of headache following treatment application to the secondary structural disorder. [19]

Headache, like other pain disorders, exhibits primary sensory, cognitive, and affective components. Pathophysiologic activation of multiple areas of the limbic system may be witnessed during functional neuroimaging of headache subjects, including the hippocampus and cingulate, insular, and orbitofrontal cortices. Beyond the emotional components innate to the pain experience, it is clear that headache patients also display higher prevalence of mood and anxiety disorders when compared to their headache-free counterparts. Subjects with TTH report significantly more daily hassles and rated the events they experienced as causing significantly more stress compared with headache-free subjects. [20] Stress is considered the most common precipitant of TTH, yet some have viewed psychological abnormalities as secondary rather than primary factors. [21] Compared with healthy controls, patients with migraine or tension-type headache have significantly higher scores on measures of anxiety, depression and hostility. [22] One recent study of psychiatric comorbidity in patients with migraine, tension-type headache, and migraine plus tension-type headache revealed significant differences in the rate of occurrence of depression, with the combined group being of highest risk. [23] The prevalence of generalized anxiety disorder is not significantly different in these headaches subgroups, while panic and obsessive-compulsive disorders seemed to correlate with the presence of migraine and not tension-type headache.

Pathophysiology of tension-type headache

The origin of tension-type headache was initially proposed as arising from excessive contraction of pericranial and cervical muscles, leading to one of the original terms of "muscle contraction headache."[24] Many believe a link to exist between these headaches and emotional distress or "life tension." Environmental influences appear to carry greater importance than genetic factors in the development of tension-type headache. [25]

Stress is a widely accepted contributing factor to tension-type headache, but the mechanisms underlying the relationship are unclear. [26] Self-reported inability to relax and poor self-health assessments, in addition to inadequate sleep, have all been reported as additional risks factors likely linked to stress. Irregular nutrition or hydration may act as trigger factors. Aside from caffeine, which may trigger TTH through excessive exposure or withdrawal, diet seems to have very little impact. A number of medications, including female hormonal supplements, certain antidepressants, and nitrates may aggravate an underlying tension-type or migraine headache disorder.

The precise cause of tension-type headache remains unknown. An inherent complexity may exist since mechanisms may vary between ETTH and CTTH populations, and also between individuals within these subgroups. [27] A number of insights on pathophysiologic aspects of TTH have been gained over the past decade implicating a multifactorial process involving both peripheral myofascial factors as well as central nervous system components. [28] Pericranial myofascial mechanisms are probably of importance in ETTH, while sensitization of central nociceptive pathways seems to contribute to the process of CTTH.

Research has implicated myofascial activity as a potential source of TTH, whereby persistent activation of trigger points might lead to peripheral nociceptor sensitization and eventual sensitization of second-order neurons in the spinal trigeminal nucleus. [29] A number of studies demonstrate increased levels of pericranial and cervical muscle tenderness in TTH patients when compared to controls. This tenderness has also been correlated directly with both frequency and intensity measures of headache. Since this abnormality has been detected on headache-free days as well as headache days, it is speculated that this represents a cause rather than an effect of headache occurrences. A series of blinded controlled studies have documented increased numbers of active and latent trigger points in patients with TTH when compared to controls, and these were associated with neck mobility and forward head posture as well as the severity of the headache disorder. [30] Although EMG-measured pericranial muscle activity is not diffusely elevated in populations of TTH patients, it is reported that EMG activity is increased in specific trigger points of these muscles. Some propose that continuous activity in a selection of motor units over a sustained period of time might excite peripheral nociceptors, perhaps through direct mechanical means, local ischemia, or through release of inflammatory mediators. [31] Although research documents deficiencies in exercise-induced increases in pericranial muscle tissue, microdialysis techniques have not yet demonstrated subsequent increased levels of lactate or inflammatory mediators in these muscles. [32]

Central mechanisms appear to be more relevant to the pathogenesis of CTTH. [33] Pain thresholds have been shown to be normal in infrequent ETTH but decreased in frequent ETTH and CTTH. Patients with CTTH have been found to be hypersensitive to stimulation via pressure, thermal, and electrical modalities as well as to intramuscular infusion of noxious substances. These sensitivities have been shown in a number of tissues (muscle, tendon, nerve) both during and between headaches and at cephalic and extracephalic sites. [34] Population-based studies demonstrate a relationship between increased pain sensitivity and both chronification and increased prevalence of tension-type headache. [35] Research has also documents deficient central nociceptive inhibitory pathways with CTTH. By means of voxel-based morphometry brain MRI scans of patients with CTTH have displayed significantly reduced density of gray matter structures along the pain matrix, including the dorsal rostral and ventral pons, the cingulate and insular and orbitofrontal cortex, the right posterior temporal lobe, parahippocampus bilaterally; and the right cerebellum. [36] This decrease in gray matter correlates positively with increasing headache duration in years.

Management of tension-type headache

The approach to the management of tension-type headache involves a combination of lifestyle, physical, and pharmacologic measures. [37] Although the scientific evidence is limited, nonpharmacological management should always be considered. Recommendations for regulation of sleep, meals and exercise are generally quite valuable. Stress management techniques and other steps towards trigger avoidance may be of great benefit. Passive physical manipulation and active cervical muscle stretching or exercise programs may be of benefit. Behavioral therapies are quite useful adjuncts in the management of episodic tension-type headache, with the most frequently advised techniques involving relaxation therapy and EMG-guided biofeedback. Cognitive behavioral therapy may provide additional benefit in cases of significant depression or anxiety. A recent set of guidelines published by the European Federation of Neurological Societies (EFNS) assessed the evidence for non-drug treatments of tension-type headache (Table 3.3). [38]

Tension-type headache is typically managed mainly through administration of medication during acute episodes. Typical analgesic remedies may be obtained over-the-counter or by prescription, and evidence is available to recommend a number of options (Table 3.4). [38] Simple analgesics, nonsteroidal anti-inflammatory drugs (NSAIDs), and combination agents are most commonly recommended. There have been many controlled studies to document the efficacy of these agents in episodes of TTH. Their use should be strictly limited to an average of 2–3 days per week to avoid the issues of medication-overuse headache and potential contribution towards transformation into chronic tension-type headache.

Aspirin is more effective than placebo and comparable to the efficacy of acetaminophen in the relief of acute tension-type headache. Given superior efficacy in comparative trials, NSAIDs are generally considered the drugs of choice for acute TTH. Ibuprofen and

Table 3.3. Non-pharmacological preventive therapies for tension-type headache

Treatment	Level of recommendation
EMG Biofeedback	A
Cognitive-behavioral therapy	C
Relaxation training	C
Physical therapy	C
Acupuncture	C

Source: Guidelines from the European Federation of Neurological Societies. A level A rating (effective) required at least one convincing class I study or two consistent convincing class II studies. A level B rating (probably effective) required at least one convincing class II study or overwhelming class III evidence. A level C rating (possibly effective) required at least two convincing class III studies.

Table 3.4. Acute therapies for tension-type headache

Agent	Dose	Level of recommendation
Acetaminophen	500–1000 mg	A
Aspirin	500–1000 mg	A
Ibuprofen	200–800 mg	A
Ketoprofen	25–50 mg	A
Naproxen	375–550 mg	A
Diclofenac	12.5–100 mg	A
Caffeine	65–200 mg	B

Source: Guidelines from the European Federation of Neurological Societies.

naproxen sodium are listed as first-line agents in the NSAID category due to better gastrointestinal tolerability. Caffeine-containing compounds may be useful in those cases that fail to respond to simple or NSAID analgesics. The addition of caffeine (130–200 mg) is shown to significantly increase the efficacy of simple analgesics and ibuprofen in controlled clinical trials. Triptans and muscle relaxants have not demonstrated consistent superiority over placebo in clinical trials of ETTH and are not recommended. Butalbital-containing compounds may be helpful in those patients who have contraindications to first-line analgesics or in those who have failed them. However, such drugs must be used with caution and their supplies limited due to an elevated risk of medication-overuse headache. Given low levels of pain severity and disability with TTH, and noting also a high risk for the development of medication-overuse headache, opioid analgesics are not recommended for the management of TTH.

Preventive pharmacologic therapy is generally advised for those patients experiencing at least 2–3 headache days each week. [39] Although analgesics may continue to be beneficial when taken at such levels, the issues of medication-overuse headache and transformation into more refractory cases of chronic tension-type headache must be considered. Progression in frequency or severity of attacks, development of adverse events with acute medications, and decline in efficacy of acute medications may all be additional indications for the institution of daily pharmacologic preventive therapy. These agents should be initiated at low doses and gradually advanced based on efficacy and tolerability. Once an effective dose is reached, treatment is typically continued for 6–12 months, at which point daily medication may be tapered and the patient followed clinically.

Although there is little well-controlled scientific evidence to support their use, most clinicians advise antidepressants and anticonvulsants to help stabilize tension-type headaches. [39] Few controlled studies have been performed, with only some demonstrating superior efficacy to placebo. The data for the tricyclic antidepressant amitriptyline is most convincing, while clomipramine, nortriptyline, and doxepin may be useful alternatives if amitriptyline is poorly tolerated. Most studies begin with amitriptyline doses of 10–25 mg per night, with the average final dose of 50–75 mg nightly for patients with CTTH. Studies of selective serotonin reuptake inhibitors do not show superiority of these drugs over placebo. Mirtazapine and the noradrenergic-serotonin reuptake inhibitor, extended-release venlafaxine, have been shown to be beneficial in single clinical trials. The centrally acting muscle relaxant tizanidine has shown efficacy in a crossover clinical trial. All data on anticonvulsants is from open-label research, and the results have been mixed. Onabotulinum toxin type A appears helpful for CTTH in a few small open-label reports, but this benefit was not confirmed by a series of double-blind placebo-controlled studies. [40] Two recent meta-analyses arrive at opposite conclusions, with one establishing benefit and the other a lack of benefit for prophylactic drugs in tension-type headache in adults. [41],[42] The EFNS guidelines have listed a

Table 3.5. Pharmacological preventive therapies for tension-type headache

Agent	Daily dose	Level of recommendation
Amitriptyline	30–75 mg	A
Mirtazapine	30 mg	B
Venlafaxine	150 mg	B
Clomipramine	75–150 mg	B

Source: Guidelines from the European Federation of Neurological Societies.

number of agents deemed effective by available data or expert consensus (Table 3.5). [38]

Prognosis of tension-type headache

Information on the prognosis of tension-type headache is fairly limited, and there is no specific data on such a prognosis among the elderly. [43] In a study of adult outpatients with tension-type headache followed over 10 years, 44% with chronic tension-type headache report significant improvement or complete resolution, while 29% of those with episodic tension-type headache converted to the chronic subtype. [44] A 2-year follow-up from a Danish cross-sectional population study reveals a 45% remission rate among those with frequent episodic or chronic tension-type headache, while 39% continued to report episodic and 16% chronic tension-type headache. Poor outcome in TTH was associated with the following variables: CTTH at baseline, coexisting migraine or sleep difficulties, and being unmarried. In this study older age (mean 57 years vs. 53 years) was reported as a positive predictive factor for remission. [45]

Conclusions

Tension-type headache is the most common headache in the general population. Due to extensive symptomatic overlap with secondary headache disorders and migraine, the diagnosis of tension-type headache first requires exclusion of these other conditions. The diagnosis is based on clinical criteria and broadly the tension-type headache category is divided into episodic (fewer than 15 days per month) and chronic (15 days per month or more) subtypes. Although attacks of TTH are generally less disabling than those with migraine, work absences are substantial and the total societal burden appears to exceed that with migraine because of the high population prevalence with TTH. Pericranial myofascial mechanisms are probably of importance in episodic tension-type headache, while sensitization of central nociceptive pathways and inadequate endogenous anti-nociceptive circuitry seem to be more relevant in chronic tension-type headache. While acute therapy with simple and NSAID analgesics is typically effective for the treatment of episodes of ETTH, chronic tension-type headache is often more difficult to manage. Although there is little scientific evidence to guide the selection of treatment modalities in CTTH, most specialists advise a combination of non-pharmacological and pharmacological therapies. The prognosis is generally favorable, with limited disability during headache occurrences and age-related improvement or resolution of episodes later in life.

References

[1] Headache Classification Committee of the International Headache Society. The International Classification of Headache Disorders, 2nd ed. *Cephalalgia* 2004; **24**(suppl 1): 9–160.

[2] Rasmussen BK. Migraine and tension-type headache in a general population: precipitating factors, female hormones, sleep patterns and relation to lifestyle. *Pain* 1993; **53**: 65–72.

[3] Sacco S, Ricci S, Carolci A. Tension-type headache and systemic medical disorders. *Curr Pain Headache Rep* 2011; **15**: 438–43.

[4] Kaniecki R. Headache assessment and management. *JAMA* 2003; **289**: 1430–3.

[5] Frishberg B, Rosenberg J, Matchar D, *et al.* Evidence-based guidelines in the primary care setting: neuroimaging in patients with nonacute headache. Available at: http://www.aan.com/professionals/practice/pdfs/gl0088.pdf Accessed December 2011.

[6] Kaniecki RG. Migraine and tension-type headache: An assessment of challenges in diagnosis. *Neurology* 2002; **58**(suppl 6): S15–20.

[7] Lipton R, Diamond S, Reed M, *et al.* Migraine diagnosis and treatment: results from the American Migraine Study II. *Headache* 2001; **41**: 638–45.

[8] Lipton R, Stewart F, Cady R, *et al.* Sumatriptan for the range of headaches in migraine sufferers: results of the Spectrum Study. *Headache* 2000; **40**: 783–91.

[9] Kaniecki R, Ruoff G, Smith T, *et al.* Prevalence of migraine and response to sumatriptan in patients self-reporting tension/stress headache. *Curr Res Med Opin* 2006; **22**: 1535–44.

[10] Tepper S, Dahlof C, Dowson A. Prevalence and diagnosis of migraine in patients consulting their physician with a complaint of headache. Data from the Landmark Study. *Headache* 2004; **44**: 856–64.

[11] Schwartz BS, Stewart WF, Simon D *et al.* Epidemiology of tension-type headache. *JAMA* 1998; **279**: 381–3.

[12] Stovner L, Hagen K, Jensen R, *et al.* The global burden of headache: a documentation of headache prevalence and disability worldwide. *Cephalalgia* 2007; **27**: 193–210.

[13] Crystal S, Robbins M. Epidemiology of tension-type headache. *Curr Pain Headache Rep* 2010; **14**: 449–54.

[14] Anttila P. Tension-type headache in childhood and adolescence. *Lancet Neurol* 2006; **5**: 268–74.

[15] Monteith T, Sprenger T. Tension-type headache in adolescence and childhood: where are we now? *Curr Pain Headache Rep* 2010; **14**: 424–30.

[16] Jensen R, Stovner L. Epidemiology and comorbidity of headache. *Lancet Neurol* 2008; **7**: 354–61.

[17] Lyngberg A, Rasmussen B, Jorgensen T, *et al.* Has the prevalence of migraine and tension-type headache changed over a 12-year period? A Danish population survey. *Eur J Epidemiol* 2005; **20**: 243–9.

[18] Ballegaard V, Thede-Schmidt-Hansen P, Svensson P, *et al.* Are headache and temporomandibular disorders related? A blinded study. *Cephalalgia* 2008; **28**: 832–41.

[19] Sacco S. Diagnostic issues in tension-type headache. *Curr Pain Headache Rep* 2008; **12**: 437–41.

[20] Ficek S, Wittrock D. Subjective stress and coping in recurrent tension-type headache. *Headache* 1995; **35**: 455–60.

[21] Jensen R. Mechanisms of tension-type headache. *Cephalalgia* 2001; **21**: 786–9.

[22] Bag B, Hacihasanoglu R, Tufecki F. Examination of anxiety, hostility and psychiatric disorders in patients with migraine and tension-type headache. *Int J Clin Pract* 2005; **59**: 515–21.

[23] Beghi E, Bussone G, D'Amico D, *et al.* Headache, anxiety and depressive disorders: the HADAS study. *J Headache Pain* 2010; **11**: 141–50.

[24] Jensen R, Bendtsen L, Olesen J. Muscular factors are of importance in tension-type headache. *Headache* 1998; **38**: 10–17.

[25] Ulrich V, Gervil M, Olesen J. The relative influence of environment and genes in episodic tension-type headache. *Neurology* 2004; **62**: 2065–9.

[26] Cathcart S, Winefield A, Lushington K, *et al.* Stress and tension-type headache mechanisms. *Cephalalgia* 2010; **30**: 1250–67.

[27] Ashina M. Neurobiology of chronic tension-type headache. *Cephalalgia* 2004; **24**: 161–72.

[28] Fumal A, Schoenen J. Tension-type headache: current research and clinical management. *Lancet Neurol* 2008; **7**: 70–83.

[29] Bendtsen L, Fernandez-de-la-Penas C. The role of muscles in tension-type headache. *Curr Pain Headache Rep* 2011; **15**: 451–8.

[30] Fernandez-de-la-Penas C, Cuadrado M, Pareja J. Myofascial trigger points, neck mobility, and forward head posture in episodic tension-type headache. *Headache* 2007; **47**: 662–72.

[31] Ashina M, Stallknecht B, Bendtsen L, *et al.* In vivo evidence of altered skeletal muscle blood flow in chronic tension-type headache. *Brain* 2002; **125**: 320–6.

[32] Ashina M, Stallknecht B, Bendtsen L, *et al.* Tender points are not sites of ongoing inflammation – in-vivo evidence in patients with chronic tension-type headache. *Cephalalgia* 2003; **23**: 109–16.

[33] Rossi P, Vollono C, Valeriani M. The contribution of clinical neurophysiology to the comprehension of the tension-type headache mechanisms. *Clin Neurophysiol* 2011; **122**: 1075–85.

[34] Lindelof K, Ellrich J, Jensen R, *et al.* Central pain processing in chronic tension-type headache. *Clin Neurophysiol* 2009; **120**: 1364–70.

[35] Buchgreitz L, Lyngberg A, Bendtsen L, *et al.* Increased prevalence of tension-type headache over a 12-year period is related to increased pain sensitivity: a population study. *Cephalalgia* 2007; **27**: 145–52.

[36] Schmidt-Wilcke T, Leinisch E, Straube A, *et al.* Gray matter decrease in patients with chronic tension-type headache. *Neurology* 2005; **65**: 1483–6.

[37] Loder E, Rizzoli P. Tension-type headache. *BMJ* 2008; **336**: 88–92.

[38] Bendtsen L, Evers S, Linde M, *et al.* EFNS guideline on the treatment of tension-type headache – report of an EFNS task force. *Eur J Neurol* 2010; **17**: 1318–25.

[39] Bendtsen L, Jensen R. Treating tension-type headache – an expert opinion. *Expert Opin Pharmacother* 2011; **12**: 1099–109.

[40] Naumann M, So Y, Argoff CE, *et al.* Assessment: Botulinum neurotoxin in the treatment of autonomic disorders and pain (an evidence-based review). Report of the Therapeutics and Technology Assessment Subcommittee of the Amercian Academy of Neurology. *Neurology* 2008; **70**: 1707–14.

[41] Jackson J, Shimeall W, Sessums L, *et al.* Tricyclic antidepressants and headaches: a systematic review and meta-analysis. *BMJ* 2010; **341**: c5222 doi:10.1136/bmj.c5222.

[42] Verhagen A, Damen L, Berger M, *et al.* Lack of benefit for prophylactic drugs of tension-type headache in adults: a systematic review. *Fam Pract* 2010; **27**: 151–65.

[43] Couch J. The long-term prognosis of tension-type headache. *Curr Pain and Headache Rep* 2005; **9**: 436–41.

[44] Mork H, Jensen R. Prognosis of tension-type headache: a 10-year follow-up study of patients with frequent tension-type headache. *Cephalalgia* 2000; **20**: 434.

[45] Lyngberg A, Rasmussen B, Jorgensen T, *et al.* Prognosis of migraine and tension-type headache: a population-based follow-up study. *Neurology* 2005; **65**: 580–5.

Chapter 4

Mood disorder and headache

Mallika Lavakumar, Philip R. Muskin, and Peter A. Shapiro

Introduction

Mood disorders encompass a group of syndromes in which pathological mood episodes dominate the clinical presentation. Mood episodes are characterized by either depressed or elevated mood accompanied by a cluster of typically associated signs and symptoms. In the fourth century BC Hippocrates used the terms "melancholia" and "mania" to label mood disturbances. He identified melancholia as a distinct entity of despondency with persisting mental and physical symptoms, which is known today as depression.

The *Diagnostic and Statistical Manual of Mental Disorders* (DSM-IV-TR), [1] the most widely used diagnostic criteria for mental disorders in the United States, organizes mood abnormality into mood episodes. The mood episodes listed in the DSM-IV-TR include major depressive episode, manic episode, hypomanic episode, and mixed episode. A major depressive episode is defined as a period lasting at least 2 weeks during which one has either depressed mood or a significant lack of interest in activities (anhedonia) with four other associated findings. Associated findings can include sleep disruption, changes in weight or appetite, psychomotor agitation or retardation, loss of energy, feelings of guilt or worthlessness, impaired concentration, and recurrent thoughts of death or suicidal behavior. A manic episode is defined as a period lasting at least one week during which one has a persistently euphoric or irritable mood. During the period of mood destabilization three (four if the mood is only irritable) of the following associated symptoms need to be present: heightened self-esteem, decreased need for sleep, more talkative than usual, a subjective experience of racing thoughts or observation of "flight of ideas," increase in goal-directed activity, and excessive hedonistic activity with potential for harm. The symptoms observed in hypomanic episodes are identical to manic episodes. The duration of a hypomanic episode can be as brief as 4 days. The presence of psychosis (i.e., delusions, hallucinations, gross thought disorder), the need for psychiatric hospitalization, and/or the persistence of symptoms for at least a week distinguish manic episodes from hypomanic ones. Mixed episodes occur when the criteria are met for a manic episode and a major depressive episode.

The DSM-IV classifies mood disorders as major depressive disorder, dysthymic disorder (mild chronic depression), bipolar I disorder, bipolar II disorder, and cyclothymic disorder, on the basis of the types of mood episodes present in the patient's history. The DSM-IV also distinguishes mood disorders that are secondary to a general medical condition or a substance as a set of diagnoses distinct from these primary mood disorders.

The presence of a single major depressive episode, in the absence of a history of mania or hypomania, and in the absence of evidence for a diagnosis of a secondary mood disorder, is diagnostic of Major Depressive Disorder. In most affected individuals depressive episodes are recurrent. Depressive episodes are characterized as mild, moderate, or severe. Severe depression can be accompanied by psychotic symptoms such as delusions or hallucinations consistent with depressive themes. Delusions of guilt (e.g., being responsible for illness or death of a loved one), delusions of deserving punishment (being punished because of a personal failure), nihilistic delusions (believing that oneself or the world is destructing) and somatic delusions (e.g., that one's organs are decaying and that death is imminent) are typical.

A diagnosis of Bipolar I Disorder requires at least one episode of mania. Manic episodes cause marked

The Neuropsychiatry of Headache, ed. Mark W. Green and Philip R. Muskin. Published by Cambridge University Press.

impairment in functioning and often require hospitalization. Patients can become psychotic during a manic episode. Bipolar II disorder requires a history of a major depressive episode and a hypomanic episode without a history of mania. The presence of psychosis (i.e., delusions, hallucinations, gross thought disorder), the need for psychiatric hospitalization, and/or the persistence of symptoms for at least a week distinguish manic episodes from hypomanic episodes. Cyclothymic disorder is characterized by at least 2 years of numerous periods of hypomanic symptoms and numerous periods of depressive symptoms that do not meet criteria for a major depressive episode.

Epidemiology

The association between headaches and mood disorders has been demonstrated for many years across various cultures. Numerous cross sectional studies have demonstrated a high prevalence of major depressive disorder in those with migraines. In a cohort of 457 Swiss adults 27–28 years of age, the 1-year prevalence of major depressive disorder in those with migraines (14.7%) is twice that of patients without migraines (7.3%, odds ratio 2.2, 95% CI 1.1–4.8). [2] Psychiatric diagnoses are based on research interviews and made according to contemporaneous standardized operational criteria such as the Feighner Criteria. [3] the Research Diagnostic Criteria for Schizophrenia and Affective Disorders [4] and the DSM-III [5], and the diagnosis of migraines is likewise based on contemporaneous standardized criteria. [6] Similarly, a larger (n = 36 984) and more recent (2008) study, using the standardized Comprehensive International Diagnostic Interview (CIDI) and DSM-IV criteria for mood disorders, finds that the lifetime prevalence of depression is 18.8% in migraineurs (95% CI 17.0–20.5) and 9.8% (95% CI 9.3–10.3) in patients without migraines. [7]

The association of migraine with major depressive disorder in cross-sectional studies has led to investigations of whether the presence of either headaches or mood disorders predisposes to the development of the other condition. These studies have yielded conflicting results. Breslau and colleagues examine the association between migraine and depression in a prospective sample of 1007 young adult (age 21–30) members of a large HMO in southeast Michigan. The hazard ratio for new-onset migraine in subjects with major depression is 3.1 (95% CI 2.0–5.0). Conversely, the hazard ratio for new-onset major depression in subjects with migraine is 3.2 (95% CI 2.3–4.6). [8] In another prospective cohort, including 1186 middle-aged adults. [9] similar bidirectional relationships are detected. The risk of first-onset migraine in persons with pre-existing major depression is threefold higher than in persons with no history of major depression. The risk of first-onset major depression in persons with pre-existing migraine is more than fivefold higher than the risk for persons with no history of headaches. A retrospective cohort study from the Canadian National Population Health Survey, with 12 years of follow-up data, finds that respondents with migraines are 1.6 times more likely to develop major depressive episodes than those without migraines. [10] There is no association of major depressive disorder history in this study with an increased incidence of migraines. The Baltimore Epidemiological Catchment Area Study finds no prospective relationship between the two conditions. [11] In summary, longitudinal studies suggest a bidirectional relationship between migraine and major depressive disorder, but further investigation to confirm this is necessary.

Differences in mood pathology and associated behaviors seem to exist between migraineurs with aura and those without aura. In a prospectively studied cohort in whom migraine is strongly associated with the development of major depression, the association is stronger in migraineurs with aura (odds ratio 4.9; 95% CI 3.34–7.19) than in migraineurs without aura (odds ratio 3.0; 95% CI 2.23–4.14). [12] Patients with migraine with aura are more likely to attempt suicide than those without aura. [13] Compared to those with no aura, migraineurs with aura are more likely to be depressed, nervous, and inhibited, and less likely to be resilient. [14] These studies suggest that the presence of an aura should raise suspicion and vigilance for affective pathology.

In addition to the association with major depressive disorder, migraine is also associated with bipolar affective disorder. Merikangas *et al.* find that the 1-year prevalence of bipolar spectrum disorders is nearly three-fold higher in migraine sufferers compared with those without migraines. [2] In another study of migraine patients, the lifetime prevalence rates of bipolar disorder type I and type II are 4.9% and 7.8%, respectively, [15] both rates are substantially higher than the overall prevalence of bipolar disorder in the general population (1%). In a large Canadian community health survey the lifetime presence of bipolar disorder in migraine sufferers is 2.8% (95% CI 2.2–3.4) compared to 0.7% (95% CI 0.6–0.9) in patients without migraines.

[7] The results of the above studies indicate that bipolar disorder appears to be more prevalent in those with migraines compared to those without migraines.

Turning the relationship on its head, migraines are also more common in those with bipolar disorder than in the general population. [16] Within the bipolar spectrum migraines seem to be more prevalent in those with bipolar II disorder than in bipolar I disorder. [15,17]. Low *et al.* report an overall lifetime migraine prevalence of 39.8% among outpatients with bipolar disorder. [18] The subgroup of patients attending their clinic with bipolar II disorder have a lifetime migraine prevalence of 64.7%; however, the ascertainment of information is based on retrospective recall by patients of migraines diagnosis, which could have resulted in a recall bias and could account for the extraordinarily high prevalence reported. Longitudinal studies that examine whether having either bipolar disorder or migraines impacts the incidence of the other condition are lacking.

Co-occurrence of bipolar disorder and headaches has a substantial impact on psychosocial function and health care utilization. Patients with bipolar disorder who suffer from migraine are more likely than those without migraine to be single, to receive social welfare benefits, and to live in a low-income household, and they have more severe psychosocial impairments. [19] The Canadian Community Health Survey finds that bipolar men with migraine are more likely than those without migraine to utilize primary and mental health care services, and that bipolar women with comorbid migraine are more likely to require help with personal or instrumental activities of daily living when compared to bipolar women without migraine. [16] There is a growing body of evidence that implicates psychiatric comorbidity as a risk factor for the transformation of episodic headache into chronic and daily headache syndromes, including medication overuse headache. [20,21]

Patients with mood disorders are at higher risk for attempting suicide than the general population. Whereas the lifetime risk of suicide in people without a psychiatric disorder is 0.72% in men and 0.26% in women, the corresponding risks of suicide for those with unipolar depression are 6.67% in men and 3.77% in women, and for bipolar disorder, 7.77% in men and 4.78% in women. [22] The presence of a headache in patients with mood disorders further increases this risk. Suicide is attempted more often when a patient has comorbid mood disorder and headache than when he or she has either alone. Breslau and Davis find that the risk of suicide attempts is much higher in patients with MDD and comorbid migraine (OR 16.2, 95% CI 6.7–39.4) compared to those with either MDD (OR 7.6, 95% CI 3.4–16.8) or migraines (OR 3.0, 95% CI 1.2–8.0). [23]

Bipolar disorder patients with comorbid migraine have a higher rate of previous suicide attempts than those without migraines (40% vs. 27%, $P = 0.03$). [15] Neurologists should be aware that suicide risk is higher in bipolar patients and perhaps higher in patients with comorbid migraines and bipolar disorder. One study evaluates the relationship between suicide risk and quality of life in patients affected by chronic daily headache. An instrument assessing suicide intent evaluates past and current suicide behavior and ideation and classifies subjects into four groups: no suicidal risk, low suicidal risk, moderate suicidal risk, and high suicidal risk. Suicidal intent is inversely correlated with quality of life (standardized regression coefficient $= -0.55$; $t = -3.06$; $P<0.01$). [24]

Screening and diagnosis

The high prevalence of depression in patients with migraines warrants screening for depression during the evaluation of a new patient with migraine. Because mood disorders are episodic, euthymia (normal mood) during a clinical encounter does not preclude the diagnosis of a mood disorder. Since being diagnosed with migraines predicts new onset of major depressive disorder, it is advisable to annually screen for depression in patients with migraines. The index of suspicion for depression should be higher when routine inquiries regarding sleep and appetite problems or fatigue during a patient's visit yield affirmative responses. This should be followed up with questions regarding depressed mood and anhedonia, the cardinal symptoms of depression.

Various screening tools for depression have been validated in medically ill patients, though not specifically in patients with migraines. These include the Center for Epidemiologic Studies Depression Scale (CES-D), the Beck Depression Inventory II (BDI-II), and the Patient Health Questionnaire depression module (PHQ-9 and PHQ-2). The PHQ-2 is particularly attractive since it is a very brief rating scale. It includes the first 2 items of the PHQ-9, which is based directly on the diagnostic criteria for major depressive disorder in the DSM-IV-TR. In a study in primary care and Ob-Gyn clinics, the PHQ-2 is validated against a mental health professional interview as a screening tool for

Table 4.1. PHQ2 (Kroenke *et al.* 2003)

"Over the past two weeks, how often have you been bothered by any of the following problems?"
1. "little interest or pleasure in doing things?" 2. "feeling down, depressed, or hopeless?"
For each item, the response options are "not at all," "several days," "more than half the days," and "nearly every day," scored as 0, 1, 2, and 3, respectively. Thus, the PHQ-2 score can range from 0 to 6.

depression. [25] A score of 3 or greater has a sensitivity of 83% and a specificity of 92% for major depression. Thus, a PHQ-2 score of 3 or greater is strongly suggestive of major depressive disorder and should be followed by more detailed inquiry into symptoms diagnostic of a major depressive episode. Administration of the PHQ2 is outlined in Table 4.1.

The high prevalence of bipolar disorder in patients with migraine calls for screening during the initial visit and annually. In those found to have depression it is especially important to screen for a history of mania, since depressive episodes can represent the depressive pole of bipolar disorder, and patients with bipolar disorder typically experience more lifetime days with depressive symptoms than with manic symptoms. Some investigators believe that antidepressant treatment without a concomitant mood stabilizer in those with bipolar disorder can precipitate a switch to mania. An accurate diagnosis should be made before initiating treatment. Limitations to achieving an accurate diagnosis stem from patients' reluctance to divulge information due to the stigma associated with the illness. Mania represents an altered mental state, and patients' recollections of manic episodes may be impaired, making bipolar illness difficult to diagnose retroactively. The Mood Disorders Questionnaire is a validated self-report screening instrument for Bipolar Disorder; however, it has a sensitivity of only 70%, less than optimal for screening. [26] The best way to screen for bipolar disorder is systematic inquiry, using a curious and non-judgmental approach by the physician, about experiences reflecting the diagnostic criteria for mania and hypomania.

Treatment

The treatment of depression is broadly divided into psychopharmacological and psychological therapies. The major categories of biological therapies include selective serotonin reuptake inhibitors (SSRIs), serotonin

Table 4.2. Effective dose range of antidepressants

Drug	Dose range (mg)
Fluoxetine (Prozac)	20–80
Sertraline (Zoloft)	50–200
Paroxetine (Paxil)	20–60
Citalopram (Celexa)	20–80
Escitalopram (Lexapro)	10–30
Venlafaxine XR (Effexor XR)	75–225
Desvenlafaxine (Pristiq)	50
Duloxetine (Cymbalta)	40–120
Bupropion XL (Wellbutrin XL)	150–450
Mirtazapine (Remeron)	15–45
Trazodone (Desyrel, Oleptro)	150–600
Nefazadone (Nefazadone)	300–600
Amitriptlyne (Elavil)	50–300
Nortriptyline (Pamelor)	75–300
Imipramine (Tofranil)	75–300
Desipramine (Norpramin)	75–300
Phenelezine (Nardil)	45–90
Tranylcypromine (Parnate)	30–60
Vilazodone (Viibryd)	40

norepinephrine reuptake inhibitors (SNRIs), tricyclic antidepressants (TCAs), and monoamine oxidase inhibitors (MAOIs). In addition to these classes of antidepressants, mirtazapine, bupropion, nefazodone, and trazodone each has unique mechanisms of action and are effective for the treatment of depression. Table 4.2 lists commonly used antidepressants and their doses.

While use of older antidepressants, especially tricyclic antidepressants and monoamine oxidase inhibitors, is often limited by side effects, the relatively benign side effect profile of SSRIs, introduced into the United States market in 1988, has led to their adoption as first-line antidepressant therapies. The United States Food and Drug administration (USFDA) has approved the use of fluoxetine, sertraline, paroxetine, citalopram, escitalopram, and vilazodone for the treatment of major depressive disorder. There is also fair support for the effectiveness of some SSRIs in migraine prophylaxis. [27]

SSRIs act on the serotonin transporter to prevent serotonin reuptake into the presynaptic cell body, resulting in increased intra-synaptic serotonin and increased binding to post-synaptic receptors. The side effects of

SSRIs include gastrointestinal distress, headaches, anxiety, and sexual dysfunction. Gastrointestinal distress, headaches and anxiety may occur for the first few days following initiation of the medication and typically resolve within a week. The most common sexual side effects of SSRIs are decreased libido, anorgasmia in women, and delayed ejaculation in men. These effects tend to persist, and may interfere with treatment adherence. Treatment for SSRI-induced sexual dysfunctions includes decreasing the dose, switching to an alternative antidepressant, and adding bupropion. The benefit of antidepressant switching or dose reduction to mitigate sexual dysfunction must be weighed against the potential loss of clinical effectiveness. Abruptly stopping paroxetine, which has a short half-life, may result in an unpleasant discontinuation syndrome. Paroxetine should be gradually tapered. Other less common adverse events associated with SSRIs include abnormal bleeding due to platelet effects and the syndrome of inappropriate antidiuretic hormone.

The SNRIs are venlafaxine, its active metabolite, desvenlafaxine, and duloxetine. They act on the serotonin and the norepinephrine transporters to inhibit reuptake of these neurotransmitters, effectively increasing intra-synaptic serotonin and norepinephrine available for post-synaptic transmission. The side effects of SNRIs are similar to those of SSRIs at low doses. At high doses they have the added potential side effect of hypertension. Like paroxetine, venlafaxine and duloxetine have short half-lives; abrupt discontinuation may result in a withdrawal syndrome.

Since the first randomized trial in which a TCA was shown to improve major depression, [28] many subsequent randomized controlled trials have demonstrated their efficacy as treatment for major depressive disorder. [29] Mechanistically, these medications inhibit reuptake of serotonin and/or norepinephrine. They are also anticholinergic, anti-histaminergic and anti-α-adrenergic to varying degrees, which accounts for many of their side effects. TCAs have cardiovascular side effects such as increased heart rate, AV nodal blockade, PR and QT prolongation with accompanying risk of ventricular arrhythmias, and orthostatic hypotension. They act similarly to class I antiarrhythmics such as quinidine, disopyramide, and procainamide. Combinations of TCAs with other class I antiarrhythmics can exert toxic effects on cardiac conduction. Patients can have a range of anticholinergic side effects from the relatively benign, such as dry mouth and mild blurring of vision, to the more serious, such as paralytic ileus, hyperpyrexia, urinary retention, increased intra-ocular pressure, and delirium. SSRIs and TCAs have similar efficacy for the treatment of mild to moderate depression, with SSRIs being better tolerated. [30] There is some evidence to support the use of TCAs over SSRIs in severe depression [31] although there is also evidence to the contrary. [32] There is robust evidence that amitriptyline is successful in preventing migraine and in treatment of chronic tension-type headaches. [27] It is often effective for migraine prophylaxis at doses of 25 mg/day, while those with depression might need up to 300 mg/day. Since amitriptyline serves the dual purpose of an antidepressant and a prophylactic agent for migraines, its use can obviate polypharmacy.

Headaches are potential side effects of antidepressants such as SSRIs, SNRIs, TCAs, MAOIs, bupropion, and mirtazapine. There is not much information on the characteristics of antidepressant-related headaches or how frequently they occur. Trazodone can potentially cause migraines via its active metabolite, *m*-chlorophenylpiperazine (*m*CPP), an agent implicated in migraines. While the evidence for this is limited to a case report, patients who are started on trazodone who complain of increased headaches or anxiety may be producing larger amounts of the metabolites than is typical. [33] In general, headaches produced by antidepressants resolve within 2 weeks. When patients report that their headache is worse after the initiation of antidepressants, it is worthwhile to recommend that they stay the course for 2 weeks in anticipation that headache symptoms will likely improve.

In 2006 the USFDA issued a public health advisory stating that the combined use of SSRIs or SNRIs with serotonin agonists such as triptans can lead to serotonin syndrome. Serotonin syndrome is a potentially life-threatening adverse drug reaction that results from the use of serotonergic agents. The syndrome occurs with a spectrum of severity; features include tachycardia, shivering, hyperthermia, diaphoresis, mydriasis, tremor, hyperreflexia, clonus, and myoclonus. [34] The Hunter Serotonin Toxicity Criteria, which requires the observation of clonus and hyperreflexia in the setting of a serotonergic drug, are diagnostic of serotonin syndrome with 84% sensitivity and 97% specificity. [35] The USFDA warning was based on case reports with diagnostic criteria that are not validated. Other limitations include the lack of peer review of several cases and confounding factors that accounted for the presentation. [36] SSRIs and SNRIs are not contraindicated for use with triptans. Awareness of diagnostic classification and maintaining vigilance for the syndrome when these medications are used concurrently are recommended.

For patients with mood disorders, failure to achieve remission has been associated with adverse outcomes such as increased risk of relapse [37] and greater impairment in work, family roles, and economic functioning. [38] When patients who no longer met criteria for a major depressive episode, but had subsyndromal symptoms were compared to asymptomatic patients, they tended to have a shorter time to recurrence, a greater number of future depressive episodes, and more chronic depressive episodes. [39] Partial resolution of depression seems to predict a more severe and chronic future course. Thus attempting to achieve complete resolution of symptoms should always be the goal in treatment.

Achieving remission is a considerably more stringent outcome to achieve than simple response. The first step in this endeavor is to reliably quantify and track symptoms. This has led to the widespread use of rating scales to monitor symptoms in current clinical practice. The Beck Depression Inventory (BDI)-II is a widely accepted self-rating scale used to measure depressive distress. A BDI-II score of 0–13 indicates minimal depression, 14–19 mild depression, 20–28 moderate depression, and 29–63 severe depression.

When patients do not respond or remit, clinicians should inquire about adherence to the prescription. This should be followed by diagnostic reassessment in order to confirm whether the diagnosis is indeed major depression. The possibility of bipolar disorder should be entertained. Also one should consider the possibility that psychiatric comorbidity is complicating treatment. The two most common types of psychiatric comorbidity associated with failure to improve are personality disorders and substance use disorders. Medical comorbidities such as coronary artery disease, heart failure, ESRD, hypothyroidism, cancer, Parkinsons's disease, stroke, and multiple sclerosis should also be considered as potential contributors to the patient's depressive presentation. Finally, prescribed substances such as corticosteroids, interferon-alpha, and progestin-releasing contraceptives may lead to depressive symptoms. The classical teaching that beta-blockers, which are used for migraine prophylaxis, cause depression is not supported by a recent review of 15 randomized trials. [40]

Three broad psychopharmacological approaches are available for treating patients who have insufficient response to an antidepressant. When a patient does not achieve a sufficient clinical response, the possible treatment strategies include increasing the dose of the antidepressant, switching to a different antidepressant, or augmenting the original antidepressant with a second agent. If the patient has been on an antidepressant for 8 weeks and has not had any clinical response, then it is advisable to switch to a different agent. If partial response occurs, then it is worthwhile to increase the dose. If at 12 weeks the patient still only experiences partial response, then one may augment with various agents. When choosing between switching and augmentation consider the tolerability of the first-line agent, the potential loss of partial benefit from the first-line antidepressant, and the potential added side effects of adding a second agent.

The greatest evidence for the efficacy of switching has been studied in newer antidepressants. In one study patients who are taking an SSRI are switched to either venlafaxine (SNRI) or paroxetine (SSRI). Remission rates are 42% for venlafaxine and 20% for paroxetine. [41] In another study venlafaxine is more effective than citalopram in the subset of people with severe depression who had already been treated with an SSRI. [42] There are studies to the contrary, which show no difference in remission of symptoms when one is switched from an SSRI to either an SNRI or a different SSRI. [40] A study that examines switching between older antidepressants demonstrates that switching imipramine (TCA) non-responders to phenelzine (MAOI) is superior to switching phenelzine non-responders to imipramine. [43] In another study that investigates switching between classes, sertraline (SSRI) non-responders are switched to imipramine and imipramine non-responders are switched to sertraline. [44] Switch to sertraline demonstrates higher response rates and better tolerability. One study investigates a depressed population, which fails to remit after several different treatment attempts. In this population the effects of switching to tranylcypromine (MAOI) are no different than those of switching to a combination of mirtazapine and venlafaxine. [45]

The most intensively studied treatment strategy for non-response or partial response is augmentation with atypical antipsychotics including aripiprazole, olanzapine, quetiapine, and risperidone. A meta-analysis of ten randomized, double-blind studies indicated that antipsychotics are more effective than placebo as augmenting agents with pooled remission rates of approximately 47% vs. 22%. [46] Only aripiprazole and quetiapine have USFDA approval for use as augmentation with antidepressants for major depressive disorder. Augmentation with mirtazapine, mianserin, and omega-3 fatty acids is also supported by considerable efficacy. [46] The evidence for augmenting with desipramine, modafinil, bupropion, triiodothyronine, and lithium has yielded mixed results. [46] While there are some data to support the use of lithium and triiodothyronine as augmenting agents to TCAs, there are no data to support these medications as adjuncts to newer antidepressants such as SSRIs and SNRIs. Preliminary data suggests that testosterone may augment antidepressants in the subset of depressed men who have low serum free testosterone. [47]

Medication interventions are more likely to be successful when patients are aware of what to expect. Informing patients that it takes up to 2 weeks for symptoms to begin to improve and can take up to 12 weeks for full clinical benefit can prevent early discontinuation. False beliefs about medications contribute to poor adherence. Among these are the beliefs that antidepressants are addicting, that one is a weak person if one uses antidepressants, and that one's personality will change. Patients may need to be educated that these ideas are untrue. Typically, the first depressive symptoms to improve after initiating antidepressant therapy are the neurovegetative symptoms, such as sleep disruption, appetite changes, and fatigue. These are followed by the neurocognitive symptoms such as dysphoria, feelings of worthlessness, and hopelessness. It is common in the treatment of depressed patients for loved ones and physicians to notice an improvement before the patient notices a change.

Denial is a frequent psychological defense in medical and psychiatric illness. A frequent manifestation of denial of illness is non-adherence to medication. Patients may also try to negotiate lowering the antidepressant dose. For patients with recurrent major depression, efforts should be made to maintain the patient at the dose at which he or she attained remission, as lowering the dose is associated with a greater likelihood of relapse. [48,49] If the patient has a single episode of mild, uncomplicated depression, then one might attempt discontinuation of antidepressant therapy following a year of treatment with close follow-up.

As an alternative, or in addition, to medication treatments for depression, there is considerable evidence for the benefits of psychotherapy in the treatment of depression. Moreover, for the myriad problems in living associated with mild to moderate depressed mood, but not with all the symptoms needed to establish a diagnosis of major depressive disorder or bipolar disorder, antidepressant drugs are less likely to be of substantial benefit, and psychotherapy may be more appropriate.

The evidence-based psychotherapies for treatment of depression are cognitive therapy (CT), behavior therapy (BT), and interpersonal psychotherapy (IPT). Cognitive therapy proposes that irrational beliefs and distorted attitudes toward oneself, one's surroundings, and the future are responsible for depressive symptoms. For example, a core belief in many depressed patients is that they are bad or unworthy. Negative automatic thoughts are conclusions based on negatively valenced core assumptions drawn without conscious reflection as to their validity, and have the effect of reinforcing depressive symptoms. For example, the patient who unconsciously believes himself to be a bad person may conclude that no one would be willing to help him when he has a problem, leading to feelings of sadness and hopelessness. The goal of cognitive therapy is to identify and alter cognitive distortions that maintain depressive symptoms. Cognitive therapy is generally conducted as a once- to twice-weekly highly structured psychotherapy of several months duration, focusing on improving one's ability to identify and test irrational and erroneous negative thoughts, and to "reframe" one's experiences more realistically. Since CT was first developed in the 1960s, many clinical trials have demonstrated its efficacy for the treatment of depression. A meta-analysis that includes 48 high-quality controlled trials and a total of 2765 patients with depression of mild–moderate severity demonstrates that CT is an effective treatment in patients with mild to moderate depression. [50]

The term "cognitive behavioral therapy" (CBT) refers to the combination of cognitive therapy with specific behavioral therapy strategies. The behavioral model postulates that during depressed states normal behavior patterns are disrupted and one is prone to social withdrawal and to avoidance of pleasant experiences. Consequently, one misses the opportunity to have positive experiences which lift mood. Behavior therapy for depression involves promoting pleasant and productive activities. Examples of behavioral activation include prescriptions to shower, exercise, leave home on a daily basis, and schedule pleasant activity with a friend or a loved one. Behavior therapy has been studied and demonstrated to be an effective treatment for depression. A meta-analysis including 1109 subjects shows that behavioral therapies are superior to controls. [51]

In a pilot study evaluating the effect of CBT group treatment on headache frequency in patients with chronic, disabling headaches, 62 individuals undergo ten sessions of group CBT and are evaluated 1 month post-treatment. Overall, 50% of participants experience at least a 50% reduction in headache frequency from pre- to post-treatment. [52] The major limitation of this study is the lack of a control group, and additional studies are needed to confirm this effect. Nevertheless, the appeal of such a treatment approach as an adjunct to other headache treatments is clear. Whether an effect of CBT on headache frequency and severity is correlated with effects on mood, or depends on the presence of a mood disorder at baseline, has not been ascertained.

Interpersonal psychotherapy theory is based on the axiom that depression occurs in the context of interpersonal problems, and proposes that treatment aimed at finding solutions for these interpersonal difficulties will be associated with alleviation of depression symptoms. Specific interpersonal difficulties are understood as falling into the general categories of loss (that is mourning the death of an important person), role disputes, role transitions, and interpersonal deficits. [53] Interpersonal psychotherapy (IPT) is as effective for treatment of major depressive disorder as antidepressant medication, and significantly more effective than placebo, in the landmark NIH Collaborative Study of Depression clinical trial. [54] A recent large meta-analysis examines 38 studies of interpersonal psychotherapy with total sample size of 4356 patients. This meta-analysis demonstrates superiority of IPT compared with a control group (NNT = 2.9). Although in the acute treatment phase, pharmacotherapy is more effective than IPT, combination treatment is not more effective than IPT alone. However in the maintenance phase, combination treatment with pharmacotherapy and IPT is more effective in preventing relapse than pharmacotherapy alone (NNT = 7.6). [55]

The mainstay of treatment for bipolar disorder is treatment with a mood stabilizer. There are decades of data to support the use of lithium as a preventive agent in bipolar disorder, especially bipolar I disorder. Valproic acid, carbamazepine, and lamotrigine are alternative mood stabilizers to lithium. [56–58] In addition, recent studies support the use of aripiprazole and olanzapine as monotherapy for maintenance treatment of bipolar disorder. [59,60] Quetiapine, ziprasidone, and risperidone are effective as adjuncts to other mood stabilizers but not as monotherapy. [61] Table 4.3 lists dosing of mood stabilizers and desirable

Table 4.3. Mood stabilizer doses

Drug	Usual dose (mg)	Goal blood level
Lithium	900–1800	0.8–1.2 mmol/L
Valproic acid	1500–2500	50–100 mg/L
Carbamazepine	400–1200	8–10 mcg/mL
Lamotrigine	100–400	NA
Olanzapine	10–30	NA
Aripiprazole	10–30	NA
Quetiapine	400–800	NA

blood levels. Carbamazepine, risperidone, ziprasidone, quetiapine, paliperidone, asenapine, and haloperidol have all been studied and shown to be efficacious for treatment of acute mania. [61] In clinical practice it is efficient to initiate treatment for acute mania with an agent that can also be used for maintenance treatment. For this reason, lithium, valproic acid and olanzapine are attractive agents. In patients with delusions or hallucinations, antipsychotic interventions are necessary. Evidence-based treatments for bipolar depression include treatment with lamotrigine, olanzapine, the combination of olanzapine plus fluoxetine, and quetiapine. [62–64] There is controversy in the mood disorder literature as to whether antidepressants can precipitate treatment-emergent hypomania or mania. There is some evidence to support that antidepressant-associated switch into mania is more common in patients with migraines compared to those without migraines. [18]. This "switching" phenomenon has not been associated with lamotrigine, olanzapine, combined olanzapine plus fluoxetine, and quetiapine. If antidepressants are used, they should be used along with a mood stabilizer. ECT should be considered for patients who are suicidal, psychotic, catatonic or pregnant. Interpersonal and cognitive therapies are useful when added to pharmacotherapy.

Several treatments that are effective for mood disorders also are efficacious in headache treatment. There is robust evidence that amitriptyline is successful in preventing migraine and in chronic tension-type headaches. [27] It is effective for migraine prophylaxis at doses of 25 mg/day, while for depression doses may range up to 300 mg/day. In a randomized trial, participants with chronic tension-type headaches are randomly assigned to receive an antidepressant (amitriptyline or nortriptyline), placebo, stress management plus antidepressant, or stress management plus placebo. Both TCAs and stress management result in clinical improvement. Combined TCA and stress management produce larger reductions in headache activity, analgesic medication use and disability than either treatment alone. [65] A meta-analysis of randomized placebo-controlled trials in which patients are administered TCAs and SSRIs for prevention of migraine and tension headaches finds that administration of these antidepressants is a highly effective prophylaxis strategy. [66] The effect size in this study is large (standardized mean difference is 0.94, 95% CI 0.65–1.2). This analysis also supports the effectiveness of SSRIs in migraine and chronic tension headache prophylaxis, although the effect size is smaller than for TCAs. There is more recent evidence to support the use of venlafaxine for prophylaxis of migraines and tension headaches. [67] Valproic acid is a well-known migraine prophylactic agent. Numerous small open label trials provide robust evidence for the use of valproic acid in migraine prophylaxis. [68] Topiramate is widely used for migraine prophylaxis and occasionally for mood stabilization. Controlled studies supporting its use as a mood stabilizer are lacking. [69]

As mood disorders and headaches overlap, the medications to treat these conditions are used concomitantly. Potential drug–drug interactions between these agents are listed Table 4.4. Pharmacologic interventions

Table 4.4. Relevant drug–drug interactions of headache agents with mood disorder medications and their neuropsychiatric side effects

Headache medication	Interactions and side effects
TCAs	Levels increased by topiramate, valproic acid, fluoxetine and paroxetine Contraindicted with MAOIs due to risk of serotonin syndrome Risk of switch to mania
Valproic acid	Decreases carbamazepine levels Increases lamotrigine and amitriptyline levels Hyperammonemia and hypothermia when administered with topiramate
Carbamazepine	Levels increased by fluoxetine, trazadone, olanzapine, quetiapine, ibuprofen, verapamil, and valproic acid Decreases levels of lamotrigine, bupropion, citalopram, olanzapine, trileptal, risperidone, topiramate, trazadone, TCAs, valproic acid, and ziprasidone MAOIs should be discontinued for 14 days before initiation of carbamazepine due to risk of serotonin syndrome Coadministration with nefazadone (antidepressant mechanistically similar to trazadone) is contraindicated Concomitant administration with lithium may increase neurotoxic effects Renders oral contraceptives less effective
Lamotrigine	Levels increased by valproic acid; dose must be lowered by 50% when used concomitantly with valproic acid; if dose adjustment is not made there is a risk of toxic epidermal necrolysis Levels decreased by OCPs and carbamazepine
Propranolol	Levels increased by fluoxetine and paroxetine Increases levels of triptans Exacerbates hypotensive effects of TCAs and MAOIs
Ibuprofen	Increases plasma lithium levels
Triptans	Levels increased by MAOIs; coadministration with MAOIs is contraindicated Risk of serotonin syndrome with other serotonergic agents
Verapamil	Concurrent use with lithium may increase neurotoxicity Increases carbamazepine levels
Topiramate	Levels decreased by carbamazepine, valproic acid, and lamotrigine Concomitant administration with valproic acid can cause hyperammonemia and hypothermia At high doses can increase lithium levels
Ergotamines	Rare reports of weakness, hyperreflexia, and incoordination when used with SSRIs
Lithium	Levels increased by NSAIDs Concurrent use with SSRIs can cause diarrhea, confusion, tremor, dizziness and agitation Increased likelihood of neurotoxic effects when administered with carbamazepine
Aspirin	Increases valproate levels

(antidepressants and anticonvulsants) that simultaneously treat both headaches and mood disorders would be attractive options if efficacious. Secondary to differential dosing requirements and resulting side effect profiles, treating comorbid mood disorders and headaches with a single agent is often more effective in theory than in practice. No studies exist that assess the effects of treating mood disorders on migraine symptoms. Clinical trials of pharmacologic headache interventions typically exclude individuals with significant mood disorders. Drug studies that examine efficacy of headache agents that included depressed patients have produced mixed results as to whether headache agents have a favorable impact on depression. It is important to keep in mind that antiepileptic agents, whether prescribed for mood disorders or migraines, increase the seizure threshold and might need to be held temporarily when a patient is undergoing ECT. The USFDA has issued a warning regarding the increased risk of suicidality associated with AEDs. As a class, however, AEDs do not increase risk of suicide attempts in patients with bipolar disorder relative to patients not treated with an AED. Use of AEDs reduces suicide attempt rates in patients with bipolar disorder, both relative to patients not receiving any psychotropic medication and relative to their pretreatment levels. [70]

It is helpful for the physician treating patients with headache to develop a working relationship with a psychiatrist in order to facilitate the care of patients with comorbid migraines and mood disorders. Brief phone "curbside consultation" with a psychiatrist regarding psychiatric problems that arise in the clinic can save time and facilitate high-quality care. In emergencies, the psychiatrist may be able to assist in psychiatric hospitalization of the patient. Table 4.5 lists situations in which referral to a psychiatrist are indicated.

Table 4.5. When to refer patients with mood disorders to a psychiatrist

Patients in whom suicide is a concern
Patients whose depression does not respond to first or second-line interventions
Patients who have poorly controlled bipolar disorder
Patients who are psychotic
Patients who have comorbid substance abuse and personality disorders

References

[1] American Psychiatric Association: *Diagnostic and Statistical Manual of Mental Disorders*, 4th edn, Text Revision. Washington, DC, American Psychiatric Association, 2000.

[2] Merikangas KR, Angst J, Isler H. Migraine and psychopathology: Results of the Zurich Cohort Study of Young Adults. *Arch Gen Psychiatry* 1990; **47**: 849–53.

[3] Feighner JP, Robins E, Guze SB, Woodruff RA, Winokur G, Munoz R. Diagnostic criteria for use in psychiatric research. *Arch Gen Psychiatry* 1972; **26**: 57–63.

[4] Spitzer RL, Endicott J, Robbins E. Research Diagnostic Criteria. *Arch Gen Psychiatry* 1978; **35**: 773–82.

[5] American Psychiatric Association: *Diagnostic and Statistical Manual of Mental Disorders*, 3rd edn. Washington, DC, American Psychiatric Association, 1980.

[6] Ad Hoc Committee on Classification of Headache. *Arch Neurol* 1962; **6**: 173–6.

[7] Jette N, Patten S, Williams J, Becker W, Wiebe S. Comorbidity of migraine and psychiatric disorders-A national population-based study. *Headache* 2008; **48**: 501–16.

[8] Breslau N, Davis GC, Schultz LR, Peterson EL. Migraine and major depression: a longitudinal study. *Headache* 1994; **34**: 387–93.

[9] Breslau N, Lipton RB, Stewart WF, Schultz LR, Welch KMA. Comorbidity of migraine and depression: investigating potential etiology and prognosis. *Neurology* 2003; **60**: 1308–12.

[10] Modgill G, Jette N, Wang JL, Becker WJ, Patten SB. A population-based longitudinal community study of major depression and migraine. *Headache* doi: 10.1111/j.1526-4610.2011.02036.x.

[11] Swartz KL, Pratt LA, Armenian HK, Lee LC, Eaton WW. Mental disorders and the incidence of migraine headaches in a community sample: results from the Baltimore Epidemiologic Catchment Area Follow-up Study. *Arch Gen Psychiatry* 2000; **57**: 945–50.

[12] Breslau N, Schultz LR, Stewart WF, Lipton RB, Lucia VC, Welch KMA. Headache and major depression: is the association specific to migraine? *Neurology* 2000; **54**: 308–13.

[13] Oedegaard KJ, Angst J, Neckelmann D, Fasmer OB. Migraine aura without headache compared to migraine with aura in patients with affective disorders. *J Headache Pain* 2005; **6**: 378–86.

[14] Merikangas KR, Stevens DE, and Angst J. Headache and personality: results of a community sample of young adults. *J Psychiatry Res* 1993; **27**: 187–96.

[15] Ortiz A, Cervantes P, Zlotnik G, *et al.* Cross-prevalence of migraine and bipolar disorder. *Bipolar Disord* 2010; **12**: 397–403.

[16] McIntyre RS, Konarski JZ, Wilkins K, Bouffard B, Soczynska JK, Kennedy SH. The prevalence and impact of migraine headache in bipolar disorder: results from the Canadian Community Health Survey. *Headache* 2006; **46**: 973–82.

[17] Fasmer OB. The prevalence of migraine in patients with bipolar and unipolar affective disorders. *Cephalalgia* 2001; **21**: 894–9.

[18] Low NC. Du Fort GG. Cervantes P. Prevalence, clinical correlates, and treatment of migraine in bipolar disorder. *Headache* 2003; **43**: 940–9.

[19] Mahmood T, Romans S, Silverstone T. Prevalence of migraine in bipolar disorder. *J Affect Disord* 1999; **52**: 239–41.

[20] Radat F, Swendsen J. Psychiatric comorbidity in migraine: A review. *Cephalalgia* 2005; **25**: 165–78.

[21] Scher AI, Lipton RB, Stewart W. Risk factors for chronic daily headache. *Curr Pain Headache Rep* 2002; **6**: 486–91.

[22] Nordentoft M. Mortensen PB. Pedersen CB. Absolute risk of suicide after first hospital contact in mental disorder. *Arch Gen Psych* 2011; **68**: 1058–64.

[23] Breslau N, Davis GC. Migraine, physical health and psychiatric disorder: a prospective epidemiologic study in young adults. *J Psychiatry Res* 1993; **27**: 211–221.

[24] De Filippis S, Erbuto D, Gentili F, *et al.* Mental turmoil, suicide risk, illness perception, and temperament, and their impact on quality of life in chronic daily headache. *J Headache Pain* 2008; **9**: 349–57.

[25] Kroenke K, Spitzer RL, Williams JBW. The Patient Health Questionnaire-2: validity of a two-item depression screener. *Med Care* 2003; **41**: 1284–92.

[26] Hirschfeld RM, Williams JB, Spitzer RL, *et al.* Development and validation of a screening instrument for bipolar spectrum disorder: the Mood Disorder Questionnaire. *Am J Psychiatry* 2000; **157**: 1873–5.

[27] Colombo B, Annovazzi POL, Comi G. Therapy of primary headaches: the role of antidepressants. *Neurol Sci* 2004;25: S171–5.

[28] Kuhn KU. The treatment of depressive disorders with G22 355 (Imipramine Hydrochloride). *Am J Psychiatry* 1958; **115**: 459–64.

[29] Rogers SC, Clay PM. A statistical review of controlled trials of imipramine and placebo in the treatment of depressive illnesses. *Br J Psychiatry* 1975; **127**: 599–603.

[30] Anderson IM. Selective serotonin reuptake inhibitors versus tricyclic antidepressants: a meta-analysis of efficacy and tolerability. *J Affect Disord* 2000; **58**: 19–36.

[31] Joyce PR, Paykel ES. Predictors of drug response in depression. *Arch Gen Psychiatry* 1989; **46**: 89–99.

[32] Paykel ES. Treatment of depression: the relevance of research for clinical practice. *Br J Psychiatry* 1989; **155**: 754–63.

[33] Workman EA, Tellian F, Short D. Trazadone induction of migraine through mCPP. *Am J Psychiatry* 1992; **149**: 712–13.

[34] Boyer EW, Shannon M. The Serotonin Syndrome. *N Engl J Med* 2005; **352**: 1112–20.

[35] Dunkley EJ, Isbister GK, Sibbritt D, Dawson AH, Whyte IM. The Hunter Serotonin Toxicity Criteria: simple and accurate diagnostic decision rules for serotonin toxicity. *QJM* 2003; **96**: 635–42.

[36] Gillman PK. Triptans, serotonin agonists, and serotonin syndrome (serotonin toxicity): a review. *Headache* 2010; **50**: 264–72.

[37] Paykel ES. Ramana R. Cooper Z. Hayhurst H. Kerr J. Barocka A. Residual symptoms after partial remission: an important outcome in depression. *Psychol Med* 1995; **25**(6): 1171–80.

[38] Papakostas GI, Petersen T, Denninger JW, *et al.* Psychosocial functioning during the treatment of major depressive disorder with fluoxetine. *J Clin Psychopharmacology* 2004; **24**: 507–11.

[39] Judd LL, Paulus MJ, Schettler PJ, *et al.* Does incomplete recovery from first lifetime major depressive episode herald a chronic course of illness? *Am J Psychiatry* 2000; **157**: 1501–4.

[40] Ko DT, Hebert PR, Coffey CS, Sedrakyan A, Curtis JP, Krumholz HM. Beta-blocker therapy and symptoms of depression, fatigue, and sexual dysfunction. *JAMA* 2002; **288**: 351–7.

[41] Poirier MF, Boyer P. Venlafaxine and paroxetine in treatment-resistant depression. Double-blind, randomised comparison. *Br J Psychiatry* 1999; **175**: 12–16.

[42] Lenox-Smith AJ, Jiang Q. Venlafaxine extended release versus citalopram in patients with depression unresponsive to a selective serotonin reuptake inhibitor. *Int Clin Psychopharmacol.* 2008 May;**23**: 113–19.

[43] McGrath PJ, Stewart JW, Nunes EV, *et al.* A double-blind crossover trial of imipramine and phenelzine for outpatients with treatment-refractory depression. *Am J Psychiatry* 1993; **150**: 118–23.

[44] Thase ME, Rush AJ, Howland RH, *et al.* Double-blind switch study of imipramine or sertraline treatment of antidepressant-resistant chronic depression. *Arch Gen Psychiatry* 2002; **59**: 233–9.

[45] McGrath PJ, Stewart JW, Fava M, *et al.* Tranylcypromine versus venlafaxine plus mirtazapine

following three failed antidepressant medication trials for depression: a STAR*D report. *Am J Psychiatry* 2006; **163**: 1531–41.

[46] Papakostas GI. Strategies for major depressive disorder. *J Clin Psychiatry* 2009;[**70**suppl6]: 16–25.

[47] Pope HG, Cohane GH, Kanayama G, Siegel AJ, Hudson JI. Testosterone gel supplementation for men with refractory depression: a randomized, placebo-controlled trial. *Am J Psychiatry* 2003; **160**: 105–11.

[48] Papakostas GI, Perlis RH, Seifert C, Fava M. Antidepressant dose reduction and risk of relapse in major depressive disorder. *Psychother Psychosom* 2007; **76**: 266–70.

[49] Ellen F, Kupfer DJ, Perel JM, *et al.* Comparison of full-dose versus half-dose pharmacotherapy in the maintenance treatment of major depressive disorder. *J Affect Disord* 1993; **27**: 139–45.

[50] Gloaguen V, Cottraux J, Cucherat M, Blackburn IM. A meta-analysis of the effects of cognitive therapy in depressed Patients. *J Affect Disord* 1998; **49**: 59–72.

[51] Ekers D, Richards D, Gilbody S. A meta-analysis of randomized trials of behavioural treatment of depression. *Psychol Med* 2008; **38**: 611–23.

[52] Nash JM, Park ER, Walker, BB, Gordon N, Nicholson RA. Cognitive-behavioral group treatment for disabling headache. *Pain Med* 2004; **5**: 178–86.

[53] Klerman GL, Weissman MM, Rounsaville B, Chevron E. *Interpersonal Psychotherapy of Depression*. New York, NY, Basic Books, 1984.

[54] Elkin I, Shea MT, Watkins JT, *et al.* National Institute of Mental Health Treatment of Depression Collaborative Research Program. General effectiveness of treatments. *Arch Gen Psychiatry* 1989; **46**: 971–82.

[55] Cuijpers P, Geraedts AS, van Oppen P, Andersson G, Markowitz JC, van Straten A. Interpersonal psychotherapy for depression: a meta-analysis. *Am J Psychiatry* 2011; **168**: 581–92.

[56] Bowden CL, Calabrese JR, McElroy SL, *et al.* A randomized, placebo-controlled 12-month trial of divalproex and lithium in treatment of outpatients with bipolar I disorder. Divalproex Maintenance Study Group. *Arch Gen Psychiatry* 2000; **57**: 481–9.

[57] Calabrese JR, Bowden CL, Sachs G, *et al.* Lamictal 605 Study Group. A placebo-controlled18-month trial of lamotrigine and lithium maintenance treatment in recently depressed patients with bipolar I disorder. *J Clin Psychiatry* 2003; **64**: 1013–24.

[58] Ketter TA. Kalali AH. Weisler RH. SPD417 Study Group. A 6-month, multicenter, open-label evaluation of beaded, extended-release carbamazepine capsule monotherapy in bipolar disorder patients with manic or mixed episodes. *J Clin Psychiatry* 2004; **65**: 668–73.

[59] Keck PE Jr, Calabrese JR, McQuade RD, *et al.* Aripiprazole Study Group. A randomized, double-blind, placebo-controlled 26-week trial of aripiprazole in recently manic patients with bipolar I disorder. *J Clin Psychiatry* 2006; **67**: 626–37.

[60] Tohen M, Calabrese JR, Sachs GS, *et al.* Randomized, placebo-controlledtrialofolanzapine as maintenance therapy in patients with bipolar I disorder responding to acute treatment with olanzapine. *Am J Psychiatry* 2006; **163**: 247–56.

[61] Sachs GS. Dupuy JM. Wittmann CW. The pharmacologic treatment of bipolar disorder. *J Clin Psychiatry* 2011; **72**: 704–15.

[62] Tohen M, Vieta E, Calabrese J, *et al.* Efficacy of olanzapine and olanzapine-fluoxetine combination in the treatment of bipolar I depression. *Arch Gen Psychiatry* 2003; **60**: 1079–88.

[63] van der Loos ML, Mulder PG, Hartong EG, *et al.* LamLit Study Group. Efficacy and safety of lamotrigine as add-on treatment to lithium in bipolar depression: a multicenter, double-blind, placebo-controlled trial. *J Clin Psychiatry* 2009; **70**: 223–31.

[64] Calabrese JR, Keck PE Jr, Macfadden W, *et al.* A randomized, double-blind, placebo-controlled trial of quetiapine in the treatment of bipolar I or II depression. *Am J Psychiatry* 2005; **162**: 1351–60.

[65] Holroyd KA, O'Donnell FJ, Stensland M, Lipchik GL, Cordingley GE, Carlson BW. Management of chronic tension-type headache with tricyclic antidepressant medication, stress management therapy, and their combination: a randomized controlled trial. *JAMA* 2001; **285**: 2208–15.

[66] Tomkins GE, Jackson JL, O'Malley PG, Balden E, Santoro JE. Treatment of chronic headache with antidepressants: a meta-analysis. *Am J Med* 2001; **111**: 54–63.

[67] Adelman LC, Adelman JU, Von Seggern R, Mannix LK. Venlafaxine extended release (XR) for the prophylaxis of migraine and tension-type headache: A retrospective study in a clinical setting. *Headache* 2000; **40**: 572–80.

[68] D'Amico D. Pharmacological prophylaxis of chronic migraine: a review of double-blind placebo-controlled trials. *Neurol Sci* 2010; **31**Suppl 1: S23–8.

[69] Chengappa KN, Gershon S, Levine J. The evolving role of topiramate among other mood stabilizers in the management of bipolar disorder. *Bipolar Disord* 2001; **3**: 215–32.

[70] Gibbons R, Hur K, Hendricks Brown C, Mann JJ. Relationship between antiepileptic drugs and suicide attempts in patients with bipolar disorder. *Arch Gen Psychiatry* 2009; **66**: 1354–60.

Chapter 5

Anxiety disorders and primary headache

Justin M. Nash, Rabin Chandran, and Lucy Rathier

Anxiety is an aversive state of nervousness, apprehension, worry, and fear accompanied by unpleasant experience of physiological arousal. The accompanying symptoms can include fatigue, muscle tension, tachycardia, restlessness, sweating, lightheadedness, and dyspnea. The experience of anxiety can be a common and normal reaction when faced with situations (e.g., problems with health, finances, evaluations) that are difficult to predict, control, or obtain a desired outcome. In some cases, anxiety can be adaptive, helping individuals to prepare for an anticipated event or engage in effective problem-solving and coping efforts. In other cases, anxiety can be a problem, occurring without a known trigger, or out of proportion to what normally would be expected in a situation.

The patterns of thinking occurring with anxiety commonly relate to perceived danger and vulnerability. To the anxious person, the world can generally be viewed as unsafe or fraught with problems. Worry, concern, or fear is often associated with particular symptoms, situations, places, or people [1]. Individuals with anxiety can overestimate the likelihood that feared events will occur and will be "catastrophic." Considering the aversive nature of anxiety, it is common to engage in avoidance of feared stimuli to reduce the discomfort associated with anxiety. Avoidance can be subtle, including attempting to distract from thoughts or physical sensations associated with the feared stimuli, or more obvious, including avoiding situations, places, people, or activities that elicit the anxiety. Avoidance can also take the form of engaging in ritualistic behaviors to ward off anxious thoughts, or seeking reassurance through reliance on trusted others or through the use of anxiolytic medications. Through the process of negative reinforcement, excessive and repeated avoidance ultimately maintains and escalates anxiety. Although providing temporary relief from the unpleasant state of anxiety, avoidance provides no opportunity for individuals to learn that feared objects are relatively harmless. The result is continued vigilance of, and acute sensitivity to, anxiety-eliciting stimuli.

When anxiety persists for six months and interferes with the ability to function, it becomes a disorder. [2] Anxiety disorders take many forms with each having a different constellation of symptoms; all disorders cluster around excessive, irrational worry, fear and dread. *The Diagnostic and Statistical Manual of Mental Disorders-IV-TR* [2](DSM-IV-TR) identifies several types of anxiety disorders, including panic disorder, generalized anxiety disorder (GAD), obsessive-compulsive disorder (OCD), post-traumatic stress disorder (PTSD), specific phobia, and social phobia. Anxiety disorders commonly co-occur with other mental or physical disorders, including alcohol or substance abuse, which may mask or worsen symptoms of anxiety. Anxiety disorders are the most common class of psychiatric disorder in the general population [3] with many who suffer from anxiety disorders presenting in medical settings.

The association between primary headache and anxiety is well established. Although much attention has been focused on the relationship between depressive symptoms and headache, anxiety may be even more prevalent among headache sufferers [4–6]. Anxiety and stress are commonly cited as headache triggers and exacerbators of pain severity [4,5]. Individuals with headache disorders are two to five times more likely to suffer from certain anxiety disorders than those without headache disorders, with panic disorder and phobias being particularly prevalent [7–9]. Over half of individuals with migraine will meet criteria for at least one anxiety disorder, with panic disorder and phobias being most prevalent [7,9–11]. The associations between headache and anxiety disorder are stronger in chronic than in episodic headache [9,10,12–14]

The Neuropsychiatry of Headache, ed. Mark W. Green and Philip R. Muskin. Published by Cambridge University Press.

and more likely in migraine than in tension-type headache [13].

This chapter describes the major anxiety disorders and their associations with headache, the increased burden of comorbid anxiety and headache, the mechanisms hypothesized to explain the connection between anxiety and headache, and the behavioral treatments and strategies for managing anxiety and headache. Assessing headache patients for anxiety disorders, as well as other common psychiatric conditions, can be helpful in informing treatment options that can address both the headache and anxiety conditions.

Major anxiety disorders and associations with primary headache

Anxiety disorders are a separate category of psychiatric disorders in the DSM-IV-TR, which contains six major anxiety disorders.

Generalized anxiety disorder (GAD)

Generalized anxiety disorder (GAD) is diagnosed in people who experience constant and excessive worry about a variety of everyday problems for at least 6 months. [2] The anxiety is difficult to control and interferes with work, school, family, and social activities. The worry in GAD is associated with three or more of the following symptoms: feeling restless or keyed up; being easily fatigued; difficulty concentrating; irritability; muscle tension; and sleep disturbance. [2] Some of the symptoms of GAD overlap with symptoms of depression including agitation, dysphoria, restlessness, irritability, sleep problems, fatigue, and impaired concentration. The distinguishing features of GAD are worry, anxiety, and tension, whereas distinguishing features of depression are depressed mood, changes in appetite, feelings of worthlessness or inappropriate, excessive guilt, markedly diminished interest or pleasure in almost all activities, and recurrent thoughts of death or suicide.

GAD affects about 6.8 million American adults [15] and twice as many women as men. [16] The disorder generally develops gradually and can begin at any point in the life cycle, although the years of highest risk are between childhood and middle age. [16] Those with milder forms of GAD can function socially and be gainfully employed, while those with more severe levels have difficulty carrying out basic daily activities. While some studies suggest that individuals with migraine are 5.7 times more likely to suffer from generalized anxiety disorder (GAD), [17] the associations between migraine and GAD are not consistently reported, particularly in studies conducted with methodological rigor. [11]

Panic disorder

Panic Disorder is diagnosed in people who experience a panic attack and become preoccupied with the fear of a recurring attack. [2] A panic attack, or an abrupt onset of intense anxiety that reaches a peak within a few minutes, includes at least four of the following symptoms: a feeling of imminent danger or doom; the need to escape; heart palpitations; sweating; trembling or shaking; shortness of breath or a feeling of choking or smothering; chest pain or discomfort; nausea or abdominal distress; dizziness, lightheadedness, or feeling faint; a sense of things being unreal or feeling detached from oneself; a fear of losing control or going crazy; a fear of dying; tingling sensation; and chills or hot flushes. [2] Panic Disorder with agoraphobia occurs when there are both panic attacks and anxiety about, or avoidance of, being in places or situations from which escape may be difficult or embarrassing or help may not be available in the event of a panic attack (e.g., being in a crowd, traveling on public transportation). Many of the symptoms of panic disorder mimic symptoms of medical conditions such as heart disease, thyroid problems, and breathing disorders. Individuals with undiagnosed panic disorder often seek medical attention because they believe they have a serious illness. Anxiety about the unexplained physical symptoms is also a common symptom of panic disorder. [2]

Panic disorder affects about six million American adults [15] and women are twice as likely to experience panic disorder as men. [16] Panic attacks often begin in late adolescence or early adulthood, but not everyone who experiences panic attacks will develop panic disorder. [16] People who suffer from a high frequency of panic attacks and agoraphobia may become disabled by their condition resulting in an avoidance of situations and restricting travel. About one-third of such people become housebound or can only confront an anxiety-provoking situation when with a trusted companion. [16]

A correlation between migraine and panic disorder is frequently reported [18,19] with a bidirectional association postulated. [20] Individuals with migraine are 3.7 to 6.6 times more likely to suffer from panic disorder. [20] The association between migraine and panic disorder is stronger in migraine when compared with tension-type headache or migraine plus tension-type headache [12] and also stronger in chronic migraine than in episodic migraine. [9] The reported prevalence of panic disorder among patients with chronic migraine ranges from 25% to 30%, whereas its prevalence among patients with episodic migraine ranges from 5% to 17%. [17] The prevalence of panic disorder is even higher when both migraine and tension-type headache are present. [12]

Specific phobias

Specific phobias are marked and persistent fears that are excessive or unreasonable and elicited by the presence or anticipation of a specific object or situation. [2] Specific phobias commonly focus on animals, heights, water, flying, dental or medical procedures, and closed-in places such as elevators. Symptoms of having a specific phobia often include situationally bound or predisposed panic attacks and the recognition that the fear is excessive or unreasonable. [2] Those with specific phobias work hard to avoid the feared situation or endure it with intense psychological distress which can result in disruptions in one's personal, vocational, and social activities.

Specific phobias affect an estimated 19.2 million adult Americans and are twice as common in women as men. [15] While some children develop specific phobias, most seem to arise during adolescence or early adulthood with sudden onset and sometimes in situations that previously did not cause any anxiety. Individuals with migraine are 2.6 times more likely to have a diagnosed phobia. [20]

Social anxiety disorder

Social anxiety disorder is characterized by a marked and persistent anxiety associated with one or more social or performance situations. In these situations, individuals may be scrutinized by others and/or exposed to unfamiliar people and are fearful that they will act in a way that will be humiliating or embarrassing. [2] Exposure to the feared social situation will provoke anxiety which may have physical symptoms consistent with a panic attack. Social anxiety exceeds shyness in social situations. The social anxiety may be situation specific, such as delivering a presentation, or it may be more generalized to situations that involve any person who is not a family member. Feared situations often provoke anticipatory anxiety that may last days or weeks. The situations may be avoided or endured with severe psychological distress which in turn interferes significantly with daily life, occupational functioning, and social activities and relationships. [2] Social phobia affects about 15 million American adults. [15] It usually begins in childhood or early adolescence and, unlike other anxiety disorders, women and men are equally likely to develop social anxiety. [16] Among young adults, with the exception of GAD, social anxiety has the greatest association with migraine (OR 3.4, 95% CI 1.1 to 10.9). [21]

Obsessive-compulsive disorder

Individuals with obsessions experience unwanted and intrusive thoughts or images that are recurrent and persistent. The thoughts are not simply excessive concern about real-life problems. [2] Compulsions are the ritualistic behaviors or mental acts that occur in an effort to reduce anxiety provoked by an obsession or to prevent or ward off a dreaded situation. [2] The obsessions and compulsions may consume 1 or more hours in a day and can interfere with a person's normal routine, occupation, and social relationships. Examples of common obsessions relate to dirt, germs, or contamination; order or symmetry; harm to oneself or a loved one; and discarding objects with little or no value. Common compulsions relate to cleaning (e.g., handwashing, cleaning household items); checking (e.g., locked door, oven); repeating (e.g., name, phrase, or simple activity); hoarding useless items (e.g., newspapers, rubber bands); and mental rituals (e.g., counting).

Consistent associations are not always observed between migraine and OCD in studies, particularly in studies that use more stringent methods. [11] Some studies show that individuals with migraine are over five times more likely to suffer from OCD. [17] Other studies show that OCD is more closely associated with migraine than to tension-type headache, [11,12] and a higher prevalence of OCD occurs in patients with both migraine and tension-type headache when compared with the presence of migraine or tension headache alone. [12]

Post-traumatic stress disorder (PTSD)

Approximately 90% of individuals in the general population are exposed to traumatic life events of some type. [22] Approximately 25%–30% of victims of traumatic events develop symptoms of post-traumatic stress disorder (PTSD). [22] With PTSD, in response to either experiencing or witnessing an event that involves actual or threatened death or physical injury to self or others, individuals develop emotional and physical symptoms of re-experiencing the event, engage in efforts to avoid reminders of the trauma, and become hyperaroused. [2] In terms of re-experiencing, individuals with PTSD can have recurrent and intrusive distressing recollections of the event, or flashbacks or nightmares. They also can experience physiological and/or psychological distress upon exposure to external or internal cues that symbolize or resemble the traumatic event. In their effort to cope, individuals with PTSD typically avoid places, people, and activities that are reminders of the trauma. Alternatively, they can experience numbing or restricted emotions, diminished interest in significant activities, or feeling estranged from others. PTSD is accompanied by increased arousal such as difficulty sleeping and concentrating, hypervigilance, and being easily irritated, startled, or angry. The distressing experiences associated with the event impair functioning and last for at least a month, and often for years. [2]

PTSD affects about 7.7 million American adults [15] with a lifetime prevalence of approximately 8%. PTSD is twice as common in women as men. [22,23] In its association with headache, PTSD has received less research attention than the other mental disorders, but this trend is beginning to change. There is recent recognition of elevated rates of PTSD in patients with recurrent headache. [17] PTSD occurs more commonly in those with migraine (whether episodic or chronic) than in those without migraine. [22] The combination of PTSD and depression is suggested to be a risk factor for the transformation of episodic to chronic migraine. [22,24] The presence of PTSD in migraine sufferers also contributes to higher levels of disability and greater utilization of health care resources. [22,23] Identification and treatment of PTSD in migraine sufferers is an important and potentially modifiable part of their care that may reduce migraine-related disability and progression to chronic daily headache. [23] The association between migraine and PTSD is complex and probably multifactorial. [22]

Burden of comorbid anxiety and headache

The presence of comorbid anxiety increases the burden of headache. Increased anxiety among headache sufferers is associated with greater disability, worse quality of life, more compromised treatment response, and increased cost of care. [5,6,11,17,25,26] Migraine patients with anxiety symptoms report significantly more migraine related disability, as measured by the Migraine Disability Assessment (MIDAS) scale than migraineurs without elevated levels of anxiety or depression. [6] Health-related quality of life is also more compromised in migraineurs with anxiety symptoms than in migraineurs without anxiety. [6]

Individuals with migraine and comorbid anxiety disorders experience poorer initial treatment response and worse long-term outcomes than migraineurs without comorbid psychopathology. Patients also experience less relief and slower resumption of activities from migraine abortive agents, have less tolerance to abortive migraine agents, and are overall less satisfied with acute medication treatment. [6]

Anxiety and chronic headache

Relative to episodic headache disorders, chronic headache conditions are more disabling, costly, and difficult to manage. Chronic headache conditions are also associated with increased risk for psychiatric disorders, including anxiety disorders, [10–14] particularly when chronic headache exists for more than 5 years. [14] The addition of chronic substance abuse in individuals with chronic migraine furthers the likelihood of anxiety disorders, and in particular, panic disorder and social phobia. [11] Comorbid anxiety, in turn, is implicated as a risk factor in the transformation of episodic headache into costly and intractable chronic headache conditions, including medication overuse headache. [9,10,27] Identifying factors that contribute to the transformation of episodic into chronic headache is important in efforts to better prevent and manage chronic headache.

Understanding the interconnectedness of anxiety and headache

Despite the extensive examination of the comorbidity between migraine and psychiatric disorders (including anxiety disorders), the direction of the association and the mechanisms that underlie the connection remain unclear. The association could result from chance, one disorder causing the other, or shared etiology or risk factors underlying both disorders. Some evidence supports a bidirectional relationship between migraine and anxiety disorders, with the presence of one condition increasing the risk of the other. [11] For example, in regards to panic disorder and migraine,

Breslau and colleagues [20] report a bidirectional relationship with the influence being primarily from headaches to panic disorder, although a weaker, yet significant influence is observed in the reverse direction. Associations between migraine and anxiety disorders are observed even after controlling for major depression and gender, suggesting that common etiological mechanisms are shared between headache and anxiety. [12,20] Shared neurobiological factors and psychological factors are implicated in the association between anxiety and headache.

Neurobiological connections

Common neurobiological determinants are also not well identified; hypothesized connections, however, help to account for both the co-occurrence of headache and anxiety disorders. [11,25] Interconnected brain centers involving both pain modulation and anxiety can help explain how anxiety and anxiety disorders are associated with headache disorders. [28] Brain regions associated with pain processing are tied to circuitry involved with psychological phenomena, including anxiety. [29]

The central level mechanism that modulates pain is a circuit involving the periaqueductal gray and paraventricular hypothalamic nucleus, where anxiety and stress are hypothesized to trigger activation of a series of events in the superior salivatory nucleus and trigeminovascular system that contributes to migraine pain. [30,31] This circuit receives input from multiple forebrain regions, particularly the amygdala and limbic system, which play a role in both emotions and pain regulation. Other areas of the brain that are implicated in pain modulation (e.g., the anterior cingulate cortex, orbitofrontal cortex, insula, and hippocampus) are also affected by anxiety and anxiety-related constructs, including attention, expectations, and perceptions of controllability. [5,32]

Potential neurochemical links between anxiety and headache include serotonin and GABA dysregulation. Dysregulated GABA is implicated in anxiety [33] and medications that enhance GABA-nergic function are useful in preventing cortical excitability. [34] Migraine, as well as anxiety disorders, is understood to be at least partly a disorder of altered serotonergic functioning. [35,36,37] Selective serotonin agonists (triptans) are efficacious for migraine and selective serotonin reuptake inhibitors (SSRIs) are the conventional treatment for most anxiety disorders. [17]

At a peripheral level, anxiety can instigate a series of responses that could contribute to headache attacks. For example, anxiety could trigger adrenal release, change blood lipid levels, infuse sugar into the blood stream, and increase heart rate, respiration, and muscle tension. [5]

Psychological connections

Anxiety-related psychological constructs also help to explain the association between anxiety and headache. [17] Anxiety sensitivity and pain-related anxiety have been implicated in headache and in other forms of chronic pain. [4,5,17,26,38] Individuals with higher anxiety sensitivity misinterpret and react fearfully to unpleasant physical sensations. For example, individuals with panic disorder can interpret heart palpitations to be evidence of an impending heart attack, leading to sudden sympathetic discharge, fear, panic attacks, and subsequent avoidance of behaviors and situations that are likely to produce an attack. [5] Individuals with headache who are high in anxiety sensitivity can misinterpret innocuous sensations in negative ways (e.g., as signs of a brain tumor or indications that a headache is imminent), leading them to become fearful of pain or other related bodily sensations. Fear of pain can lead to unnecessary engagement in behaviors in an attempt to escape and avoid situations or activities that are thought to produce pain and pain-related sensations (e.g., seeking medical assurance, early and often use of narcotic analgesics, disengaging from work and other responsibilities). [5,17,26,38] Anxiety sensitivity is a significant contributor to fear of pain (accounting for about 40% of the variance), serving as a stronger predictor than severity of headache or depression level. [5,38] Although the exact mechanism is unclear, anxiety sensitivity and associated fear of pain can also increase the likelihood of having a headache attack and exacerbate pain intensity. [5,38]

Connections between anxiety and chronic headache

No single mechanism explains the association between anxiety and chronic headache. It is plausible that the constant struggle with pain, suffering, and compromised quality of life and functioning associated with chronic headache can contribute to the development of an anxiety disorder, particularly in individuals with preexisting anxiety vulnerability. It is also plausible that anxiety and its disorders can contribute to the transformation from episodic to chronic headache. Regardless of the direction of the effects, shared mechanisms can play a role.

Much of the attention is focused on identifying factors that account for the transformation from episodic headache to chronic headache conditions. Among the hypotheses proposed, many include factors already discussed (i.e., shared neurobiological and psychological factors). For example, Smitherman and colleagues and others [4,5,17,26,36,38,39] identify interrelated factors such as shared dysfunction of the serotonergic system; poor coping behaviors; anxiety sensitivity and related belief systems that magnify fear of pain and other unpleasant somatic sensations; sympathetic arousal; neuronal hyperexcitability; and medication overuse.

Medication overuse, in particular, is recognized as a leading cause of chronic headache. Medication overuse is particularly prevalent in the many patients with chronic daily headache who present to headache specialty clinics, occurring in approximately 30% of chronic migraineurs and in upwards of 50% of those who present to headache specialty clinics. [17,40,41] Elevated levels of anxiety (as well as depression) are thought to contribute to medication overuse headache, [17,42] although few longitudinal studies have explored this possibility. Anxiety sensitivity and fear of pain may lead to early and frequent use of rescue medications, resulting in medication overuse headache and chronic headache. [5,43]

Belief systems and unwarranted avoidance behaviors related to fear of pain and fear of anxiety-related sensations, while not directly implicated in headache chronification, have been associated with the persistence of headache and other forms of chronic pain. [5,17,38] Empirical attention is needed to better understand if anxiety-related belief systems can influence the development of chronic headache either directly through neuronal hyperexcitability and central pain modulation or indirectly through pathways such as medication overuse.

Behavioral approaches to co-occurring anxiety and headache disorders

Better management of anxiety in headache patients has the potential to improve response to headache treatment. [44] The heterogeneity of headache patients requires the use of a tailored approach to assessment and treatment. The clinical interview and the use of assessment measures can help determine the extent to which anxiety and related factors (e.g., self-efficacy) need to be addressed in specific headache patients. The determination can include whether anxiety is managed as part of the medical office visit or whether a referral to specialty behavioral healthcare is indicated. [10]

Anxiety screening and assessment

Anxiety screening is particularly relevant in practice settings where patients have more unusual or complex presentations, have not responded to conventional treatment regimens, or whose headache condition has persisted or progressed over time. [17] Screening for anxiety is more challenging than screening for depression due to the diffuse nature of anxiety and its numerous manifestations. Anxious patients do not always appear anxious, and symptoms of the various anxiety disorders (panic disorder, generalized anxiety disorder, obsessive-compulsive disorder, phobias, etc.) are somewhat distinct from one another. [10]

There is no simple validated verbal screening to identify the range of comorbid anxiety disorders. To identify whether anxiety may be a concern, screening procedures can start verbally with some general transitional questions about patient's sleep, energy, and stress. As needed, questions can progress to those that are more targeted regarding chronic worry (GAD), sudden rushes of fear or panic (panic disorder), uncontrollable urges to repeat certain actions (OCD), and re-experiencing of a past traumatic event (PTSD). [10] Considering the shared nature of headache and anxiety symptoms, the screening includes differentiating symptoms due to headache from those due to anxiety. For example, nausea may be a function of migraine headache or panic disorder, while muscle tension, insomnia, and concentration problems may present in chronic headache syndromes or in any number of anxiety disorders. [10]

When indicated, verbal screening can be followed up with further assessment, either through continued questioning, use of self-report measures (e.g., Patient Health Questionnaire), or a structured interview. [17] Unfortunately, most anxiety self-report screening measures inquire about global anxiety symptoms rather than about specific anxiety disorders. Examples include the Beck Anxiety Inventory and the State-Trait Anxiety Inventory. The Generalized Anxiety Disorder–7 (GAD-7) scale is designed to identify GAD among primary care patients, but can also be useful suggesting the presence of other forms of anxiety when scores exceed 8.0. The Patient Health Questionnaire (PHQ) is a longer self-report instrument that requires modest physician time and assesses multiple psychiatric disorders in addition to anxiety, including depression, somatoform, eating, and alcohol-use disorders. Numerous other screening measures and interviews for psychiatric disorders in headache patients have been reviewed and summarized, [45] along with strategies for comprehensively assessing the primary domains of interest related to anxiety disorders, such as anxiety triggers, avoidance behaviors, physical symptoms, and skills deficits. [46]

Screening for anxiety disorders are best conducted in conjunction with and not instead of screening for depression. The rationale for also screening for depression is evident in the two-fold increased risk of migraine among participants with both major depression and an anxiety disorder. [21]

Cognitive and behavioral management of anxiety

Cognitive-behavioral therapy (CBT) is an empirically validated, theory-based psychotherapeutic intervention that uses various cognitive and behavioral strategies in the treatment of both anxiety disorders and headache disorders. CBT for anxiety incorporates techniques to modify anxious patterns in thinking, regulate physiological responses associated with anxiety, and decrease avoidance behaviors. [10] CBT recognizes that thoughts have a direct influence on emotions, physiological responding, and behavior. [1] Characteristic of anxiety-related thoughts is that they can occur automatically, outside of the individual's awareness, and can distort reality. The thoughts often relate to worry, concern, or fear, and can reflect catastrophic thinking (i.e., assuming the worst). A consistent pattern of anxious thinking can emanate from underlying maladaptive core beliefs (including attitudes, expectations, and rules) that are themed around danger and vulnerability. [1] Core beliefs can develop from early learning experiences and efforts to cope with maladaptive cognitions. In addressing maladaptive cognitive processes, cognitive therapy teaches patients to identify, evaluate, and modify their maladaptive thoughts and core beliefs. Behavioral experiments can be used to help patient evaluate and test the validity of their thoughts and beliefs.

Relaxation skills can be used to reduce and self-regulate anxiety-related physiological responses. Although there are different forms of relaxation (e.g., progressive muscle relaxation, diaphragmatic breathing, meditation, guided imagery, autogenic training, cue-controlled relaxation), common among them is having the individual develop a single focus, allowing the mind to clear and the parasympathetic nervous system to become engaged, thereby reducing sympathetic tone. [47] The overall effect is producing more calming thoughts and reducing the overall level of arousal. Among the different forms of relaxation training, progressive muscle relaxation is the classic procedure that involves tensing and relaxing various muscle groups, while the mind focuses on the contrasting sensations. Because experiencing tension and relaxation at the same time is impossible, progressive muscle relaxation was useful in early desensitizing procedures in treatment of phobias. It has since been used for other anxiety disorders. At times, the anxious thoughts can interfere with the relaxation process. At those times, the relaxation process can be used to help patients better identify the types and patterns of anxious thoughts they have and their thinking patterns.

Exposure is an essential component of many behavioral approaches to managing anxiety and overcoming avoidance behaviors. Exposure involves repeated confrontation of the feared object until the patient learns that the feared stimuli are relatively harmless and no longer feared. During the exposure, patients are prevented from engaging in those responses that they seek in order to provide an escape from anxiety. Exposure may be accomplished imaginally (e.g., retelling a traumatic event) or in the actual feared context (e.g., public speaking, shopping in a crowded store). In graded exposure, patients start with engaging in activities that are associated with low to moderate anxiety, and after the anxiety level decreases significantly, they progress to the next activity in the hierarchy that produces a higher level of anxiety.

Different components of CBT are emphasized depending on the specific anxiety disorder being treated. [1] CBT for GAD teach patients to assess more realistically the threat of danger across situations and assess and fortify the patient's capacity to cope with threatening situations. Treatment for panic disorder involves the testing of the patient's catastrophic misinterpretations (usually life- or sanity-threatening erroneous predictions) of bodily or mental sensations. Therapy for social phobia emphasizes cognitive restructuring, anxiety management techniques, and guided exposure. Obsessive-compulsive disorder treatment emphasizes exposure to feared stimuli and prevention of responses (e.g., ritualistic behaviors), allowing patients to discover experimentally that the problem is thoughts rather than the possible occurrence of a real-world problem (which the patient is trying to prevent through neutralizing behavior and attempts at controlling the thoughts). In PTSD treatment, along with teaching patients techniques to manage their intense anxiety symptoms and recurrent distressing images, therapy emphasizes the identification and modification of the meaning the patient has attached to a traumatic event.

Behavioral approaches for managing both anxiety and headache

The principles and strategies of the behavioral approaches to managing headache are generally consistent with CBT for anxiety disorders. Behavioral headache management teaches self-regulation skills and stress management strategies that target physiological responses (e.g., sympathetic tone) and psychological processes (e.g., anxiety, stress-generating beliefs) that influence the onset and course of headache disorders and individual headache attacks. [48,49] Because behavioral approaches emphasize some degree of personal control over negative emotional states, behavioral management is appealing and empowering to many headache patients. [10,50]

There is a large and growing body of published evidence, including meta-analytic studies and evidence-based reviews, examining the use of behavioral approaches. Behavioral treatments, including relaxation training, biofeedback training, and cognitive-behavioral stress management, are superior to various control conditions, and the benefits are generally maintained over time. [49] In the management of chronic headache, however, behavioral treatment is understandably more challenging in its delivery and more limited in its effectiveness. The empirical evidence suggests that combined behavioral and pharmacological treatment offers the best effectiveness for chronic headache. [51,52]

Relaxation training, a self-regulation strategy, is often a primary component of behavioral management of headache. Consistent with its use in anxiety management, relaxation training has a self-regulatory function that helps patients to minimize physiological responses to stress and decrease sympathetic arousal which are common to both anxiety and headache. Relaxation skills are usually taught by clinical professionals but can be self-taught by patients using print, audio, or online resources. Relaxation strategies, including the most common form, progressive muscle relaxation, require regular, daily practice in order to become effective. [53] After practicing longer forms of relaxation (e.g., 20–30 minutes), patients can develop and then incorporate brief relaxation strategies (requiring 1–3 minutes) into their daily routine. The goal is for the patient to maintain lower levels of tension and prevent its buildup, especially when confronting stress or anxiety-provoking situations.

Biofeedback training, while not a common component of anxiety management, can be useful in support of relaxation training for headache. Biofeedback is a procedure that involves monitoring physiologic processes of which the patient may not be consciously aware or does not believe that he or she has voluntary control. [53] Through biofeedback training, patients learn to develop voluntary control and modify physiological processes, which decrease sympathetic tone and help to prevent and manage stress and headache. Biologic or physiologic information is converted into a signal that is then "fed back" to the patient, usually on a computer monitor and often with audio input. Patients are typically taught various relaxation skills, such as diaphragmatic breathing or visualization, to induce the relaxation response.

The two biofeedback responses with the strongest evidence for headache treatment are peripheral skin temperature biofeedback (i.e., thermal biofeedback) and electromyographic biofeedback. [53] Thermal biofeedback, involving increasing finger temperature using a sensitive thermometer, serves as an indirect measure of autonomic arousal. As parasympathetic activity increases and the relaxation response is activated, circulation and extremity temperature increase. Patients are taught that higher finger temperature corresponds to a more relaxed state and their goal is to raise their finger temperature. Electromyographic biofeedback uses electrodes to display muscle tension and guide the patient's efforts in producing a relaxed state, both overall as well as in particular muscle groups (e.g., frontal). Relaxation is best taught by a certified professional and requires several office visits along with home practice. Elements of cognitive behavioral-stress management are often incorporated into biofeedback sessions.

Cognitive-behavioral stress management is often a component of behavioral treatment for headache. The rationale for its use derives from the observation that the way individuals cope with everyday stressors can precipitate, exacerbate, or maintain headaches and increase headache-related disability and distress. Stress management focuses on the cognitive and affective components of headache, and it is typically administered in conjunction with relaxation training. Patients learn the role that cognitive processes play in generating the stress response and the relationship between stress, coping, and headache. Patients are taught to address maladaptive cognitive processes by identifying, evaluating, and modifying their maladaptive thoughts and beliefs, and using behavioral experiments to test the validity of their beliefs. Patients are also taught problem solving and other coping strategies to manage their headache-related stressors as well as their headaches. [48]

Behavioral treatment for headache also includes teaching patients to recognize and manage triggers in order to prevent headache attacks and to help in preventing episodic headaches from becoming chronic. [50,54,55] Having patients keep regular diaries of potential headache triggers allows the patient to see how triggers are related to headache. Specifically, patients are instructed to modify behaviors that may maintain or exacerbate headaches, and replace them with wellness behaviors, such as proper sleep habits, eating healthy foods at regular intervals, engaging regular physical activity, avoiding excessive caffeine or alcohol consumption, and smoking cessation. For patients with anxiety, it is helpful to have them recognize that being exposed to a potential trigger can set the stage for headache, but does not automatically translate into a debilitating headache.

With the considerable overlap in components in CBT for anxiety for headache, behavioral strategies for managing modest levels of anxiety can be integrated relatively easily into existing headache management protocols. [39] It is feasible for elements of these protocols to be delivered by nurses or other health professionals (e.g., care managers) in medical settings. Self-administered protocols, with support from medical professionals, can be considered as a mode of delivery for behavioral treatment of headache and management of anxiety. [50] Behavioral strategies for headache and anxiety can also be implemented in conjunction with pharmacotherapy to enhance adherence to medication and more effectively manage headaches while hopefully minimizing the potential for headache chronification.

Smitherman, Maizels, and Penzien [10] identify the strategies for behavioral management of psychopathology in headache patients. Table 5.1 outlines the strategies for behavioral management of anxiety in headache patients. More detailed information about the strategies can be found elsewhere. [10,39]

Table 5.1. Strategies for behavioral management of anxiety in headache patients

Educate the patient about the relationship between thoughts, behaviors, and emotions
Articulate that changing thoughts and behaviors can help improve anxiety
Help the patient identify overt and covert methods of avoiding feared stimuli
Decrease avoidance behavior through imaginal or in vivo exposure exercises
Have the patient write in a diary about a past traumatic experience and associated emotions
Have the patient monitor avoidance behaviors and patterns of negative thinking
Focus on generating rational alternatives to these patterns
Have the patient chart fearful predictions and the actual incidence of their occurrence
Relaxation training (such as progressive muscle relaxation commonly used with headache)
Instruct the patient to set aside 20–30 minutes each night for worry (rather than worrying throughout the entire day)
Advise the patient in initiation of a regular program of physical activity/exercise
Provide training in active coping skills and/or general stress management
Help patients realize they can live a valued life despite their chronic pain
Be alert to the potential for medication-overuse and underlying sleep disturbances

Note: Contents of table adapted from Smitherman, T.A., Maizels, M., and Penzien, D. B. (2008). Headache chronification: Screening and behavioral management of comorbid depressive and anxiety disorders, *Headache*; ***48***: 45–50.

In more complex patients, having physicians, nurses, and other medical staff incorporate behavioral strategies into medical visits will not be feasible. [10] Enlisting the services of specialty behavioral health professionals will be indicated, especially for patients with continuous or near-continuous headaches, high levels of medication overuse, and with more severe anxiety or other psychopathology. Behavioral health professionals who specialize in headache are located within academic medical centers/universities or large medical practices, although many comprehensive headache centers now employ such professionals. When behavioral health specialists are not available, referral to a general clinical psychologist or psychiatrist is appropriate. On-going collaborative care can occur between the referring physician and the psychologist or other specialist in behavioral health. If not part of this or one's own spectrum of practice, it may be helpful to refer a patient with comorbid anxiety for medical management of anxiety disorders. However, relatively few headache sufferers presenting for treatment fall into the more severe categories and thus most headache patients presenting for treatment will benefit from some form of anxiety management in the medial setting.

Concluding comment

Anxiety disorders and primary headache are commonly occurring conditions, both independently and as co-occurring conditions. The presence of anxiety and anxiety disorders in individuals with headache negatively impacts quality of life, functioning, and response to headache treatment. Effective management of headache necessitates understanding, identifying, and addressing anxiety, anxiety-related disorders, and their underlying factors that are related to headache. While no clear set of factors definitively explains the connection between anxiety and headache, a number of related neurobiological and psychological factors have been identified. Particular attention needs to be paid to the role that anxiety and anxiety-related factors play in the transformation of episodic headache conditions into costly and intractable chronic headache conditions. In particular, greater attention is needed in understanding and addressing the role of anxiety and the related factors of anxiety sensitivity and pain-related anxiety in the use and overuse of medication that can contribute to chronic headache development.

Addressing anxiety holds promise in being able to improve management of headache. A set of common behavioral strategies are helpful in addressing both headache and anxiety. These strategies, although having a different focus when treating anxiety versus headache, are cognitive-behavioral in nature and often include the components of relaxation training and cognitive-behavioral stress management. For anxiety management, a critical component is using exposure strategies. When indicated, exposure based approaches can also be used in headache management.

For patients without complex presentations, physicians, nurses, and other health professionals can learn to incorporate behavioral strategies into their medical visits in order to address anxiety and headache. The efforts of health professionals in medical settings can be supplemented with the self-administered and home-based efforts on the part of patients to learn and use behavioral skills to address their own anxiety and headache problems. For patients with complex presentations, the treatment is best conducted by a professional from the behavioral health specialty, often from psychology, who is well informed about headache, anxiety, and cognitive-behavioral therapy. The specialist from behavioral health can either work in an integrated fashion in a medical setting or work in a specialty behavioral health setting.

References

[1] Beck JS. *Cognitive Therapy: Basics and Beyoud*. New York: The Guilford Press; 1995.

[2] Association AP. *Diagnostic and Statistical Manual of Mental Disorders* 4th Edn Text Revision. Washington DC: American Psychiatric Association; 2000.

[3] Kessler RC, Berglund P, Demler O, Jin R, Merikangas KR, Walters EE. Lifetime prevalence and age-of-onset distributions of DSM-IV disorders in the National Comorbidity Survey Replication. *Arch Gen Psychiatry* 2005; **62**: 593–602.

[4] Nash JM, Thebarge RW. Understanding psychological stress, its biological processes, and impact on primary headache. *Headache* 2006; **46**: 1377–86.

[5] Nicholson RA, Houle TT, Rhudy JL, Norton PJ. Psychological risk factors in headache *Headache* [Research Support, N.I.H., Extramural Review]. 2007; **47**: 413–26.

[6] Lanteri-Minet M, Radat F, Chautard MH, Lucas C. Anxiety and depression associated with migraine: influence on migraine subjects' disability and quality of life, and acute migraine management. *Pain* 2005; **118**: 319–26.

[7] Breslau N. Psychiatric comorbidity in migraine. *Cephalalgia* 1998; **18** Suppl 22: 56–8; discussion 8–61.

[8] Hamelsky SW, Lipton RB. Psychiatric comorbidity of migraine. *Headache*. 2006; **46**: 1327–33.

[9] Radat F, Swendsen J. Psychiatric comorbidity in migraine: a review. *Cephalalgia* 2005; **25**: 165–78.

[10] Smitherman TA, Maizels M, Penzien DB. Headache chronification: screening and behavioral management of comorbid depressive and anxiety disorders. *Headache* 2008; **48**: 45–50.

[11] Antonaci F, Nappi G, Galli F, Manzoni GC, Calabresi P, Costa A. Migraine and psychiatric comorbidity: a review of clinical findings. *The Journal of Headache and Pain* [Review]. 2011; **12**: 115–25.

[12] Beghi E, Bussone G, D'Amico D, Cortelli P, Cevoli S, Manzoni GC, et al. Headache, anxiety and depressive disorders: the HADAS study. *J Headache Pain*; **11**: 141–50.

[13] Juang KD, Wang SJ, Fuh JL, Lu SR, Su TP. Comorbidity of depressive and anxiety disorders in chronic daily headache and its subtypes. *Headache* 2000; **40**: 818–23.

[14] Verri AP, Proietti Cecchini A, Galli C, Granella F, Sandrini G, Nappi G. Psychiatric comorbidity in chronic daily headache. *Cephalalgia* 1998; **18** Suppl 21: 45–9.

[15] Kessler RC, Chiu WT, Demler O, Merikangas KR, Walters EE. Prevalence, severity, and comorbidity of 12-month DSM-IV disorders in the National Comorbidity Survey Replication. *Arch Gen Psychiatry* 2005; **62**: 617–27.

[16] Robins LN, Regier DA, eds. *Psychiatric Disorders in America: The Epidemiologic Catchment Area Study.* New York: The Free Press; 1991.

[17] Smitherman TA, Penzien DB, Maizels M. Anxiety disorders and migraine intractability and progression. *Curr Pain Headache Rep* 2008; **12**: 224–9.

[18] Stewart W, Breslau N, Keck PE, Jr. Comorbidity of migraine and panic disorder. *Neurology* 1994; **44**(10 Suppl 7): S23–7.

[19] Jette N, Patten S, Williams J, Becker W, Wiebe S. Comorbidity of migraine and psychiatric disorders – a national population-based study. *Headache* 2008; **48**: 501–16.

[20] Breslau N, Schultz LR, Stewart WF, Lipton R, Welch KM. Headache types and panic disorder: directionality and specificity. *Neurology* 2001; **56**: 350–4.

[21] Merikangas KR, Angst J, Isler H. Migraine and psychopathology. Results of the Zurich cohort study of young adults. *Arch Gen Psychiatry* 1990; **47**: 849–53.

[22] Peterlin BL, Tietjen GE, Brandes JL, *et al.* Posttraumatic stress disorder in migraine. *Headache* 2009; **49**: 541–51.

[23] Kessler RC, Sonnega A, Bromet E, Hughes M, Nelson CB. Posttraumatic stress disorder in the National Comorbidity Survey. *Arch Gen Psychiatry* 1995; **52**: 1048–60.

[24] Peterlin BL, Ward T, Lidicker J, Levin M. A retrospective, comparative study on the frequency of abuse in migraine and chronic daily headache. *Headache* 2007 Mar; **47**: 397–401.

[25] Lipton RB, Scher AI, Kolodner K, Liberman J, Steiner TJ, Stewart WF. Migraine in the United States: epidemiology and patterns of health care use. *Neurology* 2002; **58**: 885–94.

[26] Nash JM, Williams DM, Nicholson R, Trask PC. The contribution of pain-related anxiety to disability from headache. *J Behav Med* 2006; **29**: 61–7.

[27] Lipton RB, Pan J. Is migraine a progressive brain disease? *JAMA*. 2004; **291**: 493–4.

[28] Cady R, Farmer K, Dexter JK, Schreiber C. Cosensitization of pain and psychiatric comorbidity in chronic daily headache. *Curr Pain Headache Rep* 2005; **9**: 47–52.

[29] Melzack R. From the gate to the neuromatrix. *Pain* 1999; **Suppl 6**: S121–6.

[30] Burstein R, Jakubowski M. Unitary hypothesis for multiple triggers of the pain and strain of migraine. *J Comp Neurol* 2005; **493**: 9–14.

[31] Fields H. State-dependent opioid control of pain. *Nat Rev Neurosci* 2004; **5**: 565–75.

[32] Ploghaus A, Becerra L, Borras C, Borsook D. Neural circuitry underlying pain modulation: expectation, hypnosis, placebo. *Trends Cogn Sci* 2003; **7**: 197–200.

[33] Lydiard RB. The role of GABA in anxiety disorders. *J Clin Psychiatry* 2003; **64** Suppl 3: 21–7.

[34] Welch KM. Brain hyperexcitability: the basis for antiepileptic drugs in migraine prevention. *Headache* 2005; **45** Suppl 1: S25–32.

[35] Silberstein SD. Serotonin (5-HT) and migraine. *Headache* 1994; **34**: 408–17.

[36] Bell CJ, Nutt DJ. Serotonin and panic. *Br J Psychiatry* 1998; **172**: 465–71.

[37] Lipton RB, Silberstein SD. Why study the comorbidity of migraine? *Neurology* 1994; **44**(10 Suppl 7): S4–5.

[38] Norton PJ, Asmundson GJ. Anxiety sensitivity, fear, and avoidance behavior in headache pain. *Pain* 2004; **111**: 218–23.

[39] Lipchik GL, Smitherman TA, Penzien DB, Holroyd KA. Basic principles and techniques of cognitive-behavioral therapies for comorbid psychiatric symptoms among headache patients. *Headache* 2006; **46** Suppl 3: S119–32.

[40] Dodick D, Freitag F. Evidence-based understanding of medication-overuse headache: clinical implications. *Headache* 2006; **46** Suppl 4: S202–11.

[41] Mathew NT. Transformed migraine. *Cephalalgia* 1993 Apr; **13** Suppl 12: 78–83.

[42] Lake AE, 3rd. Medication overuse headache: biobehavioral issues and solutions. *Headache* 2006; **46** Suppl 3: S88–97.

[43] Asmundson GJ, Wright KD, Norton PJ, Veloso F. Anxiety sensitivity and other emotionality traits in predicting headache medication use in patients with recurring headaches: implications for abuse and dependency. *Addict Behav* 2001; **26**: 827–40.

[44] Senaratne R, Van Ameringen M, Mancini C, Patterson B, Bennett M. The prevalence of migraine headaches in an anxiety disorders clinic sample. *CNS Neurosci Ther*; **16**: 76–82.

[45] Maizels M, Smitherman TA, Penzien DB. A review of screening tools for psychiatric comorbidity in headache patients. *Headache*. 2006; **46** Suppl 3: S98–109.

[46] Antony MM, Rowa K. Evidence-based assessment of anxiety disorders in adults. *Psychol Assess* 2005; **17**: 256–66.

[47] Benson H. *The Relaxation Response*. New York: William Morrow; 1975.

[48] Lipchik GL, Nash JM. Cognitive-behavioral issues in the treatment and management of chronic daily headache. *Curr Pain Headache Rep* 2002; **6**: 473–9.

[49] Rains JC, Penzien DB, McCrory DC, Gray RN. Behavioral headache treatment: history, review of the empirical literature, and methodological critique. *Headache* 2005; **45** Suppl 2: S92–109.

[50] Nicholson R, Nash J, Andrasik F. A self-administered behavioral intervention using tailored messages for migraine. *Headache* 2005; **45**: 1124–39.

[51] Holroyd KA, Cottrell CK, O'Donnell FJ, *et al.* Effect of preventive (beta blocker) treatment, behavioural migraine management, or their combination on outcomes of optimised acute treatment in frequent migraine: randomised controlled trial. *BMJ* **341**: c4871.

[52] Holroyd KA, O'Donnell FJ, Stensland M, Lipchik GL, Cordingley GE, Carlson BW. Management of chronic tension-type headache with tricyclic antidepressant medication, stress management therapy, and their combination: a randomized controlled trial. *JAMA* 2001; **285**: 2208–15.

[53] Buse DC, Andrasik F. Behavioral medicine for migraine. *Neurol Clin* 2009; **27**: 445–65.

[54] Bigal ME, Lipton RB. Modifiable risk factors for migraine progression (or for chronic daily headaches) – clinical lessons. *Headache* 2006; **46** Suppl 3: S144–6.

[55] Scher AI, Lipton RB, Stewart W. Risk factors for chronic daily headache. *Curr Pain Headache Rep* 2002; **6**: 486–91.

Chapter 6

Stress and headache

Carolyn B. Britton

Primary headache disorders are among the most prevalent conditions affecting various populations worldwide. [1] They are also an important cause of disability. A 2007 review of published population-based and other studies of headache from around the world estimate that 46% of the world's population has an active headache disorder, 11% with migraine, 42% with tension type and 3% with chronic daily headache. Disability due to headache is more prevalent for tension-type headache than for migraine. In the World Health Organization's ranking for disability, headache disorders are among the ten most disabling conditions for both genders and the top five for women. [2]

For both migraine and tension-type headache, the most common primary headache disorders, triggers are important potentially modifiable modulators of headache frequency and severity (Table 6.1). Among recognized headache triggers, stress is the most frequently cited and is thought to play a role in headache onset, frequency, severity, and progression to a chronic disorder. [3,4] In a study of German adolescents, the role of stress is evaluated by headache type, i.e., migraine, tension-type and miscellaneous headache. Migraine and mixed migraine with co-existing tension type headache are associated more with stressful experiences than tension-type headache alone in this particular study. [5] In other studies stress is an important modulator of all headache types.

Although a common term, stress is a complex concept that requires consensus about definition to evaluate its role in headache. Stress may be defined by objective or subjective criteria, external or internal factors. A comprehensive understanding of stress and stress management requires integration of varied concepts – the biological, the psycho-social-cultural and the individual or idiosyncratic.

Simply stated, some suggest that stress can be conceptualized as a strain on the system, either biological or psychological. Claude Bernard, Walter Cannon, and Hans Selye are credited with adaptation of the term stress from its use in physics to describe load on a structure to its use as a physiological/psychological construct to describe the human response to external or internal events. [6] McEwen views the stress response as an allostatic process that responds to challenge to the normal biological homeostatic system. [7,8]

The biological or physiological response to stress involves the hypothalamic–pituitary–adrenal axis (HPA) and the sympathetic nervous system. Activation of both systems is responsible for the physiological and behavioral changes that accompany stress. Stress stimulates release of corticotrophin-releasing hormone (CRH) from the paraventricular nucleus of the hypothalamus that, in turn, acts on the pituitary to release adrenocorticotropic hormone (ACTH) and beta-endorphin. ACTH acts on the adrenal gland to release cortisol. Cortisol is a steroid hormone with myriad effects, among them elevation of heart rate, blood pressure, blood sugar, immune modulation, and anti-inflammatory properties. Cortisol also sensitizes blood vessels to the effects of norepinephrine. Beta-endorphins are hormones with morphine-like properties and are anti-nociceptive in acute stress. Stress-related events also activate the autonomic nervous system causing release of epinephrine. Although all of these hormones or neurotransmitters are involved in the stress response, it is the cortisol response that is regarded as having a major role in propagation of headache.

Researchers have sought objective criteria to define stress, drawing on the analogy to stress as defined in physics. In this model, the stressor is an objective event or situation whose significance could potentially be

The Neuropsychiatry of Headache, ed. Mark W. Green and Philip R. Muskin. Published by Cambridge University Press.

Table 6.1. Headache triggers

Lifestyle:	Stress Sleep disturbance or disorder Irregular eating habits (missing meals) Alcohol Caffeine
Hormonal:	Menses Birth control pills
Environmental/ allergic:	Odors Foods Weather/barometric pressure Bright or flickering lights Loud noise

measured by an objective output, e.g., the cortisol response. Richard Lazarus and others propose valid limitations of this model. [9] In a review of the role of emotions in psychological stress, he broadens the focus to include the individual, more specifically individual motivational and cognitive variables that affect response to stress. He argues for the importance of the individual appraisal process in determining the significance of a stressor and the individual coping mechanisms that might blunt or mitigate stressor impact. His formulation moves the discussion of stress and stress responses from the biological model to the psycho-social-cultural realm. In so doing, he expands the discussion to include psychological as well as physiological stressors and emphasizes that response to psychological stressors can only be understood through the prism of the individual appraisal process, i.e., the individual determination of what is harmful.

Lazarus discusses the evolution of thinking about psychological stressors in his 1993 paper. He suggests the concept of appraisal as the cognitive mediator of stress reactions. The nature and severity of potential harm from a "stressor" is assessed through a primary appraisal process. Equally important is a secondary appraisal that assessed mitigating factors, i.e., available coping mechanisms and support. The secondary appraisal process links the stress response to the overall psychological make-up of the individual and the social context they inhabit, e.g., personality or behavior traits/habits, mood disorders, social resources, among others. He emphasizes that the process of appraisal and coping is not static, but often contextual and capable of modification over time, although some individual coping mechanisms may also be relatively stable. The concepts outlined by Lazarus are important to the development of interventions to mitigate stress and to improved understanding as to how gender (a social role), as well as sex (a biological role) influence stress responses.

The sex and gender roles in stress reactivity mediated by the HPA/cortisol axis have been examined in several studies. [10] These studies show that men and women may differ in appraisal of a particular event as stressful (gender or socio-cultural differences) and in the peak response to a commonly recognized stressor (sex or biological differences). A study by Stroud *et al.* concludes that women are more likely to perceive stress in situations characterized by social rejection, while men are more likely to perceive stress in situations where achievement is the measure. [11]

The biological basis for sex differences is, in part, attributed to differences in HPA regulation by sex hormones. For example, estrogen hormones stimulate production of corticosteroid binding globulin (CBG). CBG levels, in turn, influence the proportion of available free or active cortisol. Therefore, when CBG levels are high, stress responses may be attenuated, e.g., in pregnancy or in the follicular phase of the normal cycle. Estrogens also bind to receptors in the central nervous system and may exert effects on cortisol production via CNS feedback loops involving the hippocampus or other areas. Some question the hormonal or estrogen effect on cortisol production, suggesting that natural estrogen fluctuations are insufficient stimulus for significant changes in cortisol. Oral contraceptives, however, are shown to increase CBG levels in the blood, thereby reducing levels of free cortisol. No significant role is postulated for androgens in HPA regulation. Although this area of study is unsettled, the preponderance of studies suggests an estrogen effect in women not present in men is important to the biological basis for sex differences.

Studies of the biological responses to stressful stimuli are further complicated by the observation that various pharmacologic or physical stressors stimulate the HPA axis at different levels. Pharmacologic agents are thought to act at the level of the hypothalamus, pituitary, or adrenal cortex, physical stressors at the hypothalamus directly, and psychosocial stressors through limbic forebrain circuits that connect to the hypothalamus.

Personality traits and psychiatric disorders are important comorbid and possibly causal conditions in migraine and mediators of stress impact on migraine or tension-type headache (Table 6.2). These include

Table 6.2. Psychiatric modulators or mediators of stress susceptibility

Neuroticism
Anxiety/panic disorders
Depression
Post-traumatic stress disorder

neuroticism, anxiety, panic disorder, depression, and post-traumatic stress disorders. A prospective study of neuroticism showed increased predictive risk for migraine in women and increased lifetime incidence of migraine in both men and women, independent of depression and anxiety. [12] Neuroticism as a personality construct is postulated to confer susceptibility to stress. A Swedish study by Hedborg and colleagues looks at personality factors, stress, life events and gender in migraine. [13] This study confirms the importance of stress in migraine and notes high mean scores for stress susceptibility that correlated with perceived stress in women and men with migraine, as determined by response to a standardized personality inventory, the Karolinska Scales of Personality. Women are more likely than men to report negative life events and to endorse psychic or somatic anxiety, and depression.

The co-occurrence of depression and/or panic attacks/anxiety is well established for headache disorders, especially migraine, where the impact of these diagnoses is bidirectional. Breslau and colleagues report on a prospective study of an adult cohort from Detroit that includes persons with migraine, other severe headache and no headache, at baseline and 2-year follow up. [14] This study found a three-fold increase of migraine with major depression compared with migraineurs with no depression. Similarly, for those with a history of migraine, there is a five-fold risk for first-onset major depression. For those with severe, non-migraine headache, there is an increased risk for depression that is not statistically significant, but there is no increased risk of severe, non-migraine headache in those with depression.

A 2004 paper by McWilliams *et al.* reports on the relationship among three common pain conditions and psychopathology using data from the Midlife Development in the United States Survey (MIDUS). [15] This large, population-based study is important because the potential bias of evaluations based on select clinical populations is eliminated. The sample included 3032 adults, aged 25 to 74, who completed a 30-minute telephone interview and two questionnaires. The participants report on medical conditions that occurred within the previous year. These included three pain conditions: arthritis, migraine, and back pain. Psychiatric diagnoses are determined by analysis of diagnostic specific measures from the Composite International Diagnostic Interview-Short Form (CIDI-SF). [16,17]

Results of the MIDUS study show that, for migraine headache, odds ratios are increased for generalized anxiety disorder, panic attacks, and depression, and remain significant after multivariate analysis for demographic or medical variables. The association of headache with anxiety disorder was stronger than for depression, although both were significant. Lanteri-Minet and colleagues report on a French population-based study (FRAMIG 3) that evaluates anxiety and depression associated with active migraine. [18] This study also looks at the influence of these diagnoses on disability and quality of life. The results are similar to the American MIDUS study. Anxiety and/or depression are found in 50.6% of subjects, 28.0% anxiety alone, 3.5% depression alone, and 19.1% both anxiety and depression. Migraine-associated disability and reduced quality of life are more likely with anxiety alone or anxiety with depression. None of these studies addresses post-traumatic stress disorder.

Post-traumatic stress disorder (PTSD) is a well-recognized risk for and modulator of headache. It describes a clinical syndrome that follows a significant traumatic event that results in a series of disabling clinical symptoms, among them flashbacks, nightmares, avoidance of circumstances associated with the event, sleep problems, and irritability. [19] These symptoms must be present for more than 1 month and result in clinically significant impairment of social, occupational, or other important functional areas. The criteria for diagnosis are outlined in the American Psychiatric *Association Diagnostic and Statistical Manual of Mental Disorders*, 4th edition, text revision (DSM-IV-TR).

A critical element of the PTSD diagnosis is the precipitating traumatic event that is time linked or contextually linked to psychological sequelae. Traumatic events include natural disaster, rape and other assaultive behavior, military combat, and accidental injury. Although the psychological construct for PTSD is accepted, the definition is evolving, particularly with regard to the nature of the inciting trauma. In preparation for DSM-5, there is vigorous debate about this issue. It is likely that the definition will be further refined.

The lifetime prevalence of PTSD is estimated at 8%, and twice as common in women as men. [20] In a prospective study at six headache centers, Peterlin and colleagues evaluate the relative frequency of PTSD in episodic migraine (EM), chronic daily headache (CDH), and the impact on headache-related disability. The patients are recruited by headache specialists. The psychiatric assessment is by self-administered checklists for PTSD, depression, life events, and disability. Despite the relative limitation of the use of self-report checklists, this study confirms the observation of others that PTSD is more common in migraine populations than in the general public, 25% overall for both EM and CDH vs. 8% for the general population. Other findings include higher frequency of PTSD in CDH and depression and the independent association of PTSD with headache-related disability.

In 2011, Peterlin and colleagues report on the National Comorbidity Survey Replication (NCS-R) results. [21] Data from this survey are analyzed to examine the relationship of PTSD, episodic and chronic daily headache, drug and alcohol abuse, mood disorders, anxiety, and gender. This is a cross-sectional, general population survey of mental disorders in the United States that is conducted between 2001 and 2003. A structured, lay administered, diagnostic interview was used to assess DSM-IV disorders, the World Health Organization's Composite International Diagnostic Interview (CIDI), version 3.0. PTSD is assessed by inquiry about 27 specific traumas and any self-reported other traumatic event. Traumatic events are summed and PTSD assessed for those endorsing at least one traumatic event. Headache diagnosis is assessed for those with frequent or severe headache within the last 12 months. A limitation of this study is the restriction of headache diagnosis to active headaches within the past year while mood disorders and traumatic events were evaluated over the lifetime and within the past 12 months. Also, the headache diagnosis is not validated with physician diagnosis.

The National Comorbidity Study confirms the increased prevalence of mood disorders, major depressive disorder (MDD), and generalized anxiety disorder (GAD), in both EM and CDH for lifetime and 12-month interval, as compared with those without headache. For MDD, this holds true after adjustments, but for GAD the increased prevalence was for EM alone after adjustments. The significant findings of this study are: increased odds ratio of PTSD in both EM and CDH, when adjusted for demographics, mood disorders, drug and alcohol use; poor predictive power of mood disorder diagnosis for presence of PTSD; increase of PTSD in women and men with headache but stronger association in men; no association of alcohol and migraine; association of migraine and drug use attributable to comorbid PTSD; and depression.

The National Comorbidity Study results underscore the need to be vigilant in assessing for PTSD among migraineurs, especially men. This study is especially relevant to the assessment and management of returning veterans of war conflict, some of whom have PTSD.

Many studies document the role of stress in headache conversion from episodic to chronic, the latter defined as ≥15 headache days monthly. Chronic daily headache (CDH) is estimated to affect 3%–5% of the adult population and consists of several subtypes. In a population-based study by Scher *et al.* [22] of major life changes before and after the onset of chronic daily headache, cases and controls are selected from US adults who participated in a general health telephone survey for the Frequent Headache Epidemiology Study. This nested case-control study is conducted 1 year after the initial survey and consisted of a 30–40-minute telephone interview on risk factors for CDH. These risk factors included major life events adapted as a shortened version of the Life Events Inventory used in other studies. Six types of major life changes are assessed for the year prior to onset of CDH, the year of CDH, and the year after onset of CDH. The Primary Care Evaluation of Mental Disorders mood module is used to assess current depression.

Analysis of the data shows that stressful life events are more likely to occur in the 2 years prior to CDH onset than for episodic migraine. This is true for both men and women and for migraine and non-migraine headache. The effect of stressful life events is attenuated by correction for other risk factors for CDH such as snoring, excessive caffeine intake, obesity, and head and neck injury. However, when stratified by age, antecedent life events remained significant for those over 40. There is no effect of major life events in the year after CDH onset.

For migraine headache, many factors, in addition to stress, also contribute to transformation to chronic migraine. [23] These include possible genetic factors, high attack frequency, medication overuse, obesity, caffeine overuse, snoring, and other pain syndromes. Medication overuse is an especially important and potentially modifiable cause of migraine transformation. This is especially likely to occur when there is a need to treat a concomitant pain condition. Bigal and Lipton [23] summarize selected clinic and population studies that address this issue. They conclude that data show a two-fold increased incidence or risk for chronic migraine in those using opiates and barbiturates but not for triptans, NSAIDs or acetaminophen. The odds for transformation to chronic migraine increase with days of exposure, more than 5 days per month for barbiturates, 8 days a month for opiates. It is important to note that both triptans and NSAIDs are associated with migraine progression in those with high frequency headache, more than ten headache days/month.

The successful management of stress in headache requires attention to three areas:

- Physician or provider knowledge of the patient
  - Headache diagnosis
  - Comorbid diagnosis: personality disorders; mood or anxiety disorders; post-traumatic stress disorder; medically important diagnoses
  - Habits and behaviors: diet; sleep (snoring); exercise; weight; alcohol/drug use; medication use and beliefs (prescription, over the counter and supplements)
- Patient self-awareness or self-knowledge, disease knowledge, coping skills, support environment
- Multifaceted approach for shared goal by physician or provider and patient, i.e., the amelioration of stress and improvement in headache outcome.

Effective stress management may require both pharmacologic and behavioral treatment. Pharmacologic treatment should be appropriate to the headache diagnosis and associated comorbid conditions, and limited to medications necessary to treat identified problems. An equally important part of management requires patient self-direction and adherence, i.e. patient education and behavioral management. In some cases, formal psychotherapy may also be needed.

There are many pharmacologic options for treatment of acute and chronic headache, among them medications that may serve a dual purpose of treatment for anxiety or depression, as well as pain reduction. The American Academy of Neurology (AAN) published a Practice parameter for migraine management that reviews evidence for efficacy or lack thereof for all the classes of medication used in treatment of acute and chronic migraine. [24] Several medications listed in the Practice Parameter have class A or B efficacy for frequent migraine headache and may have cross-efficacy for mood disorder. These include: anti-depressants – amitriptyline, fluoxetine; anti-convulsants that are potential mood stabilizers – valproate, carbamazepine, and topiramate. The following anti-depressants are rated as class C: nortriptyline; protriptyline; and imipramine. Some studies also show efficacy in chronic tension-type headache for combination tricyclic anti-depressant therapy with stress management techniques, the combination superior to either alone. [25]

Behavioral management techniques are well-established interventions for both headache and stress. [26,27] Techniques include relaxation therapy, cognitive/behavioral therapy, biofeedback (temperature, EMG, EEG, cephalic vasodilatation), or hypnotherapy. Modalities may be combined, e.g., relaxation therapy with cognitive behavioral therapy and /or biofeedback. Multiple studies over more than three decades have shown efficacy for these modalities that range from 30 to 50% reduction in headache frequency, in adolescents and adults, and in varied populations. [28] The efficacy of behavioral management is also confirmed by meta-analysis.

It is argued that the beneficial impact of cognitive/behavioral therapy is mediated through changes in locus of control beliefs and self-efficacy. [29,30] Locus of control refers to the belief that external events or either within or beyond an individual's personal control, i.e., the locus of control is internal or external. Persons with a high internal locus of control have better headache treatment outcomes and are more likely to experience success with behavioral management. Persons with low internal locus of control are more likely to believe that external events beyond their control are the driver in their headache severity and that self-management is ineffective. Self-efficacy is the belief that a desired outcome can be achieved through personal or individual actions. Successful efforts often reinforce self-efficacy. Self-efficacy is an important modulator of stress impact and mediator of successful behavioral management strategies. Both anxiety and depression negatively impact response to stressful events in those with low internal locus of control and low self-efficacy. This means that stress is more likely to trigger headache, increase pain severity, or result in disability.

In a study of 114 persons with headache, Marlowe designs a self-efficacy scale that was correlated with stressful events and headache activity. [29] He finds that stressful events correlated with headache frequency and severity and that this relationship was moderated by self-efficacy. Higher self-efficacy reduces the correlation between stressful events and headache. Nicholson and colleagues note that data on mechanisms underlying behavioral management effectiveness supported improved self-efficacy as a major cause of change rather than physiological mechanisms such as improved blood flow or muscle relaxation. [30] Maladaptive coping behaviors and stress are associated with anxiety and poor headache outcome in a large prospective observational study of headache patients in primary care in France (SMILE study). [31]

Behavioral management may involve a single modality, combined modalities or a behavioral modality with pharmacotherapy. The US Headache Consortium and the AAN Practice Parameter guidelines conclude that relaxation therapy, thermal biofeedback combined with relaxation, electromyographic feedback and cognitive behavioral therapy all have Grade A evidence for efficacy in the treatment of headache. Despite the substantial evidence for efficacy, there are significant challenges for behavioral management that are both scientific and procedural with regard to ease of accessibility.

The challenges for behavioral management are: the need for hypothesis-driven controlled clinical trials that identify characteristics of patient populations for specific treatments and that identify prospective measurable mechanisms predictive of treatment efficacy; increased diversity of patient populations selected for study; development of cost-effective, less labor-intensive adaptations of treatment that can be implemented across diverse populations; development of effective management protocols suitable for use in a broad array of practice environments; and sustainability of patient adherence. Cognitive/behavioral therapy particularly requires trained personnel and regular visits to a provider that may prove costly and difficult to sustain long term. Some studies suggest that shorter duration, less intensive training is as effective as many of the longer interventions. Self-administered materials have the disadvantage of possible poor utilization and adherence.

Nicholson and colleagues report their results on the effectiveness of a Self-Administered Behavioral Intervention using Tailored Messages (SEABIT) for migraine. [32] This is a small study of 25 people, 95% female, 90% Caucasian, 21 of whom completed the 8-week study. This study seeks to address the issue of poor adherence to self-administered behavioral and cognitive-behavioral therapy through the integration of individually tailored messages. The patients are interviewed and complete a questionnaire for confirmation of headache diagnosis, assessment of outcomes of interest and information for tailored feedback. Participants complete a baseline 28-day, daily recording of headache pain, medication usage, and lifestyle behavior.

The SEABIT consists of eight weekly educational and skills components that included tailored messages. The educational materials are basic written materials from various sources about headache. Skills training included self-management skills for relaxation and/or coping using audiotapes for home-based learning. Tailored messages are derived from the weekly diary and might address headache triggers, headache-related disability, emotional factors (anxiety or depression) or headache management self-efficacy. At week 5, participants are updated on progress. At the conclusion of the intervention, participants complete another 28-day daily diary and a questionnaire. Overall, 62% (13/21) report at least 50% reduction in headache frequency. The study also finds improvement for other measures that include headache-related disability, behavioral/emotional factors, and headache-management self-efficacy.

Although SEABIT is a provocative first step in determining if there are low cost, effective alternatives to frequent provider contact for behavioral management, the study's limitations are small, uniform participant population, open-treatment design subject to outcome bias and lack of validation of participant utilization of materials provided. The value of this exploration is that, if validated further, this model could be developed for more diverse populations, including varied written materials accessible to a lower level of education or for different languages, and use of internet models that may offer maximal flexibility for language and message tailoring, as well as feedback to an evaluator.

Merelle and colleagues in the Netherlands evaluate lay trainers for home-based behavioral therapy. [33] This study uses lay trainers with migraine headache to provide home-based behavioral therapy to study participants with migraine. This is a randomized controlled study of a group who receive behavioral therapy (BT) compared with a waitlist-control group (WLC) who receive their usual care. Lay trainers with migraine had received BT as part of their care and were additionally trained in small group BT. Participants receive written materials, assignments, diary ratings and self-evaluation tools and CD-ROM with auditory relaxation exercises. BT consists of seven 2-hour sessions over 10 weeks in small groups of two to four.

The lay trainer study showed a modest effect on headache frequency, but a more robust effect on self-efficacy and locus of control. Quality of life and disability are unchanged. Although lay trainers with migraine show effectiveness in BT, the intensity of the task had the potential for adverse consequences for some in their personal struggle with migraine. A second study by the same group looks at 6-month follow-up after the waitlist-control group received BT. [34] This study shows modest improvement in headache frequency and headache quality of life and more robust and sustained improvement in locus of control and self-confidence in headache management. Headache attack frequency is more improved for those with high attack frequency. This study suggests that lay trainers may be employed in a continuum of care for migraine patients, but the most effective protocol for their use that considers health needs of trainer and trainee is not yet established.

Although not extensively studied, available evidence suggests that behavioral treatments such as relaxation therapy and biofeedback are effective in children and adolescents. [35] Trautmann and colleagues performed a meta-analysis on 23 studies of tension-type and migraine headache in adolescents and children from 1966 to 2004. [36,37]. They find that significantly more patients were benefited by treatment (≥50% headache frequency reduction) than by wait-list conditions. Clinical improvement is durable and lasts up to 1 year.

Cottrell and colleagues report on behavioral training of 34 adolescents by telephone-administered training. [35] A 2-month telephone behavioral training is compared with standard triptan management. Treatment effect is large for both telephonic training and triptan. Both treatment groups show clinically significant improvements in migraine frequency, disability and quality of life. An important observation is the excellent adherence of adolescents to the telephone protocol and their preference for this method to clinic follow-up. This suggests that use of social media platforms might be very effective adjuncts in headache behavioral management, particularly for this patient population.

A comprehensive review of biofeedback by Nestoriuc and colleagues includes meta-analysis of 94 studies that confirms the efficacy of biofeedback for adult migraine and tension-type headache patients. [38] There are various biofeedback modalities that are chosen for use dependent on the headache mechanism under consideration, i.e., vascular (migraine) or musculo-skeletal (tension type) (Table 6.3). These modalities include: peripheral temperature feedback (TEMP-FB); blood–volume–pulse feedback BP (BVP-FB); electromyographic feedback (EMG-FB); electroencephalogram feedback (EEG-FB); and galvanic skin response training (GSR-FB).

Table 6.3. Stress management techniques

Relaxation Techniques -Progressive muscle relaxation -Guided imaging
Cognitive/Behavioral Modification
Biofeedback -Peripheral temperature feedback -Blood-volume-pulse feedback -Electromyographic feedback -Electroencephalographic feedback -Galvanic skin response training
Hypnotherapy

The review demonstrated that, for migraine headache, TEMP-FB in combination with relaxation training or EMG-FB are the most frequently used modalities. TEMP-FB alone and BVP-FB alone is also used, but much less often. EMG-FB alone, EEG-FB, and GSR-FB were seldom used. Of all the methods used for migraine, GSR-FB is the most effective compared with others and EEG-FB, the least, but differences among the modalities overall are insignificant. For tension-type headache, 92% of biofeedback treatments were EMG-FB. The average number of treatments ranged from 3 to 24, average 11. Treatment duration was 20 to 95 minutes, average 43 minutes. This meta-analysis showed that biofeedback was effective in migraine headache and in tension-type headache. The effect of EMG-FB in tension-type headache is particularly robust and specific in that it shows additional significant effects over placebo and relaxation therapies. Treatment effects for both headache types are enduring and stable for an average follow-up of 14 months. For migraine, however, additional home training and treatment manuals boosted treatment effects. The short duration of treatment and the long duration of benefit make biofeedback an attractive and cost-effective stress management tool.

Although the meta-analysis shows that EEG-FB is seldom used for migraine headache, a recent study reported quantitative EEG-guided neurofeedback for recurrent migraine headache. [39] This is an open enrollment therapy offered to 71 patients in a single practice who complete a quantitative EEG that showed excessive beta activity. Forty-six elected neurofeedback to reduce beta activity, 25 continued usual care. The excessive beta activity was noted in parietal, central, and frontal regions. QEEG neurofeedback was given to reduce beta activity in those regions, five 30-minute sessions for each site of elevation. The author reports complete remission of headache in 54%, reduction of headache frequency more than 50% in 39% of participants and < 50% in 4%. Although the results are intriguing, they require validation in a properly powered controlled clinical trial.

The goal of behavioral management for stress must be to improve headache frequency and severity and to improve quality of life by increasing patient self-knowledge, disease knowledge, and sense of control and self-efficacy. The provider's role is to provide useful and usable information, support, targeted, and effective stress management interventions, appropriate pharmacotherapy or psychotherapy, and guidance for a multifaceted approach.

Gaul and colleagues report a study in the West German Headache Center in 2008 that evaluate the benefit of a multidisciplinary treatment program for adherence to treatment recommendations. [38] The multidisciplinary team is composed of neurologists, behavioral psychologists, physical and sports therapists, headache nurses and consultants from psychosomatic medicine, psychiatry, and dentistry. The patient population consists of difficult headache patients with high headache frequency, medication overuse headache and difficult to treat primary headache. The program lasts 5 days with a daily program of headache education for 60 minutes, group session with behavioral psychologist for 90 minutes, relaxation training for 60 minutes, aerobic exercise for 60 minutes with professional physiotherapist, two appointments with a neurologist, and one appointment with a psychologist. Stress management tools and lifestyle modifications are important messages in the education and counseling program.

The multidisciplinary approach yields significant improvement in this difficult to manage patient population. Forty-three % achieve a reduction in headache days after 12–18 months. Of note, 51/56 medication overuse headache patients improved. Other findings included: patient adherence medication prophylaxis in 35%; adherence to relaxation therapy in 61%; and adherence to aerobic exercise in 71%. The significance of this multidisciplinary approach is that significant gains can be achieved for chronic and difficult patients in a short-duration, intensive program and that these gains can be maintained over time. [40]

Summary

The role of stress as a modifier or trigger of headache should be actively evaluated in all patients with recurrent or chronic headache disorders. Patient education with a focus on understanding specific headache disorders and coping skills for stress, in conjunction with cognitive/behavioral therapy with relaxation or with biofeedback, biofeedback alone, with pharmacotherapy or psychotherapy where necessary, will improve headache frequency, severity and quality of life in most patients.

References

[1] Stovner LJ, Hagen K, Jensen R, *et al.* The global burden of headache: a documentation of headache prevalence and disability worldwide. *Cephalalgia* 2007; **27**: 193–210.

[2] Leonardi M, Steiner TJ, Scher AT, *et al.* The global burden of headache: Measuring disability in headache disorders with WHO's classification of functioning, disability and health (ICF). *J Headache Pain* 2005; **6**: 429–40.

[3] Kelman L. The triggers or precipitants of the acute migraine attack. *Cephalalgia* 2007; **27**: 394–402.

[4] Andress-Rothrock P, King W, Rothrock J. An analysis of migraine triggers in a clinic-based population. *Headache* 2010; **50**: 1366–70.

[5] Milde-Busch A, Blaschek A, Heinen F, *et al.* Associations between stress and migraine and tension-type headache: Results from a school-based study in adolescents from grammar schools in Germany. *Cephalalgia* 2011; **2**: 774–85.

[6] Selye H. What is Stress? *Metabolism* 1956; **5**: 525–30.

[7] Nash JM, Thebarge RW. Understanding psychological stress, its biological processes, and impact on primary headache. *Headache: J Head Face Pain* 2006; **46**: 1377–86.

[8] McEwen BS. Protection and damage from acute and chronic stress: Allostasis and allostatic overload and relevance to the pathophysiology of psychiatric disorders. *Ann N Y Acad Sci* 2004; **1032**: 1–7.

[9] Lazarus RS. From psychological stress to the emotions: a history of changing outlooks. *Annu Rev Psychol.* 1993: **44**: 1–21.

[10] Dedovic K, Wadiwalla M, Engert V, *et al.* The role of sex and gender socialization in stress reactivity. *Devel Psychol* 2009; **45**: 45–55.

[11] Stroud LR, Salovey P, Epel ES. Sex differences in stress responses: social rejection versus achievement stress. *Biol Psychiatry* 2002; **52**: 318–27.

[12] Breslau N, Chilcoat HD, Andreski P. Further evidence on the link between migraine and neuroticism. *Neurology* 1996; **47**: 663–7.

[13] Hedborg K, Anderberg UM, Muhr C. Stress in migraine: personality-dependent vulnerability, life events, and gender are of significance. *Uppsala J Med Sci* 2011; **116**: 187–99.

[14] Breslau N, Lipton RB, Stewart WF, *et al.* Comorbidity of migraine and depression: Investigating potential etiology and prognosis. *Neurology* 2003; **60**: 1308–12.

[15] McWilliams LA, Goodwin RD, Cox BJ. Depression and anxiety disorders associated with three pain conditions: Results from a nationally representative sample. *Pain* 2004: **111**: 77–83.

[16] World Health Organization. *Composite International Diagnostic Interview. Geneva*. Switzerland: World Health Organization.

[17] Kessler RC, Andrews G, Mroczek D, *et al.* The World Health Organization composite international diagnostic interview short form (CIDI-SF). *Int J Methods Psychiatry Res* 1998; **7**: 171–85.

[18] Lanteri-Minet M, Radat F, Chautard MH, *et al.* Anxiety and depression associated with migraine: Influence on migraine subjects disability and quality of life, and acute migraine management. *Pain* 2005; **118**: 319–26.

[19] North CS, Suris AM, Davis, *et al.* Toward validation of the diagnosis of posttraumatic stress disorder. *Am J Psychiatry* 2009; **166**: 34–41.

[20] Peterlin BL, Tietjen GE, Brandes JL, *et al.* Posttraumatic stress disorder in migraine. *Headache* 2009; **49**: 541–51.

[21] Peterlin Bl, Rosso AL, Sheftell FD, *et al.* Post-traumatic stress disorder, drug abuse and migraine: new findings from the National Comorbidity Survey Replication (NCS-R). *Cephalalgia* 2011; **31**: 235–44.

[22] Scher AI, Stewart WF, Buse D, *et al.* Major life changes before and after the onset of chronic daily headache: a population-based study. *Cephalalgia* 2008; **28**: 868–76.

[23] Bigal ME, Lipton RB. What predicts the change from episodic to chronic migraine? *Curr Opin Neurol* 2009; **22**: 269–76.

[24] Silberstein, SD. Practice parameter: evidence-based guidelines for migraine headache (an evidence-based review): Report of the Quality Standards Subcommittee of the American Academy of Neurology. *Neurology* 2000; **55**: 754–65.

[25] Holroyd, KA, O'Donnell FJ, Stensland N, *et al.* Management of chronic tension-type headache with tricyclic antidepressant medication, stress management therapy, and their combination: a randomized controlled trial. *JAMA* 2001; **285**: 2208–15.

[26] Penzien DB, Rains JC, Andrasik F. Behavioral management of recurrent headache: Three decades of experience and empiricism. *Appl Psychophys Biofeedback* 2002; **27**: 163–81.

[27] Sauro KM, Becker WJ. The stress and migraine interaction. *Headache* 2009; **49** 1378–86.

[28] Nicholson RA, Houle TT, Rhudy JL *et al.* Psychological risk factors in headache: *Headache* 2007; **47**: 413–26.

[29] Marlowe, N. Self-efficacy moderates the impact of stressful events on headache. *Headache* 1998: **38**: 662–7.

[30] Nicholson RA, Hursey KG, Nash JM. Moderators and mediators of behavioral treatment for headache. *Headache* 2005; **45**: 513–19.

[31] Radat F, Mekies C, Geraud G, *et al.* Anxiety, stress, and coping behaviours in primary care migraine paitents: results of the SMILE study. *Cephalalgia* 2008; **28**: 1115–25.

[32] Nicholson R, Nash J, Andrasik F. A Self-administered behavioral intervention using tailored messages for migraine. *Headache* 2005; **45**: 1124–39.

[33] Merelle, SYM, Sorbi MJ, van Doornen LJP, *et al.* Migraine patients as trainers of their fellow patients in non-pharmacological preventive attack management: short-term effects of a randomized controlled trial. *Cephalalgia* 2007; **28**: 127–38.

[34] Merelle SYM, Sorbi MJ, van Doornen LJP, *et al.* Lay trainers with migraine for a home-based behavioral training: a 6-month follow-up study. *Headache* 2008; **48**: 1311–25.

[35] Baumann RJ. Behavioral treatment of migraine in children and adolescents. *Pediatr Drugs* 2002; **4**: 555–61.

[36] Trautmann E, Lackschewitz H, Kroner-Herwig B. Psychological treatment of recurrent headache in children and adolescents – A meta-analysis. *Cephalalgia* 2006; **26**: 1141–246.

[37] Cottrell C, Drew J, Gibson J, *et al.* Feasibility assessment of telephone-administered behavioral treatment for adolescent migraine. *Headache* 2007; **47**: 1293–302.

[38] Nestoriuc Y, Martin A Rief W, *et al.* Biofeedback treatment for headache disorders: a comprehensive efficacy review. *Appl Psychophysiol Biofeedback* 2008; **33**: 125–40.

[39] Walker J. QEEG-guided neurofeedback for recurrent migraine headaches. *Clin EEG Neurosci* 2011; **42**: 59–61.

[40] Gaul, C, Van Doorn C, Webering N, *et al.* Clinical outcome of a headache-specific multidisciplinary treatment program and adherence to treatment recommendations in a tertiary headache center: an observational study. *J Headache Pain* 2011; **12**: 475–83.

Chapter 7

Drug dependence in headache patients

Margaret E.M. Haglund and Eric D. Collins

Introduction

Headache patients frequently seek analgesic and other medications, many of which are controlled substances, to provide symptomatic relief. Approximately 2% of the American population suffers from chronic migraine, and about one-third of these patients overuse their symptom-relief medications. [1] Of patients who have chronic headaches related to medication overuse ("medication overuse headaches"), approximately two-thirds meet DSM-IV criteria for dependence on their analgesic. [2] The prevalence of addiction to any substance in pain populations is estimated to be around 10%. [3] As a result, physicians often confront a range of questions and concerns about prescribing controlled substances for headaches. Will the patient requesting opioids or other potentially abused medications develop a dependence problem with the medication? Does the patient already has a dependence problem? Are symptoms feigned(malingering) or exaggerated in order to obtain the medications? It is beyond the scope of this chapter to address the medical evidence regarding the use of opioids and other controlled substances in the management of headache pain. Rather, this chapter will focus on the issues that arise when prescribing opioids and other controlled substances for chronic headache pain. This chapter addresses the use of opioids for chronic non-cancer pain (CNCP), the occurrence of opioid dependence in the management of headaches, special considerations related to specific medications (tramadol, butorphanol, barbiturates, benzodiazepines, cannabis, and caffeine), malingering, and management of the patient with suspected addiction.

The topic of substance dependence cannot be addressed without first clarifying the terminology, some of which is confusing and much of which is frequently misused. For the purposes of this chapter, the term dependence (as in "substance dependence") will be used synonymously with addiction. Confusion around terminology arises when people mistake physiologic or physical dependence on a substance with addiction. Physical or physiologic substance dependence refers simply to the neuronal adaptations to regular, often daily, substance use occurring over a period of usually 2 weeks or more. These manifest as a substance or substance-class specific withdrawal syndrome when the drug is stopped or markedly reduced in dosage or when an antagonist is administered. Tolerance (a reduction in medication response that accompanies regular use of a substance) usually accompanies physical dependence, as it also results from neuronal adaptations to regular substance ingestion. Conceptually, particularly for pain patients, the most useful definition of addiction may be the consensus definition that "addiction is a primary, chronic, neurobiologic disease, with genetic, psychosocial, and environmental factors influencing its development and manifestations. It is characterized by behaviors that include one or more of the following: impaired control over drug use, compulsive use, continued use despite harm, and craving. [4]" While the authors generally favor the criteria for substance dependence found in the *Diagnostic and Statistical Manual of Mental Disorders*, Fourth Edition (DSM-IV), these criteria may not be optimally suited to make diagnoses among patients whose addictions involve prescribed medications and will not be employed in this chapter.

Several other terms referring to substance-related problem behaviors are often misused in any of several ways; these will be discussed here and avoided throughout the remainder of the chapter. The terms *substance abuse* and *drug abuse* are used commonly in many clinical settings, but they are not precise and can be confused with the DSM-IV diagnosis "substance

The Neuropsychiatry of Headache, ed. Mark W. Green and Philip R. Muskin. Published by Cambridge University Press.

abuse," a less severe clinical condition than the DSM-IV substance dependence (addiction) diagnosis, which is generally much less predictive of significant long-term consequences related to substance use. The term *medication misuse* is also vague and may refer to any non-medical use of a substance, including use of the substance in combination with other substances, whether illicit or prescribed, usually for a purpose other than intended (e.g., to obtain a euphoric effect). The term *medication overuse* is generally not used in addiction settings, though it is used to describe "medication overuse headache," a specific diagnostic entity [5] used to denote headaches that occur on at least 15 days each month and are likely caused by regular and frequent (at least twice weekly for at least 3 months) use of headache medications. The term *drug-seeking* (or *drug seeking behavior)* will be avoided here. While it could describe requests for medication for symptom relief, it is often employed with the negative connotation that the requests are made in the service of supporting an addiction. This is unfortunate, because individuals with pain understandably and rationally make requests, sometimes irritably, for medications to relieve their suffering. Individuals with undertreated pain are often described as *drug seeking* when they do seek relief, and are susceptible to another phenomenon, *pseudoaddiction.* This occurs when pain is inadequately treated and a patient engages in aberrant medication use behaviors: using more medication than prescribed, using the medication by a different route than prescribed, or obtaining the medication or other similar medications from multiple physicians and/or from illicit sources.

Use of opioids for chronic non-cancer pain

Opioids are prescribed frequently for different types of commonly occurring chronic non-cancer pain (CNCP), including low back pain, headaches, fibromyalgia, and osteoarthritis. Most issues that arise related to prescribing opioids for CNCP also apply to the prescription of opioids for headaches. As there is a much smaller literature devoted to opioid use for headaches, this section frames the use of opioids for headache pain in the broader context of the prescription of opioids for all types of CNCP and addresses some of the issues associated with the use of opioids for CNCP. These issues include the controversy surrounding the use of opioids for CNCP, the dramatic increase in opioid prescribing in the United States starting in the 1990s, the addiction-related problems these patients may develop, and the possibility that opioids actually worsen chronic pain through a phenomenon known as opioid-induced hyperalgesia.

The prescription of opioids for CNCP is highly controversial, in large part because the evidence for the efficacy of long-term opioid therapy in chronic pain is limited, while the risks of chronic opioid therapy for CNCP are significant and include the possibilities of addiction, overdose deaths, and diversion. The headache community remains strongly divided over the use of opioids for headache pain, [6], as does the broader pain management community. [7] While it is beyond the scope of this chapter to review opioid use in chronic pain, it is worth observing that, prior to the 1980s, opioids were generally used primarily for acute pain and for chronic pain secondary to malignancy. Beginning in the 1980s and rapidly escalating through the 1990s, opioid prescribing for non-cancer pain began to increase. Between 1990 and 2011, there was a greater than ten-fold increase in opiates prescribed, [8] and currently over 90% of opiates prescribed are for CNCP. [9] Opponents of the widespread use of opioids for CNCP cite the concurrent dramatic increases in fatal accidental opioid-related drug overdoses, emergency room visits related to opioid use, and opioid use disorder treatment program admissions. [10] While these problems are not necessarily caused by the increased prescription of opioids, they do raise serious questions and appear likely to result in potentially sweeping changes in the federal and state regulation of opioid prescribing. These changes, if they materialize, raise some concerns that pain patients will be undertreated and therefore suffer unnecessarily. Unfortunately, there is scant and weak evidence to guide practice in this area. A recent Cochrane review of 26 studies of opioid treatment of at least 6 months' duration, only one of which was a randomized controlled trial, finds that patients on long-term opioid therapy do experience clinically significant pain relief, but whether these patients improve on quality of life measures or functional status is inconclusive. [11] The occurrence of opioid addiction in these patients when it was reported, was 0.27%, but this quite low rate must be interpreted with the understanding that most of the studies reviewed screened out patients with a history of addiction.

With respect to addiction-related problems in patients with CNCP, the prevalence of problematic or aberrant drug behavior (i.e., using larger doses than prescribed, reporting lost or stolen prescriptions, visiting multiple providers) is reported to be as high as 24% of CNCP patients taking prescribed opioids. [12] Several studies find that, for patients prescribed opioids chronically, there is a strong association between a personal history of a substance use disorder or comorbid psychiatric disorders and the development of abuse of or dependence on prescribed opioids. [13] A study of 15,160 individuals treated in the Veterans Administration health care system finds that, in patients prescribed opioids for CNCP, a history of non-opioid substance abuse (as defined by ICD-9 criteria) is the strongest predictor of the development of ICD-9 defined opioid abuse or dependence, with an odds ratio (OR 2.34, $P < 0.005$). Comorbid mental health disorders (specific diagnoses not available) are moderately strong predictors (OR 1.46, $P < 0.005$). Men, younger adults, and individuals with greater supplies of prescription opioids are more likely to develop opioid dependence. [14]

One additional issue related to long-term opioid therapy should be considered. People can potentially develop increased pain sensitivity, or opioid-induced hyperalgesia (OIH), in response to regular ingestion of opioids. [15] OIH seems to develop independent of tolerance and likely involves neuronal adaptation to chronic opioid exposure, activating proprioceptive pathways. The prevalence of OIH is unknown. Patients who develop OIH complain of more pain as their opioid dosing increases. The increased pain may be an exacerbation of their primary pain syndrome and/or may involve diffuse pain sensitivity, even to usually non-painful stimuli (allodynia). The possibility of OIH should be considered whenever the analgesic effects of opioids seem to wear off, particularly when the underlying disease does not progress. It can be extremely difficult to distinguish patients with OIH from those with opioid addiction because both sets of patients often improve when opioids are reduced or even completely discontinued.

Opioid dependence in headache patients

Although the literature suggests that chronic opioid therapy is ineffective for chronic headaches, may exacerbate headache pain, and can lead to dependence [16], opioid prescriptions for headaches are common. A 2009 review of a medical insurance claims database in the United States finds that 19% of chronic opioid prescriptions (defined as greater than 180 days per year) are for treatment of headache. [17]

The use of opioid medications for the treatment of headache is associated with a significant risk of dependence. A 2009 US epidemiologic study of migraine patients finds a prevalence of opioid dependence, per DSM-IV criteria, of nearly 17% among patients using any opioids in the three months prior to the survey. [18] Of those individuals, those who take opioids daily or nearly daily have rates of DSM-IV dependence close to 50%. Other studies of headache patients with regular opioid use find a similar prevalence of dependence, whether measuring dependence by DSM-IV criteria or presuming dependence by assessing aberrant drug-related behaviors [19].

Regular opioid use exacerbates pre-existing headaches and is implicated in the development of medication overuse headache. [9,20] Regular opioid use may even cause headaches in patients who did not suffer from them prior to exposure. In a study of 1051 individuals who reported abusing variety of substances including opioids, 27% report chronic headaches, and 95% of these patients report onset of the headaches after substance use. [21] Headache patients may increase their opioid use because of worsening headache pain, possibly related to OIH, and/or because of addiction and tolerance.

The majority of headache patients who overuse or develop dependence on opioids and opioid-containing compounds suffer from migraine-type headaches. Headache patients who demonstrate opioid dependence also report the most severe pain, the highest frequency of headaches, the longest duration of illness, [18,22] and have the highest rates of headache-related disability. The 2009 American Migraine Prevalence and Prevention Study finds that migraine sufferers with probable opioid dependence (per DSM-IV criteria) report far more headache-related disability than non-opioid users and opioid users without dependence. On the Migraine Disability Assessment Scale (MIDAS), which measures loss of productivity caused by migraines, current opioid users with dependence score 44.4 on average indicating high levels of migraine-related disability. Non-users score 7.8 ($P < 0.001$) and current non-dependent users score 19.1 ($P < 0.001$). [23] Opioid-using headache patients use significantly more health care resources as measured by visits to outpatient providers, emergency department visits and inpatient hospitalizations. Estimates are that opioid-dependent headache patients make 6–11 times more visits to primary care physicians, obstetricians, neurologists, mental health providers, physician assistants, and nurse practitioners. This difference in number of visits remains statistically significant even when controlling for migraine-related disability. [18] Because studies of level of pain, disability rates, and health care utilization associated with opioid use are cross-sectional, the causal direction is unknown. Patients who make more health care visits may ultimately be more likely to be prescribed an opioid, independent of their headache severity, and those interested in obtaining opioids are likely to make more visits to their physicians in order to obtain opioids.

As with other types of chronic pain, individual factors linked with opioid over-use or dependence in headache patients include a personal history of any substance abuse or dependence [24,25] and comorbid psychiatric illness. Multiple studies have found that headache and other chronic pain patients who regularly use or over-use opioids are more likely (on the order of two to five times increased risk) to suffer from major depression, anxiety, or personality disorders. [18,26–29] Depression is the most prevalent comorbid psychiatric condition, but patients who over-use analgesics also have increased rates of anxiety, neuroticism, hypochondriasis and hysteria (excessive displays of emotion, attention seeking and sensitivity to criticism and rejection). [30,31] Personality disorders are also associated with treatment failure when prescribing opioids in chronic daily headache patients. [32]

Clinicians are typically unable to determine which patients are at the highest risk of developing opioid dependence. [33] There are a number of tools designed to facilitate screening for risk of opioid addiction, however, these are not entirely reliable. Most have been used in patients with chronic non-cancer pain, and none exists specifically for headache patients. The Opioid Risk Tool, developed in 2005, is one of the most widely used assessments. Studies of its accuracy in detection are mixed. While initial validation studies show a sensitivity of 91% and specificity of 94%, [34] more recent research suggests that the Opioid Risk Tool is not reliable across methods of administration, with clinician administration yielding significantly higher sensitivity than patient self-report. [35] Other measures designed to identify patients potentially at risk to develop opioid dependence include the Screener and Opioid Assessment for Patients with Pain, revised (SOAPP-R, 2008), and the Pain Medication Questionnaire, revised (PMQ, 2009). [3,36] Both of these measures also show relatively low sensitivity and specificity in later validations (SOAPP-R, sensitivity 81% and specificity 68%; PMQ sensitivity 82%, specificity 56%). [37] A direct comparison of these commonly used measures with each other and with clinical interview finds that clinical interview yields highest sensitivity overall, and that among the screening assessments (SOAPP-R, ORT, PMQ), SOAPP-R has the highest sensitivity. [38] As noted above, SOAPP-R has relatively low specificity and thus over-rates the risk of dependence.

Other measures are proposed to detect opioid addiction among patients already taking opioids. The Current Opioid Misuse Measure (COMM, 2006) is commonly used in chronic pain patients; it shows approximately 80% sensitivity and specificity. [39,40] Other less commonly used measures include the Pain Assessment and Documentation Tool (PADT, 2004), the Prescription Drug Use Questionnaire (PDUQ, 1998), the Screening Instrument for Substance Abuse Potential (SISAP, 1996) and the Addiction Severity Index (ASI 5th edn, 1992). Overall, screening tools have weak predictive value for identifying aberrant drug behaviors or dependence for pain patients receiving opioids. [41]

Clinical interview, history, and demographic factors should be taken into account when assessing patients for treatment with opioids. When using screening measures, clinicians should keep in mind the low specificity and high false-positive rates of most measures, which may lead to under-treatment of pain in patients not at risk for dependence. Another limitation of these measures is the risk that patients may provide false information with respect to past substance abuse, particularly when a "high risk" score may lead to a denial of a request for opioids. Given the importance of identifying individuals at high risk of developing dependence, the authors favor the use of the SOAPP-R to screen individuals for whom a trial of opioids is being considered, and to consider the results carefully before initiating opioid use and during any opioid trials. To assess possible opioid misuse in patients currently treated with opioids, the authors recommend the use of the COMM tool together with careful history and attention to "red flags," such as unwillingness to participate in urine screening, requests for specific opioids or immediate release formulations, and reluctance to follow recommendations for further evaluation by specialists. The identification and management of suspected opioid abuse are further discussed in the section on malingering at the end of this chapter. The authors ultimately favor the use of "Universal Precautions" in managing patients with headache and other pain syndromes using opioids. [42] These precautions include thorough investigation and attempts to treat the underlying cause of pain; evaluation for any untreated comorbid medical or psychiatric disorders; a careful assessment of current and past substance use, with active untreated addiction a contraindication to prescription of opioids; informed consent of the risks of opioid treatment; an explicit treatment agreement regarding appropriate use of prescribed medications; and regular assessments of pain levels to provide rationale for continuation of treatment.

Tramadol dependence in headache patients

Tramadol is an analgesic that produces norepinephrine and serotonin reuptake inhibition [43] and has weak opioid effects at the mu receptor. The metabolite, O-desmethyl tramadol produces greater mu-agonist activity. [44] The mechanism of analgesia is not fully understood, but seems to result from activity at non-opioid receptors: studies of naloxone treatment in patients taking daily tramadol for 3 or more weeks have not precipitated opioid withdrawal. [45] Adrenoreceptor antagonism with yohimbine reverses the analgesic effects. [46] Tramadol withdrawal often includes symptoms not typically seen in pure opioid withdrawal, such as extreme anxiety, panic or paranoia, hallucinations, and feelings of numbness and tingling in extremities. [47] The literature is mixed regarding the potential for dependence in patients prescribed tramadol, and there is insufficient evidence to draw conclusions about the risk of dependence in headache patients. The existing literature on tramadol dependence in headache patients consists primarily of case reports. [48–50] Far more literature exists concerning tramadol abuse and dependence among CNCP patients; however, the evidence is mixed, and no definitive conclusions can be drawn. A 2006 randomized trial of analgesic agents used in CNCP found that, after 1 year of treatment, patients randomized to the tramadol arm are no more likely to develop dependence, as measured by inappropriate use and self-reported withdrawal symptoms, than are patients randomized to treatment with NSAIDs. Patients randomized to the tramadol arm were also significantly less likely to develop suspected dependence than patients randomized to hydrocodone (2.7% vs 4.9%, n = 8139). [51] Supporting the evidence that the abuse and dependence potential of tramadol is low, post-marketing surveillance studies find that diversion of the drug is rare, [52] and a risk-management program analyzing patterns of use in the United States between 1994 and 2004 estimates rates of both abuse and withdrawal at less than 1 case per 100 000 patients exposed to the drug. [53] The authors of that study acknowledge that the data were imprecisely gathered and relied on spontaneous reports. Others argue that among certain populations, tramadol abuse and dependence is relatively common; physicians have been identified as a higher risk group. A review of the records of all physicians enrolled in drug monitoring programs in Alabama and Michigan between 1994 and 2002 (n = 595) find that tramadol is a frequently abused drug, and that it comprises 10% of all reported cases of opioid dependence, ranking third (after hydrocodone and meperidine) with respect to the number of physicians who report abusing it. [54] Of the physicians who report abusing tramadol (n = 33), 32 have a diagnosis of tramadol dependence and one has a diagnosis of tramadol abuse (per DSM-IV). [55] As with full opioid agonists, it is thought that the strongest risk factor for developing tramadol dependence is a history of other substance abuse or dependence. [56,57]

Butorphanol

Butorphanol, an opioid with partial mu-agonist effects, was first developed in injectable form and initially used in hospital settings mainly for postoperative and labor pain. It was formulated as a nasal spray in 1992 and marketed for the treatment of acute pain, particularly migraine headaches, and the majority of prescriptions were for migraines (60% within the first 3 years). [58] Butorphnaol nasal spray was an unscheduled drug until 1995. During these first 3 years of its availability, there are many reports of addiction, dependence and even deaths, both in medical journals and in the popular press; prevalence of dependence is estimated as at least 24%, based on reports to the FDA of adverse drug reactions. In 1995 it was reclassified as a schedule IV drug. Since then, it is prescribed far less frequently, and current rates of butorphanol dependence among headache patients are not available. An American managed care study of controlled substance use among insured patients finds that, in 2000, among nearly 3 million insured patients under the age of 65, the prevalence of probable butorphanol dependence, including tablet, injection, and spray formulations, is 1.5%. [59] This estimate is generated, based on the number of patients requesting four or greater butorphanol prescriptions sequentially, for any type of pain. As with tramadol, it is difficult to draw conclusions from these data regarding dependence risk in headache patients; however it is likely that both drugs have some risk of dependence, but less than that with pure mu-opioid agonists.

Barbiturate dependence in headache patients

The only barbiturate indicated specifically for the treatment of headache is butalbital, prescribed in the various combination medications. Butalbital has a rapid onset of action, a duration of action of 3–6 hours, and a plasma half-life of 20–80 hours. Various combinations of butalbital and other analgesic substances exist (including aspirin, acetaminophen, codeine, phenacetin, aminophenazone, propyphenazone, caffeine). The most commonly used combinations for treatment of headache are acetaminophen, caffeine, and butalbital (Fioricet) and aspirin, caffeine, and butalbital (Fiorinal). These are available over the counter in many countries, though not in the United States. In randomized clinical trials, butalbital-containing compounds are shown to be efficacious in the treatment of tension-type headache. [60] They are thought to be effective in treating migraine headaches as well, though there is no clear evidence to support this view. In a 2006 American epidemiologic study of 9694 migraine patients, 6% of episodic migraine patients regularly use butalbital-containing compounds, with average use at 7.3 days per month; in patients with chronic migraine, 13.5% use butalbital-containing compounds, and average use is 15.9 days per month. [61] There are many anecdotal reports of problematic drug-related behaviors in patients using butalbital-containing compounds for headache, and over-use of the drug is frequently reported. [1] There are also case reports documenting withdrawal syndromes from butalbital used for headache, [62,63] a serious risk given that barbiturate withdrawal can be life threatening.

As with opioids, over-use of butalbital is associated with the exacerbation of existing headaches in severity, duration, and resistance to treatment. For butalbital-containing compounds, it is estimated that the dose at which exacerbation of headache begins is approximately 5 days of use per month. [64] This phenomenon tends to lead to increasing use, and overdose on barbiturates is a significant danger. [65,66]

As with opioids, the risk factors for dependence on barbiturates include a prior history of any substance abuse or dependence and psychiatric comorbidity, including anxiety and mood disorders and personality disorders. [67] A 1987 study of headache patients finds that study subjects assigned to treatment with butalbital report significant reductions in anxiety and psychological tension, [68] and the authors conclude that patients with underlying anxiety may seek and abuse the drug. However, there is too little data on risk factors for butalbital dependence among headache patients to draw meaningful conclusions.

Benzodiazepines used in patients with tension-type headaches

Benzodiazepines are not indicated for the treatment of pain, including headache. However, chronic pain and headache patients are sometimes prescribed benzodiazepines, and some patients experience an analgesic effect. A 1996 study of 125 patients at a London chronic pain clinic finds that 22 (17.6%) of them took benzodiazepines to treat their pain; 5 of these individuals (4% of sample, 23% of benzodiazepine using subset) abused the medication, and 4 (3.2% of sample, 18% of benzodiazepine using subset) meet DSM-IIIR criteria for dependence. [69] The literature on the risk of benzodiazepine addiction is mixed, with some studies suggesting minimal risk [70] and others suggesting high abuse liability. [71] The disagreement about the risk of benzodiazepine dependence may be at least partly explained by authors using different definitions of dependence (i.e., not carefully distinguishing between physical dependence and addiction).

Cannabis

In the current era of "medical cannabis," (or "medical marijuana,"), which is now approved as a legal, if informal, possibility in over 15 US states, cannabis may be effective in the treatment of migraine, cluster, and/or tension-type headaches. Some headache patients, including some who are already receiving prescriptions for opioids and/or other controlled substances, report that cannabis relieves their headache pain. There is insufficient medical evidence to assert that cannabis may be effective for headaches [72] and/or for the treatment of chronic pain [73] of other types. Any patient who reports using cannabis for analgesic effects should be monitored closely and evaluated for possible cannabis dependence as well as for possible dependence on other substances, including prescribed medications. The care of cannabis-using patients may be managed best by coordinating their continuing headache care with an addiction specialist.

Caffeine

When included in mixed-analgesics medications (e.g., Fioricet/Fiorinal), caffeine is associated with medication over-use, primarily due to its butalbital component. By itself, caffeine is thought to have low addiction potential according to ICD-10 criteria for dependence, and has not been found to have an independent role in promoting abuse or dependence. [74,75] It is well known that patients with physiologic dependence on caffeine routinely develop caffeine withdrawal headaches.

Malingering in headache patients

Malingering, which is falsely complaining of some symptom (pain in this chapter) in order to obtain a desired response (the so-called secondary gain), is thought to be common. Estimates of the prevalence of malingering in patients complaining of pain vary widely, depending on many factors, notably the desired secondary gain (i.e., to obtain disability payments, or opioids or other controlled substances for personal use and/or diversion) [75], but usually fall in the range of 10% to 30%. [76,77] Most studies to date have focused on the estimated prevalence and detection of malingering in patients seeking certification of disability; much less is known about patients malingering for the purpose of obtaining controlled substances, for chief complaints of general pain or of headache, and the prevalence of this form of malingering is unknown.

Studies have shown that clinicians are generally unable to distinguish genuine pain complaints from malingering. [78,79] Further complicating the detection of malingering, patients may present with genuine pain and also exaggerate their symptoms in order to obtain controlled substances. Certain behaviors are associated with malingering in patients requesting opioids: these include requesting specific opioid-containing medications by name, reporting allergies to non-opioid analgesics, reporting lost or stolen medications, presenting frequently to the emergency department with pain, reporting 10 or >10 out of 10 pain, and requesting that pain medication be administered parenterally. These behaviors are seen less often in patients with genuine pain complaints and should raise a suspicion for malingering. [80] These behaviors may also occur with pseudoaddiction, which results from the undertreatment of pain.

There is no single reliable screening tool to identify malingering in patients presenting with pain (headache or other), though efforts to design such measures continue. The Personality Assessment Inventory has been revised to detect malingering and is widely used for that purpose. In initial validations, the measure shows high sensitivity and specificity, in the 80%–90% range, for the detection of malingered pain. [81] Sensitivity and specificity are found to vary depending on the population in which the instrument is used, and subsequent studies suggest that the measure may be less reliable than initially thought. [82] Other measures commonly used are the Minnesota Multiphasic Personality Inventory version 2 and version 2 Restructured Format (MMPI-2 and MMPI-2 RF), which measure personality traits thought to be associated with malingering, such as cynicism, low positive emotion, and feelings of persecution, and the Structured Interview of Reported Symptoms (SIRS), which captures the plausibility of symptoms reported. [83] The reliability of these and other screening assessments for detecting malingering in headache patients seeking opioids or other controlled substances (e.g., butalbital) is unknown. The use of such screening instruments is not recommended to detect possible malingering in headache patients requesting controlled substances.

Among patients receiving regular prescriptions for controlled substances, there are a number of approaches that prescribers can incorporate to detect and/or deter possible malingering for controlled substances. The combination of spot urine drug screens, random checks between visits to count pills, close tracking of prescription refills, patient observation, and, where available, utilization of prescription monitoring programs can curtail malingering. Obtaining random or spot urine drug screens is among the most reliable methods for detecting drug misuse, [84] except when the patient is only over-using the prescribed analgesic medication. Laboratory urine drug screens are more useful than point-of-care urine tests, because they have higher specificity and sensitivity and can include definitive testing for the molecular fingerprint of a substance and/or its metabolites. Additionally, phoning patients routinely for random pill counts can be an effective way to monitor a patient's use of controlled substances throughout the month. Keeping track of patient refill requests to ensure that patients do not routinely obtain medications earlier than their regimen requires will detect some cases of over-use of the prescribed medication. Physicians should also periodically examine patients for track marks that would suggest diversion of opioids to intravenous use. Prescription monitoring programs constitute a potentially effective tool to detect malingering for controlled substances. These programs are available in some states, but in different forms; they typically allow physicians to determine what controlled medications have been prescribed previously. Ideally, these programs include prescriptions filled anywhere in the country, but they should routinely include prescriptions obtained by the patient locally and in neighboring regions.

Because of the estimated high rates of malingering (including for disability payments) and the difficulty in accurate detection/diagnosis by clinicians, some practice settings have implemented regulations regarding the prescription of opioids. Some hospitals have instructed emergency department physicians to limit their prescriptions to a pre-determined number of tablets per patient per month; others have instituted algorithms and specific guidelines regarding the selection of pain medication to be used. An emergency medicine physicians' group based in North Carolina instituted guidelines for headache patients in two affiliated emergency departments, stipulating that non-opioid oral medications should be used as first-line treatment, that no patient should receive intramuscular opioid injections in the emergency department, and that for treatment-refractory headaches, intravenous medications should be used. These guidelines are posted in a location visible to patients entering the emergency department and consistently enforced. However, despite these practices, between 2003 and 2005 the emergency departments involved did not experience a decreased volume of headache patients seeking opioids; the study authors conclude that the prevalence of malingering among these patients is lower than had been assumed. [85]

Management of suspected or confirmed addiction

Any practitioner who routinely prescribes controlled substances for the management of chronic headache pain will encounter patients with comorbid addiction illnesses. When this happens, the optimal response is essentially unchanged, from that employed to address any other co-occurring chronic illness. Most practitioners evaluate co-occurring conditions as fully as possible within the scope of their usual practice and then refer the patient to a specialist for further evaluation and management of the condition. In the case of suspected addiction, the initial evaluation by the primary doctor may include a period of further observation that incorporates any or all of the following: more frequent visits for patient observation and additional pill counts, regular observed urine toxicology testing, provision of medications for short periods between regular, frequent visits, review of data from prescription monitoring programs, and a re-evaluation of the value of opioid therapy to the particular patient for pain control, optimal functioning, and the lowest side effect burden.

For many headache patients, successful treatment of co-occurring addiction may improve the underlying headache syndrome. There are many reasons for this, but sometimes the improvement may reflect diminished opioid-induced hyperalgesia that follows medically assisted withdrawal from opioids. Any practitioner who prescribes opioids (or other controlled substances) for headaches should be able to help patients safely and comfortably reduce the dosages and withdraw from opioids. This involves gradual reductions in dosages, but in some patients it may best be accomplished by use of buprenorphine, which is approved both for detoxification from opioids and maintenance therapy of opioid dependence. (This does not belong in an international book.) Detailed instructions for how to induct patients onto buprenorphine and/or to withdraw patients from opioids and other controlled substances can be found in many textbooks on addiction.

Summary

Many headache patients receive prescriptions for opioids and/or other controlled substances for pain relief, despite significant questions about the long-term efficacy of these practices and the risk of addiction among these patients. While a majority of headache patients given controlled substances do not develop addiction problems, every practitioner who prescribes controlled substances for headaches needs to consider the associated addiction risks and how to mitigate them. It is often difficult to predict which patients are at the greatest risk to develop addiction and to detect ongoing addiction in patients already taking controlled substances. Careful patient selection is helpful, and the single best predictor of opioid addiction among headache and all pain patients is a personal history of a prior addiction. Another important risk factor for the development of addiction problems in headache patients is comorbid psychiatric illness, including mood, anxiety, and personality disorders. The treating physician should conduct careful interviews to identify these risk factors and make appropriate referrals to ensure treatment of comorbid psychiatric illness. When prescribing opioids or other controlled substances for headaches, clinicians should conduct periodic assessments of treatment efficacy and evaluate whether addiction may be present. Screening methods may be of utility in these evaluations but should not replace clinical assessments. Monitoring of prescriptions, pill counts, and urine drug screens will also aid clinicians in detecting abuse and dependence. In addition, physicians should recognize that opioids are associated with heightened sensitivity to pain and must consider this possibility when evaluating a patient's continuing pain complaints in the face of escalating analgesic use. The possibilities of pseudoaddiction (aberrant analgesic use behaviors associated with undertreated pain) and of malingering (feigning or exaggerating pain symptoms to obtain controlled substance prescriptions) must also be considered, but it may be difficult to confirm pseudoaddiction and/or malingering. When clinicians suspect an addiction problem, pseudoaddiction, and/or malingering, referral to an addiction psychiatrist to help with patient management is frequently valuable.

References

[1] Evans RW, Basin SM. Why migraineurs abuse butalbital-containing combination analgesics? *Headache* 2012; **50**: 1194–7.

[2] Fuh JL, Wang SJ. Dependent behavior in patients with medication-overuse headache. *Curr Pain Headache Rep* 2012; **16**: 73–9.

[3] Butler SF, Fernandez K, Benoit C, Budman SH, Jamison RN. Validation of the revised screener and opioid assessment for patients with pain (SOAPP-R). *J Pain* 2008; **9**: 360–72.

[4] Definitions related to the use of opioids for the treatment of pain: a consensus document from the American Academy of Pain Medicine, the American Pain Society, and the American Society of Addiction Medicine, 2001. (http://www.painmed.org/Workarea/DownloadAsset.aspx?id=3204)

[5] Silberstein SD, Olesen J, Bousser MG, *et al.* (2005). *The International Classification of Headache Disorders*, 2nd edn (ICHD-II) – revision of criteria for 8.2 Medication-overuse headache. *Cephalalgia* 2005; **25**(6): 460–5.

[6] Tepper SJ, Rothrock JF. Conclusions on opioids. *Headache* 2012; **52** Suppl 1: 38–9.

[7] Schneider JP, Kirsh KL. Defining clinical issues around tolerance, hyperalgesia, and addiction: a quantitative and qualitative outcome study of long-term opioid dosing in a chronic pain practice. *J Opioid Managem* 2010; **6**: 385–95.

[8] Okie S. A flood of opioids, a rising tide of deaths. *N Engl J Med* 2010; **363**: 1981–5.

[9] Saper JR, Lake AE 3rd, Bain PA, *et al.* A practice guide for continuous opioid therapy for refractory daily headache: patient selection, physician requirements, and treatment monitoring. *Headache* 2010; **50**: 1175–93.

[10] Okie, S. A flood of opioids, a rising tide of deaths. *N Engl J Med.* 2010; **363**: 1981–5.

[11] Noble M, Treadwell JR, Tregear SJ, *et al.* Long-term opioid management for chronic noncancer pain. *Cochrane Database of Syst Rev* 2010, Issue 1.

[12] Saper JR, Lake AE. Continuous opioid therapy (COT) is rarely advisable for refractory chronic daily headache: limited efficacy, risks and proposed guidelines. *Headache* 2008; **48**: 838–49.

[13] Edlund MJ, Martin BC, Fan MY, Devries A, Braden JB, Sullivan MD. Risks of opioid abuse and dependence among recipients of chronic opioid therapy: results from the TROUP study. *Drug Alcohol Depend* 2010; **112**: 90–8.

[14] Edlund MJ, Steffic D, Hudson T, Harris KM, Sullivan M. Risk factors for clinically recognized opioid abuse and dependence among veterans using opioids for chronic non-cancer pain. *Pain* 2007; **129**: 355–62.

[15] Lee M, Silverman SM, Hansen H, Patel VB, Manchikanti L. A comprehensive review of opioid-induced hyperalgesia. *Pain Physician* 2011; **14**: 145–61.

[16] Saper JR, Lake AE 3rd, Hamel RL, *et al.* Daily scheduled opioids for intractable head pain: long-term observations of a treatment program. *Neurology.* 2004; **62**: 1687–94.

[17] Cicero TJ, Wong G, Tian Y, Lynsey M, Todorov A, Isenberg K. Co-morbidity and utilization of medical services by pain patients receiving opioid medications: data from insurance claims database. *Pain* 2009; **144**: 20–7.

[18] Buse DC, Pearlman SH, Reed ML, Serrano D, Ng-Mak DS, Lipton RB. Opioid use and dependence among persons with migraine: results of the AMPP study. *Headache* 2012; **52**: 18–36.

[19] Radat FR, Creac'h C, Guegan-Massardier E, *et al.* Behavioral dependence in patients with medication overuse headache: a cross-sectional study in consulting patients using the DSM-IV criteria. *Headache* 2008; **48**: 1026–36.

[20] Bigal ME, Lipton RB. Excessive opioid use and the development of chronic migraine. *Pain* 2009; **142**: 179–82.

[21] Beckmann YY, Seckin M, Manavgat AI, Zorlu N. Headaches related to psychoactive substance use. *Clin Neurol Neurosurg* 2012; epub ahead of print.

[22] Lake AE, Saper JR, Hamel RL. Comprehensive inpatient treatment of refractory chronic daily headache. *Headache* 2009; **49**: 555–62.

[23] Buse DC, Pearlman SH, Reed ML, Serrano D, Ng-Mak DS, Lipton RB. Opioid use and dependence among persons with migraine: results of the AMPP study. *Headache* 2012; **52**: 18–36.

[24] Ziegler DK. Opioids in headache treatment. Is there a role? *Neurol Clin* 1997; **15**: 199–207.

[25] Sullivan MD, Edlund MJ, Fan MY, Devries A, Brennan Braden J, Martin BC. Risks for possible and probable opioid misuse among recipients of chronic opioid therapy in commercial and medicaid insurance plans: the TROUP study. *Pain* 2010; **150**: 332–9.

[26] Sullivan MD, Edlund MJ, Steffick D, Unutzer J. Regular use of prescribed opioids: association with common psychiatric disorders. *Pain* 2005; **119**: 95–103.

[27] Cicero TJ, Wong G, Tian Y, Lynskey M, Todorov A, Isenberg K. Co-morbidity and utilization of medical services by pain patients receiving opioid medications: data from an insurance claims database. *Pain* 2009; **144**: 20–7.

[28] Lake AE, Saper JR, Hamel RL. Comprehensive inpatient treatment of refractory chronic daily headache. *Headache* 2009; **49**: 555–62.

[29] Manchikanti L, Giordano J, Boswell MV, Fellows B, Manchukonda R, Pampati V. Psychological factors as predictors of opioid abuse and illicit drug use in chronic pain patients. *J Opioid Managem* 2007; **3**: 89–100.

[30] Galli F, Pozzi G, Frustaci A, *et al.* Differences in the personality profile of medication-overuse headache sufferers and drug-addict patients: a comparative study using MMPI-2. *Headache* 2011; **51**: 1212–27.

[31] Radat F, Irachabal S, Swendsen J, Henry P. Analgesic abuse and psychiatric comorbidity in headache patients. *Encephale* 2002; **28**: 466–71.

[32] Ziegler DK. Opiate and opioid use in patients with refractory headache. *Cephalalgia* 1994; **14**: 5–10.

[33] Butler SF, Budman SH, Fernandez KC, *et al.* Development and validation of the current opioid misuse measure. *Pain* 2007; **103**: 144–56.

[34] Brown J, Setnik B, Lee K, *et al.* Assessment, stratification, and monitoring of the risk for prescription opioid misuse and abuse in the primary care setting. *J Opioid Managem* 2011; **7**: 467–83.

[35] Jones T, Passik SD. A comparison of methods of administering the opioid risk tool. *J Opioid Managem* 2001; **7**: 347–51.

[36] Buelow A, Haggard R, Gatchel RJ. Additional validation of the pain medication questionnaire in a heterogeneous sample of chronic pain patients. *Pain Pract* 2009; **9**: 428–34.

[37] Hojsted J, Nielsen PR, Kendall S, Frich L, Sjogren P. Validation and usefulness of the Danish version of the pain medication questionnaire in opioid-treated chronic pain patients. *Acta Anaesthesiol Scand* 2011; **55**: 1231–8.

[38] Jones T, Moore T, Levy JL, *et al.* A comparison of various risk screening methods in predicting discharge from opioid treatment. *Clin J Pain* 2012; **28**: 93–100.

[39] Butler SF, Budman SH, Fanciullo GJ, Jamison RN. Cross validation of the current opioid misuse measure to monitor chronic pain patients on opioid therapy. *Clin J Pain* 2010; **26**: 770–6.

[40] Meltzer EC, Rybin D, Saitz R, *et al.* Identifying prescription opioid use disorder in primary care: diagnostic characteristics of the Current Opioid Misuse Measure (COMM). *Pain* 2011; **152**: 397–402.

[41] Chou R, Fanciullo GJ, Fine PG, Miaskowski C, Passik SD, Portenoy RK. Opioids for chronic noncancer pain: prediction and identification of aberrant drug-related behaviors: a review of the evidence for an American Pain Society and American Academy of Pain Medicine clinical practice guideline. *J Pain* 2009; **10**: 131–46.

[42] Gourlay DL, Heit HA, Almahrezi A, *et al.* Universal precautions in pain medicine: a rational approach to the treatment of chronic pain. *Pain Med* 2005; **6**: 107–12.

[43] Raffa RB. Basic pharmacology relevant to drug abuse assessment: tramadol as example. *J Clin Pharm Ther* 2008; **33**(2): 101–8.

[44] Desmeules JA. The tramadol option. *Eur J Pain* 2000; **4**: A15–21.

[45] Richter W, Barth H, Flohe L, Giertz H. Clinical investigation on the development of dependence during oral therapy with tramadol. *Arzneimittelforschung* 1985; **35**: 1742–4.

[46] Desmeules JA, Piquet V, Collart L, Dayer P. Contribution of monoaminergic modulation to the analgesic effect of tramadol. *Br J Clin Pharmacol* 1996; **41**: 7–12.

[47] Senay EC, Adams EH, Geller A, *et al.* Physical dependence on ultram (tramadol hydrochloride): both opioid-like and atypical withdrawal symptoms occur. *Drug Alcohol Depend* 2003; **69**: 233–41.

[48] Stoehr JD, Essary AC, Ou C, Ashby R, Sucher M. The risk of tramadol abuse and dependence: findings from two patients. *JAAPA* 2009; **22**: 31–2.

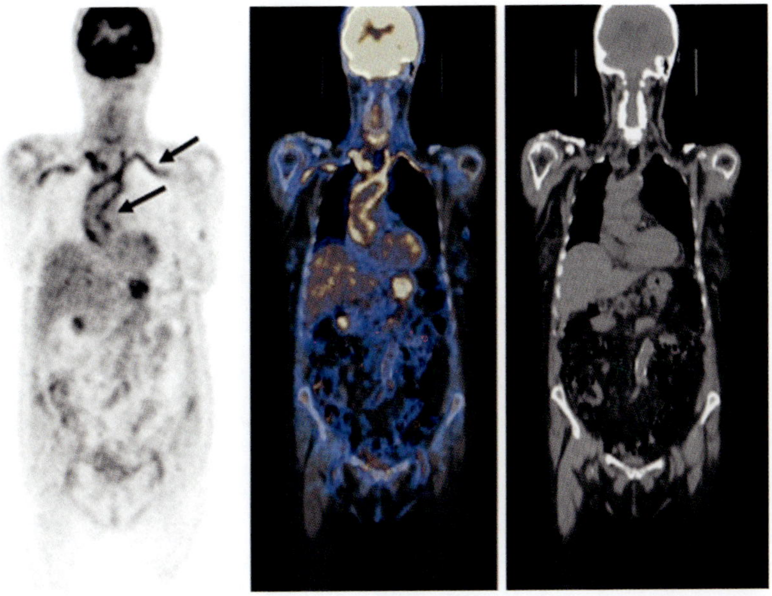

Fig. 8.3. Coronal 18F-FDG PET (left), PET/CT (center), and CT (right) slices in a 78-year-old woman who presented with a 6-week history of fever, night sweats, and weight loss, which demonstrate intense linear 18F-FDG uptake along walls of thoracic aorta and brachiocephalic and subclavian arteries (arrows) consistent with Giant Cell Arteritis [111]; adapted with permission.

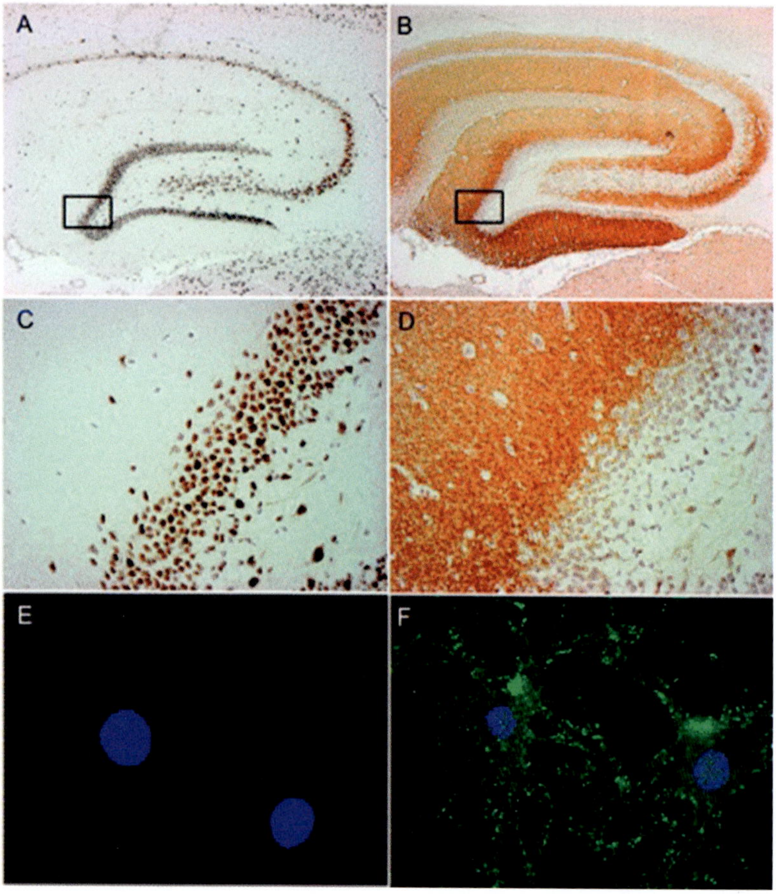

Fig. 8.4. Part 2. Consecutive sections of rat hippocampus immunostained with CSF of a patient with antibodies directed against Hu, an intracellular antigen (A) and CSF of a patient with antibodies directed against a cell surface synaptic antigen (NMDA receptor [NMDA-R] (B). (C, D) The framed areas are shown at higher magnification. Compared with the intracellular antigen, the cell surface synaptic antigen (NMDA-R) is demonstrated as robust neuropil staining, sparing neuronal cell bodies (the nuclei of neurons are mildly counterstained with hematoxylin). Using live, nonpermeabilized cultures of dissociated rat hippocampal neurons, the Hu antibody does not show reactivity due to lack of penetration into the neuron (E), whereas the NMDA-R antibody demonstrates robust neuronal cell surface immunolabeling (F), indicating the presence of an extracellular epitope (nuclei of neurons counterstained in blue with 4′,6-diamidino-2-phenylindole) [61]; reprinted with permission.

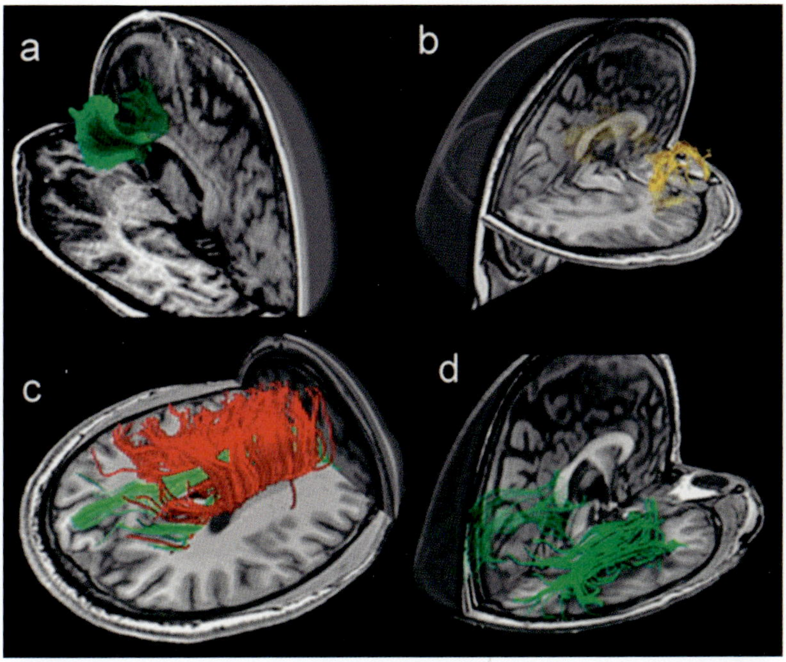

Fig. 8.7. Fiber tractography of commonly damaged tracts in mild traumatic brain injury, including: (a) anterior corona radiata and genu of corpus callosum, (b) uncinate fasciculus, (c) cingulum bundle in green and body of corpus callosum in red, and (d) inferior longitudinal fasciculus [84]; reprinted with permission.

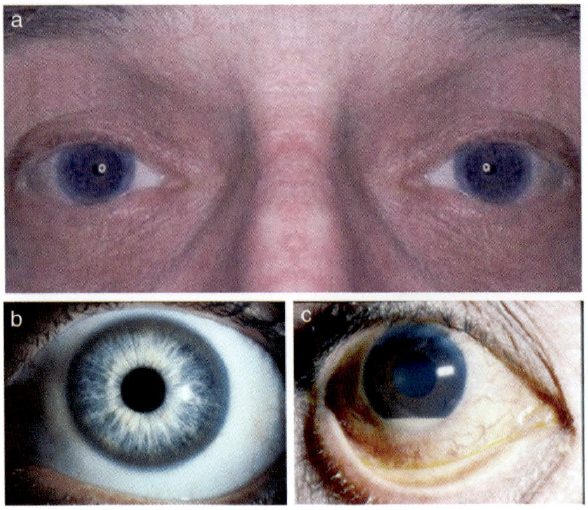

Fig. 8.8. (a) Argyll Robertson pupils (http://www.mrcophth.com/pupils/argyllrobertson.html); (b) Kayser–Fleischer ring (http://dmnemonics.blogspot.com/2011/12/wilsons-diseases.html); (c) Hypopyon and uveitis (http://medicalpicturesinfo.com/hypopyon/).

[49] Freye E, Levy J. Acute abstinence syndrome following abrupt cessation of long-term use of tramadol (Ultram): a case study. *Eur J Pain* 2000; **4**: 307–11.

[50] Robbins L. Tramadol for tension-type headache. *Headache* 2004; **44**: 192–3.

[51] Adams EH, Breiner S, Cicero TJ, *et al.* A comparison of the abuse liability of tramadol, NSAIDs, and hydrocodone in patients with chronic pain. *J Pain Symptom Managem.* 2006; **31**: 465–76.

[52] Inciardi JA, Cicero TJ, Munoz A, *et al.* The diversion of ultram, ultracet, and generic tramadol HCL. *J Addict Dis* 2006; **25**: 53–8.

[53] Cicero TJ, Inciardi JA, Adams EH, *et al.* Rates of abuse of tramadol remain unchanged with the introduction of new branded and generic products: results of an abuse monitoring system, 1994–2004. *Pharmacoepidemiol Drug Saf.* 2005; **14**: 851–9.

[54] Skipper GE, Fletcher C, Rocha-Judd R, Brase D. Tramadol abuse and dependence among physicians. *JAMA* 2004; **292**: 1818–19.

[55] Adams EH, Dart RC, Knisely JS, Schnoll SH. Tramadol abuse and dependence among physicians. *JAMA* 2005; **293**: 1977–8.

[56] Cicero TJ, Adams EH, Geller A, *et al.* A postmarketing surveillance program to monitor Ultram (trazodone hydrochloride) abuse in the United States. *Drug Alcohol Depend* 1999; **57**: 7–22.

[57] Tjaderborn M, Jonsson AK, Ahlner J, Hagg S. Tramadol dependence: a survey of spontaneously reported cases in Sweden. *Pharmacoepidemiol Drug Saf.* 2009; **18**: 1192–8.

[58] Loder E. Post-marketing experience with an opioid nasal spray for migraine: lessons for the future. *Cephalalgia* 2006; **26**: 89–97.

[59] Parente ST, Kim SS, Finch MD, *et al.* Identifying controlled substance patterns of utilization requiring evaluation using administrative claims data. *Am J Managm Care* 2004; **10**: 783–90.

[60] Silberstein SD, McCrory DC. Butalbital in the treatment of headache: history, pharmacology, and efficacy. *Headache* 2001; **41**: 953–67.

[61] Bigal ME, Borucho S, Serran D, Lipton RB. The acute treatment of episodic and chronic migraine in the USA. *Cephalalgia* 2009; **29**: 891–7.

[62] Raja M, Altavista MC, Azzoni A, Albanese A. Severe barbiturate withdrawal syndrome in migrainous patients. *Headache* 1996; **36**: 119–21.

[63] Sarrecchia C, Sordillo P, Conte G, Rocchi G. Barbiturate withdrawal syndrome: a case associated with the abuse of a headache medication [article in Italian]. *Ann Ital Med Int.* 1998; **13**: 237–9.

[64] Bigal ME, Lipton RB. Excessive acute migraine medication use and migraine progression. *Neurology* 2008; **71**: 1821–8.

[65] Buckley NA, McManus PR. Changes in fatalities due to overdose of anxiolytic and sedative drugs in the UK (1983–1999). *Drug Saf.* 2004; **27**: 135–41.

[66] Coupey SM. Barbiturates. *Pediatr Rev* 1997; **18**: 260–4.

[67] Sellers EM, Hoornweg, Busto UE, Romach MK. Risk of drug dependence and abuse posed by barbiturate-containing analgesics. *Can J Clin Pharmacol* 1996; **6**: 18–25.

[68] Friedman AP, DiSerio FJ. Symptomatic treatment of chronically recurring tension headache: a placebo-controlled, multicenter investigation of Fioricet and acetaminophen with codeine. *Clin Ther* 1987; **10**: 69–81.

[69] Kouyanou K, Pither CE, Wessely S. Medication misuse, abuse and dependence in chronic pain patients. *J Psychosom Res* 1997; **43**: 497–504.

[70] Huffman JC, Stern TA. The use of benzodiazepines in the treatment of chest pain: a review of the literature. *J Emerg Med* 2003; **25**: 427–37.

[71] Lader M. Benzodiazepines revisited – will we ever learn? *Addiction.* 2001; **106**: 2086–109.

[72] Napchan U, Buse DC, Loder EW, *et al.* The use of marijuana or synthetic cannabinoids for the treatment of headache. *Headache: J Head Face Pain* **51**: 502–5.

[73] Martín-Sánchez E, Furukawa TA, Taylor J, *et al.* (2009). Systematic review and meta-analysis of cannabis treatment for chronic pain. *Pain Med* **10**: 1353–68.

[74] Feinstein AR, Heinemann LA, Dalessio D, *et al.* Do caffeine-containing analgesics promote dependence? A review and evaluation. *Clin Pharmacol Ther* 2000; **68**: 457–67.

[75] Mittenberg W, Patton C, Canyock EM, Condit DC. Base rates of malingering and symptoms exaggeration. *J Clin Exp Neuropsychol* 2002; **24**: 1094–102.

[76] Fishbain DA, Cutler R, Rosomoff HL, Rosomoff RS. Chronic pain disability exaggeration/malingering and submaximal effort research. *Clin J Pain* 1999; **15**: 244–74.

[77] Aronoff GM, Mandel S, Genovese E, *et al.* Evaluating malingering in contested injury or illness. *Pain Pract* 2007; **7**: 178–204.

[78] Nicholson K, Martelli MF. The problem of pain. *J Head Trauma Rehabil* 2004; **19**: 2–9.

[79] Evans RW. Persistent post-traumatic headache, postconcussion syndrome, and whiplash injuries: the evidence for a non traumatic basis with an historical review. *Headache* 2010; **50**: 716–24.

[80] Grover CA, Close RJ, Wiele ED, Villarreal K, Goldman LM. Quantifying drug-seeking behavior: a case control study. *J Emerg Med* 2012; **42**: 15–21.

[81] Hopwood CJ, Orlando MJ, Clark TS. The detection of malingered pain-related disability with the Personality Assessment Inventory. *Rehabil Psychol* 2010; **55**: 307–10.

[82] Rogers R, Gillard ND, Wooley CN, Ross CA. The detection of feigned disabilities: the effectiviness of the personality assessment inventory in a traumatized inpatient sample. *Assessment* 2012; **19**: 77–88.

[83] Sellbom M, Toomey JA, Wygant DB, Kucharski LT, Duncan S. Utility of the MMPI-2-RF (Restructured Form) validity scales in detecting malingering in a criminal forensic setting: a known-groups design. *Psychol Assessm* 2010; **22**: 22–31.

[84] McCarberg BH. A critical assessment of opioid treatment adherence using urine drug testing in chronic pain management. *Postgrand Med* 2011; **123**: 124–31.

[85] Hawkins SC, Smees F, Hamel J. Emergency management of chronic pain and drug-seeking behavior: an alternate perspective. *J Emerg Med* 2008; **34**: 125–9.

Chapter 8

The neuropsychiatry of psychosis and headache

Sander Markx

Introduction

Although there may not be an immediately obvious relationship between the occurrence of headache and psychosis, a clinical association between these two symptom clusters exists. Patients can suffer from a primary psychotic disorder with headache as a direct consequence of the psychiatric disorder, the medication prescribed to treat the disorder, or both. Conversely, patients who suffer from a primary neurological condition in which headache is part of the core symptomatology can also develop psychotic symptoms, such as delusions and perceptual disturbances. The psychotic and headache symptoms can also both be the result of a separate etiology, e.g., a neurological condition, a systemic disorder, an infection, or perhaps as side effects of a medication used for an unrelated condition. Finally, headache and psychosis can also occur independently as comorbid conditions without any apparent relationship in pathophysiology. It is important for clinicians to differentiate these categories, since the treatment can vary greatly depending on the etiology.

The first use of the term "psychogenic headaches" in the psychiatric literature was made back in 1947 when it was used to refer to headache which was thought to be a symbolical expression of an unconscious conflict (e.g., feelings of hostility) in the context of a conversion disorder. [1,2] In 1962, the Ad Hoc Committee of the Classification of Headache proposed to divide psychogenic headaches up into two separate categories: "muscle contraction headaches" and "headache of delusional, conversion, or hypochondriacal states." [3] In the first version of the international classification of headaches, headache as a symptom in the context of a primary psychiatric disorder was not the subject of a separate code. [4] The temporal relation between the moment when the headache appeared or worsened and when the psychiatric disorders occurred was considered essential to establish whether a headache could be interpreted as being psychogenic. In the second version of the classification of headaches [5], specific diagnostic criteria were proposed for "headaches secondary to psychiatric disorders." These criteria include "headache, no typical characteristics known, not attributed to another cause; presence of a somatization disorder or presence of a delusional belief about the headache occurring in the context of delusional disorder, schizophrenia, major depressive episode or manic episode with psychotic features or other psychotic disorder. The headache must occur during the active phase of the psychiatric condition and resolve when the psychiatric condition remits."

In order to establish whether co-occurring psychosis and headache develop as a consequence of a primary psychiatric disorder, a primary neurological condition, or as shared symptomatology of a separate neuropsychiatric illness or condition, it is important to evaluate the temporal relationship between these two symptom clusters. If a patient has been suffering from a chronic psychotic illness, such as schizophrenia or schizoaffective disorder, and then subsequently develops a headache disorder, the link may be quite obvious. In some cases the onset of both the headache and psychosis can be insidious when they are the presenting symptoms of a separate neuropsychiatric etiology. This chapter will review the differential diagnosis of combined psychosis and headache, the required evaluation, and specific treatment considerations.

Case

Ms. A is a 45-year-old mother of three children, working as a social worker, with no previous psychiatric or neurological history, who presents in the emergency

The Neuropsychiatry of Headache, ed. Mark W. Green and Philip R. Muskin. Published by Cambridge University Press.

room with a 3-day history of a diffuse throbbing headache. Ms. A has no history of headaches and does not take any medications. She is evaluated and the physical examination, the laboratory studies and an MRI are all normal. Ms. A is sent home with an outpatient follow-up appointment at the neurology clinic. In the next several weeks, Ms. A develops hyperreligiosity (i.e., she has become increasingly preoccupied with reading Biblical texts and prays multiple times a day – a clear difference from before, since she previously identified herself as an atheist). Ms. A also states that she hears her name being called by a voice she doesn't recognize and has been noted by her husband to be increasingly paranoid. Subsequently, Ms. A experiences a generalized tonic–clonic (GTC) seizure at home and is admitted to the hospital. Upon admission, Ms. A undergoes another MRI, which again is normal, and additional laboratory studies are performed, including a lumbar puncture with CSF analysis for neuronal auto-antibodies. While on the neurological floor, Ms. A develops visual hallucinations (i.e., seeing babies crawl on the wall of her room and the room being on fire). She has two additional GTC seizures after which her post-ictal confusion progresses into a prolonged delirium with autonomic instability. Ms. A is transferred to the Intensive Care Unit. The results from the CSF analysis reveal autoantibodies against the NMDA-R receptor and she is started on intravenous IgG for the treatment of limbic encephalitis. Over the next 10 days, her vital signs stabilize, her delirium resolves, and her psychotic symptoms disappear. A whole-body PET scan is done, finding no evidence of a tumor. Ms. A has no memory of the period during which she developed symptoms and appears close to her premorbid level of cognitive functioning. After receiving a second 5-day course of intravenous IgG, Ms. A is discharged with outpatient neurological follow-up. She returns back to work with no recurrence of the neurological or psychiatric symptoms (Table 8.1).

Table 8.1. Differential diagnosis for patients with both psychosis and headache

1. **Primary psychiatric disorder with new-onset headache**
   - (a) Psychotic disorder (e.g., schizophrenia or schizoaffective disorder) or mood disorder with psychotic features with co-occurring headache disorder (e.g., tension headache, cluster headache, trigeminal neuralgia, or migraine)
   - (b) Psychotic or mood disorder with tactile hallucinations (e.g., headache as a perceptual disturbance) or delusional interpretation of headache.
   - (c) Delusional disorder – somatic delusion (e.g., headaches with psychotic interpretation of having a certain medical illness, such as a brain tumor)
   - (d) Somatoform disorder (i.e., somatization disorder or pain disorder) in patients who also suffer from a psychotic disorder
2. **Primary neurological disorder with new-onset psychosis**
   - (a) Migraine
   - (b) Seizure disorder – specifically temporal lobe epilepsy
   - (c) Cerebrovascular accidents (CVAs, including transverse sinus thrombosis)
   - (d) Brain tumor
3. **Psychosis and headache as a result from a separate etiology**
   - (a) Systemic disease
   - (b) Infectious etiology
   - (c) Endocrine disorders
   - (d) Metabolic disorders
   - (e) Traumatic brain injury
   - (f) Limbic encephalitis (e.g., neuronal autoimmunity against NMDA- or AMPA-receptors)
   - (g) Hydrocephalus (both obstructive and normal-pressure hydrocephalus)
   - (h) Idiopathic intracranial hypertension (pseudotumor cerebri)
   - (i) Demyelination disorders
   - (j) Neurodegenerative disorders
   - (k) Substance-induced psychosis and headache – both with onset during intoxication and/or withdrawal
   - (l) Medication-induced psychosis and headache
   - (m) Exposure to CNS toxins (e.g., heavy metals, organophosphates, inhalants)
   - (n) Mitochondrial disease (e.g., MELAS)

Primary psychiatric disorder with episodes of psychosis and headache

Patients who suffer from a primary psychotic disorder, such as schizophrenia or schizoaffective disorder, can experience headache like any other patient. The headache can also represent part of the psychosis when it is the result of a perceptual disturbance (e.g., a tactile hallucination) or when there is a delusional interpretation of the headache (e.g., the patient thinks that his/her headache is caused by parasites in the brain or is the consequence of a chip which was implanted into the patient's brain). These symptoms can also be seen in patients who suffer from a mood disorder with psychotic features or in bipolar disorder with psychotic features. If the patient suffers from a delusional disorder, the delusions are typically not bizarre in nature (i.e., they could in theory be real – for example, the patient believes that the headache indicates that he/she is being poisoned with gas by someone) and the level of functioning is not severely impaired. These patients can suffer from somatic delusions (e.g., head is increased in size) and can have tactile hallucinations related to the theme of the delusions (e.g., the headache is experienced as evidence that the head is increasing in size). In somatization disorder, patients typically experience multiple physical complaints for which there is no good medical explanation or which is excessive if a medical condition is present. These physical complaints consist of pain symptoms in at least four locations, two gastrointestinal symptoms, one sexual symptom, and one pseudo-neurological symptom. These patients often seek medical attention for their physical complaints. Patients with psychotic disorders can also suffer from comorbid somatization disorder. For more information regarding the symptoms of these primary psychiatric disorders, please refer to the *Diagnostic and Statistic Manual of Mental Disorders*, 4th edn, Text Revision (DSM-IV-TR). [6]

Primary neurological disorder with episodes of psychosis and headache

Migraine madness

There have been several reports of patients with a longstanding history of migraines with concurrent mental illness. For example, "dysphrenic migraine" is a term sometimes used to refer to "mental changes or psychic alterations" associated with migraine. [7],[8] This includes a wide range of neuropsychiatric manifestations, including visual, auditory, and olfactory hallucinations, ideas of references, religious or persecutory delusions, confusional states and stupor. [7–11] Cotard syndrome, where patients suffer from a delusion in which they believe that they are dead or do not exist, [12,13] has also been described in patients with migraine disorder. [14,15] Children with a history of migraines have also been found sometimes to experience auditory and visual hallucinations. What differentiates these episodes from a chronic primary psychotic disorder, such as schizophrenia or schizoaffective disorder, is that typically there is a full recovery between episodes with intact reality testing and insight. [8] There have also been reports of families who suffer from familial hemiplegic migraines (FHM) who present with paranoid delusion and hallucination. [16] Some of these patients have been found to carry missense mutations of the CACNL1A4 gene, which encodes a brain-specific P/Q-type calcium channel α1 subunit. [17] Because of this, acetazolamide has been used in patients with FHM to target the frequency and severity of the hemiplegic migraine attacks. [16] Interestingly, the treatment regimen for migraine headaches, in addition to acute treatments like sumatriptans, also includes mood stabilizers such as lithium and divalproic acid, which are considered to be first-line treatments for bipolar disorder, as well as dopamine antagonists, [18] which are typically used to treat psychotic disorders, such as schizophrenia.

Seizure disorder

In patients with a seizure disorder, headache can be a pre-ictal, ictal, or post-ictal phenomenon. Pre-ictal and ictal headache are typically brief, whereas post-ictal headache can last longer, often goes undiagnosed, and can have a more negative effect on quality of life. [19] Headache can also be the sole or the predominant clinical manifestation of a seizure, although this is considered to be relatively rare. [20,21] Psychotic symptoms can also be seen during the ictal, post-ictal, and inter-ictal phases – especially in temporal lobe epilepsy, [22] [23] which can sometime be hard to differentiate from a primary psychotic disorder with a comorbid seizure disorder.

During the post-ictal state, headache, and specifically migraines, commonly occur, as can Todd's paralysis, impaired cognition (problem with attention, concentration and memory), and confusion. Post-ictal psychosis is a rare but potentially serious complication, often characterized by perceptual disturbances, delusions, affective symptoms, and aggression. [24] After the occurrence of the seizure, the patient typically experiences confusion and lethargy during the post-ictal state, and then gradually recovers to a normal state. This is referred to as the lucid phase. In patients with post-ictal psychosis, the lucid phase usually lasts between 2 hours and a week before the onset of psychosis. In approximately 12%–50% of patients with a seizure disorder, the lucid phase is followed by a period of psychosis that can last from 12 hours up to more than 3 months (mean is ~9–10 days). [24]

Some psychotic symptoms tend to occur more frequently in patients with epilepsy (e.g., visual hallucinations and hyperreligiosty). [24] There tend to be less negative symptoms and arguably less overall functional decline. [25] Nevertheless, it can be challenging to differentiate epilepsy with psychosis from a primary psychotic disorder, such as schizophrenia. One has to evaluate the pattern of the psychotic episodes and how they relate to the occurrence of seizures (i.e., ictal, post-ictal, or inter-ictal). Furthermore, psychotic symptoms thought to be secondary to the seizure disorder typically respond to standard antipsychotic medication but in contrast to schizophrenia, both ictal, post-ictal and inter-ictal psychosis can potentially be prevented with adequate seizure control. [23,24,26,27]

Cerebrovascular disease

Post-stroke depression and cognitive deficits are among the most common neuropsychiatric disorders occurring after stroke, and are still frequently under-diagnosed, especially by non-psychiatric physicians. [28,29] Post-stroke psychosis is a rare complication of stroke; however, psychotic symptoms may be seen more commonly in cerebrovascular accidents which involve the right fronto-parietal region. [28,30] Post-stroke psychotic symptoms may indicate dementia with emerging psychosis. [30] The treatment of these psychotic symptoms is the same as the treatment of primary psychotic disorders. Headache can also accompany CVA, especially subarachnoid hemorrhage, where patients can experience an acute and intense headache, which develops over the course of seconds to minutes ("worst ever headache, like being kicked in the head"). Vomiting and seizures may also be present, along with a wide range of other neurological symptoms.

A rare, but important diagnosis to recognize is transverse sinus thrombosis, which can present with headache (a frequent symptoms in up to ~68% of patients) and psychosis (a more rare symptom). [31–33] This form of cerebrovascular disease can also manifest itself with only psychotic symptoms during the post-partum period, and is easily missed. [32,34] Assessing the mental status of women during the post-partum period is therefore important. [32] Magnetic resonance imaging (MRI) / magnetic resonance venography (MRV) imaging typically demonstrates a filling defect in the transverse sinus region (see Fig. 8.1).

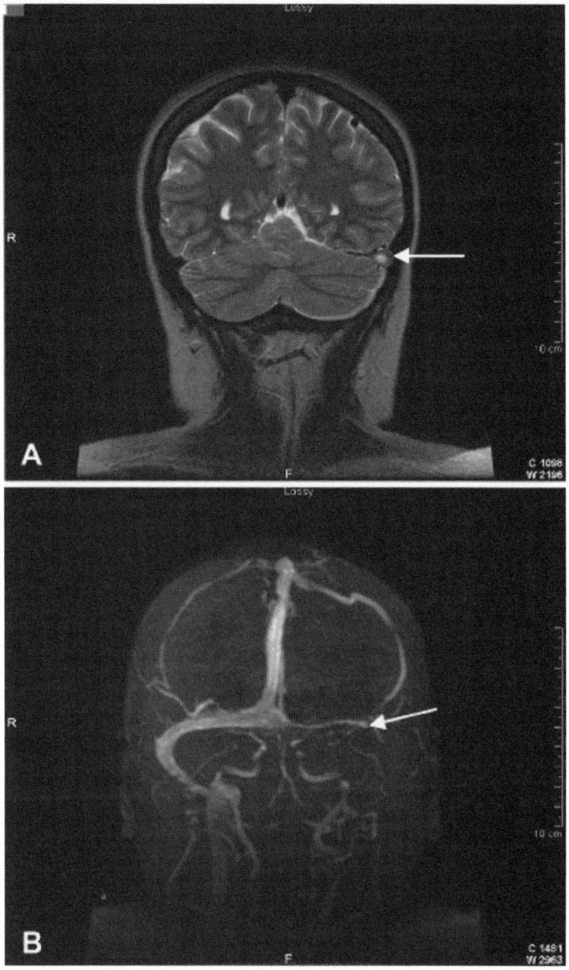

Fig. 8.1. MRI/MRV images demonstrating left transverse sinus thrombosis. (A) Coronal T2-weighted image: arrow demonstrates absence of filling void in left TS, (B) 2-D MRV image shows decreased left sagittal and TS signal [32]; adapted with permission.

Brain tumors

Any space-occupying lesion, independent of location and whether benign (e.g., meningioma, tuberous sclerosis, neurofibromatosis) or malignant (e.g., glioblastoma multiforme), potentially can cause both headache and psychosis. This is also part of the reason why all patients with a first-break psychosis should undergo neuroimaging to rule out any identifiable brain pathology, including tumors. Neoplasms are a much more common cause of psychosis in patients in later stages of life, and should always be an important differential diagnostic consideration when working up an older patient with new-onset psychosis. Headache is a common presenting symptom in patients with any kind of tumor leading to intracranial hypertension, which can also cause vomiting and altered state of consciousness. Accompanying focal neurological symptoms can sometimes point to certain brain regions where the tumor is exerting pressure on the brain parenchyma.

New-onset psychosis and headache

Systemic disease

There are several systemic diseases, which can involve the brain and which can present with both psychosis and headache. **Systemic lupus erythematosus** is a systemic autoimmune disease that can affect virtually any part of the body, and often involves the brain. Common initial and chronic complaints include fever, malaise, joint pains, myalgia, and fatigue and ~30%–50% of all patients develop the classic malar rash ("butterfly rash"). In children suffering from lupus, neuropsychiatric manifestations are found in approximately 25%, and in these patients, headache and psychosis are two of the most prevalent symptoms. [35,36] In adults, approximately 80% of all patients present with neuropsychiatric symptoms, and headache is common (~20%–40%) while a minority of the patients presents with psychosis (~2.5%–3.5%). [37,38]

Behçet's disease is a rare immune-mediated, relapsing systemic vasculitis, which almost always involves mucous membrane ulceration (i.e., mouth ulcers) and which is the first presenting symptom in ~70% of the cases. [39] Occular pathology is another common manifestation of this disease (e.g., posterior or anterior uveitis with or without hypopyon – see Fig. 8.8c; retinal vasculitis). This inflammatory eye disease, when untreated, can lead to permanent vision loss within 5 years in approximately 50% of all cases. [40,41] HLA type B51 has been found in ~60%–70% of Turkish and Japanese patients with Behçet's disease, while present in only 10%–20% of European patients. [42] Conversely, patients with HLA type B51 have an estimated six times increased risk to develop the Behçet's disease, and the disease is typically more severe in these patients. [42] The estimates of central nervous system involvement ("neuro-Behçet's disease") vary widely from as low as ~1%–3% to as high as 59%. [43] Patients with neuro-Behçet's commonly suffer from headache, and this can be an early indicator of neurological involvement, [44] although it does not necessarily imply that the brain is affected. [43] In rare cases, neuro-Behçet's disease can present with idiopathic intracranial hypertension, which can be the consequence of a cranial venous thrombosis. [45,46] Patients with neuro-Behçet's disease can also become psychotic, either as a consequence of the associated idiopathic intracranial hypertension, [45] or because of presumed parenchymal involvement. [47] Treatment can involve corticosteroids, tumor necrosis factor antagonists, infliximab, azathioprine, methotrexate, or ciclosporin A (the latter is commonly used for patients with severe ocular involvement). [43]

Sarcoidosis is a rare systemic disorder characterized by the presence of non-caseating granulomas, and involves the central nervous system ("**neurosarcoidosis**") in ~5%–15 % of the cases. [48,49] The prevalence of subclinical neurosarcoidosis has been suggested to be much higher. [49] Virtually any part of the central nervous system can be affected, but cranial nerves, the hypothalamus and pituitary gland are most commonly involved. [49] Granulomas can develop in the meninges, parenchyma of the brain, hypothalamus, brainstem, subependymal layer of the ventricular system, choroid plexuses, peripheral nerves, and blood vessels supplying the nervous structures. [49] Technically, a biopsy is needed to make a definitive diagnosis of neurosarcoidosis. [49] Headache is the most common manifestation of neurosarcoidosis after cranial neuropathy, affecting an estimated 30% of patients. [50] Psychosis is less common, but may indeed be present. These symptoms may be responsive to corticosteroids, the first drug of choice. In addition to this, cytotoxic drugs such as methotrexate azathioprine, ciclosporin, and cyclophosphamide – have all been tried. Drugs that affect the immune system, or block cytokine effect, have also been used, including the antimalarial drugs chloroquine and hydroxychloroquine, anti-tumor necrosis factor-α, and thalidomide and infliximab. In rare cases, radiotherapy or neurosurgical treatment may be indicated (Fig. 8.2). [49]

Giant cell arteritis (**GCA**) or **temporal arteritis** is a systemic immune-mediated vasculitis affecting medium- and large-size arteries. [51] It is typically associated with an acute phase response and characteristic findings include headache (especially over temples and suboccipital regions), tender scalp or temporal arteries (on palpation), jaw claudication, and constitutional symptoms (fever, weight loss, night sweats, and malaise) but may also lead to severe complications, such as visual loss, stroke, and aortic aneurysm due to vascular insufficiency and/or tissue ischemia. [51] There have been some reports of patients with GCA who present with psychosis (i.e., perceptual disturbances and delusions). [52] In rare cases, patients with GCA can also develop the Charles Bonnet Syndrome, where visual loss and possibly brain ischemia have been thought to lead to "cortical release and hyperexcitability" which, in turn, can lead to visual hallucinations – see Box 8.1. [53,54] These patients typically do not present with delusions, auditory hallucinations, or disorganized speech/behavior, and usually have intact reality testing. The diagnosis of GCA is established with temporal artery biopsy but may also be aided by blood tests (e.g., ESR, CRP, platelets) as well as several imaging modalities (e.g., ultrasound of the arteries, MRI, PET). Treatment of GCA includes high-dose corticosteroids,

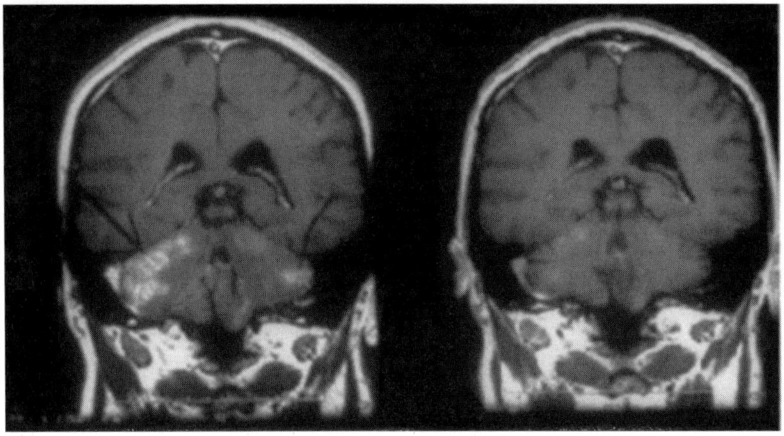

Fig. 8.2. Left: enhanced lesion in a middle aged, white man with multisystem sarcoidosis. A biopsy of the cerebellum showed noncaseating granuloma. Right: resolution of the lesion after combined prednisone and hydroxychloroquine therapy [49]; adapted with permission.

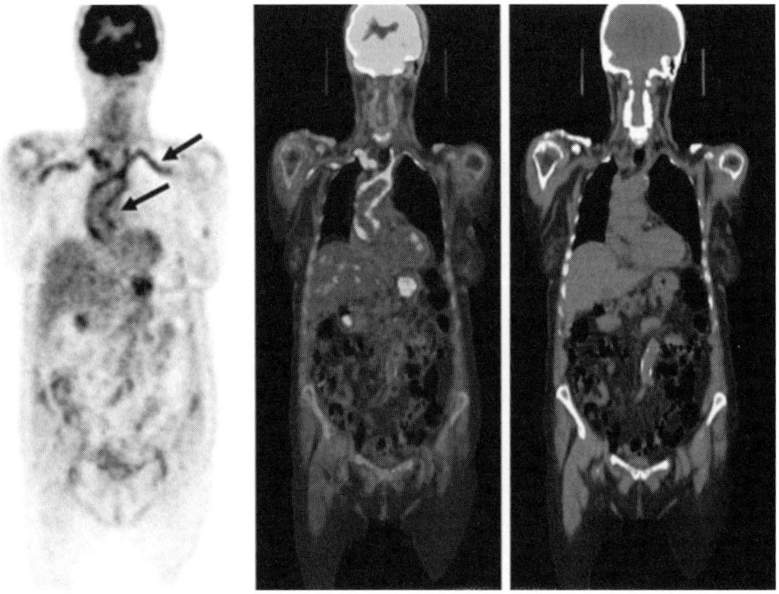

Fig. 8.3. Coronal 18F-FDG PET (left), PET/CT (center), and CT (right) slices in a 78-year-old woman who presented with a 6-week history of fever, night sweats, and weight loss, which demonstrate intense linear 18F-FDG uptake along walls of thoracic aorta and brachiocephalic and subclavian arteries (arrows) consistent with Giant Cell Arteritis [111]; adapted with permission. See color plate section.

cytotoxic drugs, antitumor necrosis factor monoclonal antibody, and antiplatelet aggregation therapy with the goal to prevent visual loss and ischemic tissue damage. [51] The symptoms of GCA, including the Charles Bonnet Syndrome, typically respond rapidly to high-dose glucocorticoid therapy, but patients may need prolonged therapy (Fig. 8.3). [53–55]

Endocrine disorders: thyroid disease

Both hypothyroidsim and hyperthyroidism have been associated with a wide-range of neuropsychiatric symptoms, including headache and psychosis. [57,58] Treatment of the hypo- and hyperthyroidism often lead to significant improvement of the associated neuropsychiatric symptoms, and psychotropic medication may not be necessary in many cases. [57,58] Thyroid storm is a rare but life-threatening syndrome characterized by extremely severe symptoms of hyperthyroidism, including severe headache, psychosis, and agitation. It is typically treated with a combination of an antithyroid drug and a β-adrenoceptor antagonist. [58] In patients where the psychosis or agitation does not respond sufficiently to this treatment regimen, the addition of an atypical antipsychotic may be necessary. There have been reports of reserpine being used with good efficacy

Box 8.1. Charles Bonnet syndrome

Charles Bonnet syndrome (CBS) is when complex visual hallucinations arise in visually impaired, but otherwise neuropsychiatrically normal patients. A lesion at any level of the visual system can lead to CBS, such as in age-related macular degeneration, cataracts, or poor bilateral visual acuity. Patients often have a loss of central visual acuity contributing to their symptoms, although this is not always the case (e.g., peripheral vision loss due to glaucoma can also cause CBS). [56] CBS can also arise in patients with a history of stroke or GCA, where headache can also be a prominent symptom.

There are two theories regarding the pathogenesis of Charles Bonnet syndrome: The "release theory" suggests that a lesion of the visual pathway results in abnormal signals being sent to the visual cortex where "phantom images" arise, akin to phantom limb pain. The "deprivation theory" postulates that reduction in sensory input leads to the production of spontaneous images from the visual association cortex, resulting in visual hallucinations. The latter theory is supported by CBS in patients with preexisting hearing loss and social isolation.

The management of CBS involves reassurance, increased social interaction, increased home lighting, efforts to improve visual acuity, and pharmacological treatment (e.g., atypical antipsychotic). [56]

in patients with thyroid storm who did not respond to propranolol or in whom this medication was contraindicated. [59]

Autoimmune disease: limbic encephalitis

Neuronal autoantibodies described in CNS disorders can target intracellular and extracellular antigens. Examples of intracellular onconeural antibodies include Hu (ANNA1), Yo (PCA1), Ri (ANNA2), CV2 (CRMP5), amphiphysin, and Ma2 antibodies and are useful to establish the diagnosis of paraneoplastic syndrome. These neuronal autoimmune disorders are typically hard to treat. [60] In contrast to this, **limbic encephalitis (LE)** involves neuronal auto-antibodies targeting cell-surface and synaptic antigens involved in synaptic transmission and plasticity, such as the NMDA-, AMPA-, and $GABA_B$- and glycine receptors as well as LGI1 and CASPR2. [61] Patients typically present with memory deficits, psychiatric symptoms (e.g., psychosis), and seizures. Sometimes, patients can experience headache preceding the onset of the more severe neuropsychiatric symptoms. For some of these forms of limbic encephalitis, there is evidence that the antibodies ultimately affect the structure and function of the antigen, which suggests a direct pathogenic effect in the associated clinical syndrome. [61] This group of disorders is an important differential diagnostic consideration as they affect both children and adults, can be severe and protracted, occur with and without tumor association, and can respond dramatically to treatment but may sometimes relapse. [61]

At the present time, there is no standard of care for patients with limbic encephalitis. However, most experts agree that the detection of autoantibodies should prompt the use of immunosuppressant therapy while screening for a tumor is initiated. [61] First-line immunotherapies which have been used successfully in the treatment of LE include corticosteroids, intravenous immunogolulin G (IV-IgG), plasma exchange, or any combination of these treatments. Between ~60% and 80% of patients with AMPA, GABA or LGI1 antibodies typically respond to these treatments. [61] For patients with CASPR2 autoantibodies, the response rate has been suggested to be lower and these patients may need more aggressive immunotherapy. [61] For patients with NMDA-R limbic encephalitis, the response rate varies, depending in part on the presence of a teratoma. [61] Classic paraneoplastic syndromes usually do not respond to immunotherapy unless the tumor is successfully treated, and even then the responses are typically limited. Limbic encephalitis cases with antibodies directed against the cell surface antigens may respond to immunotherapy before a tumor is identified and some cases may improve spontaneously. [61] Even if no tumor is found initially, patients should be followed up and screened for a tumor for at least 2 years, even if their neuropsychiatric symptoms have remitted. (Fig. 8.4) [61]

Mitochondrial disease

Mitochondrial encephalomyopathy, lactic acidosis, and stroke-like episodes (MELAS) is a member of a family of metabolic disorders, which also include MERRF, and Leber's hereditary optic neuropathy. All these disorders are caused by genetic defects in the mitochondrial genome with only maternal inheritance, although the disease can manifest in both sexes. MELAS is a debilitating multisystem syndrome characterized by progressive encephalopathy, lactic acidosis, and stroke-like episodes, leading to significantly increased morbidity and

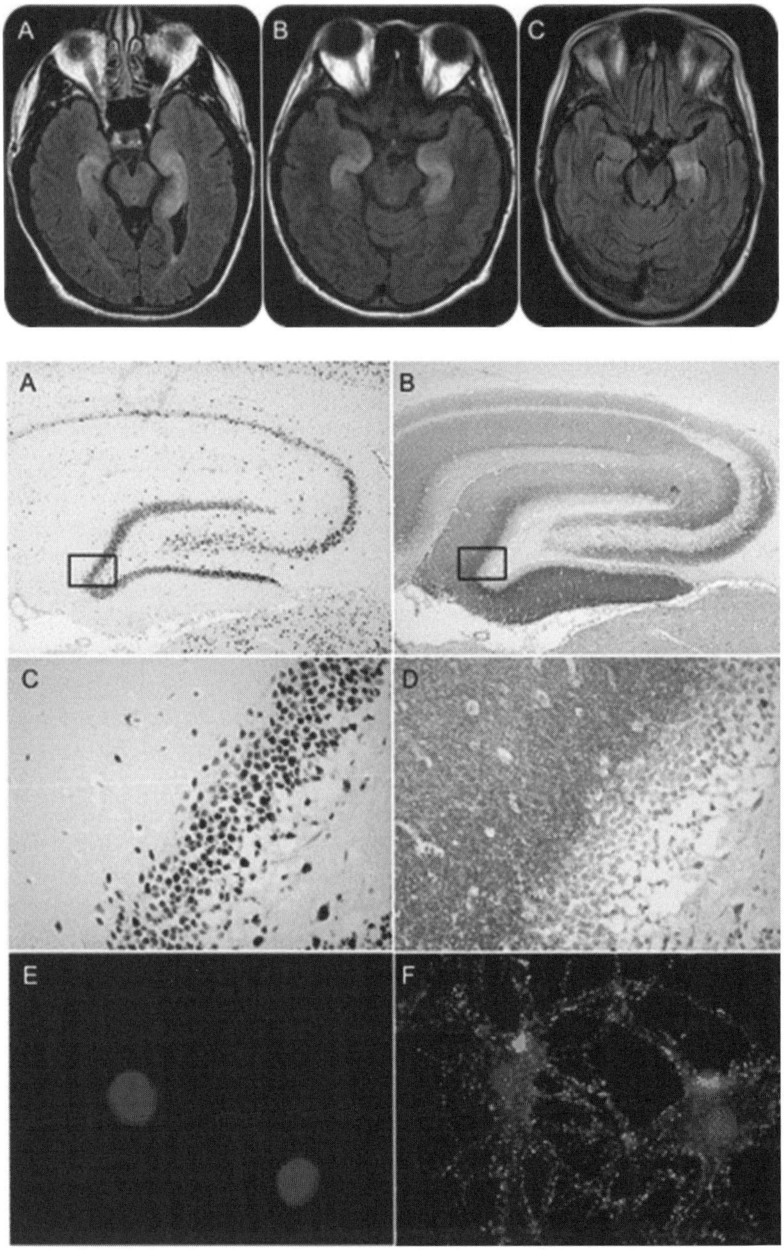

Fig. 8.4. Part 1. MRI scans of patients with antibodies directed against LGI1 (A), AMPA-R (B), and GABAB-R (C). Part 2. Consecutive sections of rat hippocampus immunostained with CSF of a patient with antibodies directed against Hu, an intracellular antigen (A) and CSF of a patient with antibodies directed against a cell surface synaptic antigen (NMDA receptor [NMDA-R] (B). (C, D) The framed areas are shown at higher magnification. Compared with the intracellular antigen, the cell surface synaptic antigen (NMDA-R) is demonstrated as robust neuropil staining, sparing neuronal cell bodies (the nuclei of neurons are mildly counterstained with hematoxylin). Using live, nonpermeabilized cultures of dissociated rat hippocampal neurons, the Hu antibody does not show reactivity due to lack of penetration into the neuron (E), whereas the NMDA-R antibody demonstrates robust neuronal cell surface immunolabeling (F), indicating the presence of an extracellular epitope (nuclei of neurons counterstained in blue with 4′,6-diamidino-2-phenylindole) [61]; reprinted with permission. See color plate section.

mortality. [62] MELAS is often associated with the mitochondrial DNA (mtDNA) A-to-G transition at nucleotide 3243 (m.3243A>G) mutation. There is considerable phenotypic variability in patients with MELAS, which has been attributed, at least in part, to heteroplasmy where there are varying proportions of mutant and wild-type mtDNA molecules in different tissues. It has been suggested that the m.3243A>G mutation is likely underrecognized in clinical populations who present with neuropsychiatric symptoms. [63]

Although the pathogenesis of the stroke-like episodes in MELAS is still unclear, oxidative phosphorylation is genetically impaired and can lead to neuronal hyperexcitability, increase in capillary permeability, and other functional changes. [64] Headache can be a presenting symptom in MELAS, sometimes followed by psychosis and a decline in neuropsychological findings, MRI abnormalities, and neurological symptoms (e.g., aphasia, hemianopsia, and eventually epileptic seizures in close association with the progression of the stoke-like lesion). [65] MRI including diffusion weighted imaging (DWI) can demonstrate a unique pattern of gradual spread of an acute brain lesion, which typically starts in one region (e.g., temporal lobe) and then subsequently evolves and spreads to surrounding cortical areas beyond the border of major vascular territories during the first few weeks following the onset of the initial symptoms (see Fig. 8.5). During the stroke-like episodes, the MRI can demonstrate a gyriform configuration of T1-weighted hyperintense signal compatible with cortical laminar necrosis in the subacute stage of the stroke-like lesions (see Fig 8.6 E). Single-photon emission computed tomography (SPECT) can demonstrate focal hyperperfusion in the affected brain regions in patients with the stroke-like episodes (see Fig. 8.6 B and D). [65] Magnetic resonance spectroscopy imaging (MRSI) typically demonstrates progressively increased ventricular lactate levels, which is thought to be the brain spectroscopic signature of MELAS. [66] Both these clinical and neuroimaging findings tend to correlate with patients with MELAS becoming progressively and often rapidly disabled by cognitive and neurologic impairment over time.

Neurodegenerative disorders: Wilson's disease

Wilson's disease or **progressive hepatolenticular degeneration** is an autosomal recessive genetic disorder of copper metabolism in which copper cannot be excreted by the liver, and subsequently accumulates in the liver, central nervous system and other tissues. It affects 1/30 000 to 1/100 000 patients. [67] A characteristic feature of Wilson's disease is the decrease in levels of serum ceruloplasmin, the main copper-transporting protein in blood. [67,68] Untreated, Wilson's disease invariably leads to severe disability or death. The diagnosis can easily be missed, but if treatment is started early, many manifestations of the disease can be prevented or reversed. [67] Wilson's disease is caused by mutations of the ATP7B gene, which encodes a transmembrane protein ATPase (ATP7B), ATP7B is highly expressed in the liver, kidney, and placenta, and functions as a copper-dependent P-type ATPase. [67] Most patients with Wilson's disease are compound heterozygotes, having two different mutations of the ATP7B gene. [67]

Wilson's disease can present with liver disease (e.g., persistently elevated serum aminotransferases, chronic hepatitis, cirrhosis, or fulminant hepatic failure), ocular findings (e.g., Kayser–Fleischer rings – see Fig. 8.8b), neurological symptoms (e.g., migraine headaches, tremor, choreiform movements, parkinsonism, pseudobulbar palsy, seizures, dysarthria), and psychiatric manifestations (psychosis, depression, and personality changes). Neuropsychiatric symptoms are the presenting features in approximately 40%–50% of patients. [67,69] MRI in patients with Wilson's disease can show widespread lesions in the putamen, globus pallidus, caudate, thalamus, midbrain, pons, and cerebellum as well as cortical atrophy and white matter changes. [67] These lesions typically demonstrate high-signal intensity on T2-weighed images and low-intensity on T1-weighed images. [67,70] MRI findings can be present in many patients, including patients without any obvious neuropsychiatric symptoms, but the lesions tend to be more severe and widespread in patients with the neurological features typically associated with Wilson's disease. [71]

The treatment of Wilson's disease is centered around the use of copper chelators (e.g., penicillamine or trientine) to promote copper excretion from the body, or zinc to reduce copper absorption, or both. In cases of acute fulminant hepatic failure or when medication therapy is ineffective, liver transplantation is indicated. The recent discovery of the Wilson's disease gene has led to research focusing on a new molecular diagnostic approach, and could perhaps form the basis of future gene therapy. [67]

Substance-induced psychosis and headache

Several substances and medications can cause psychosis and headache in both adult and pediatric patient populations. For medications, these symptoms can be known side effects which can occur within the therapeutic dose range, whereas they can also be caused by unintentional (e.g., a medication error) or intentional overdoses (i.e., a suicidal gesture or suicide attempt). It is therefore critical to take a careful history to determine which medications the patient is taking, including over-the-counter drugs. Examples of medications that can

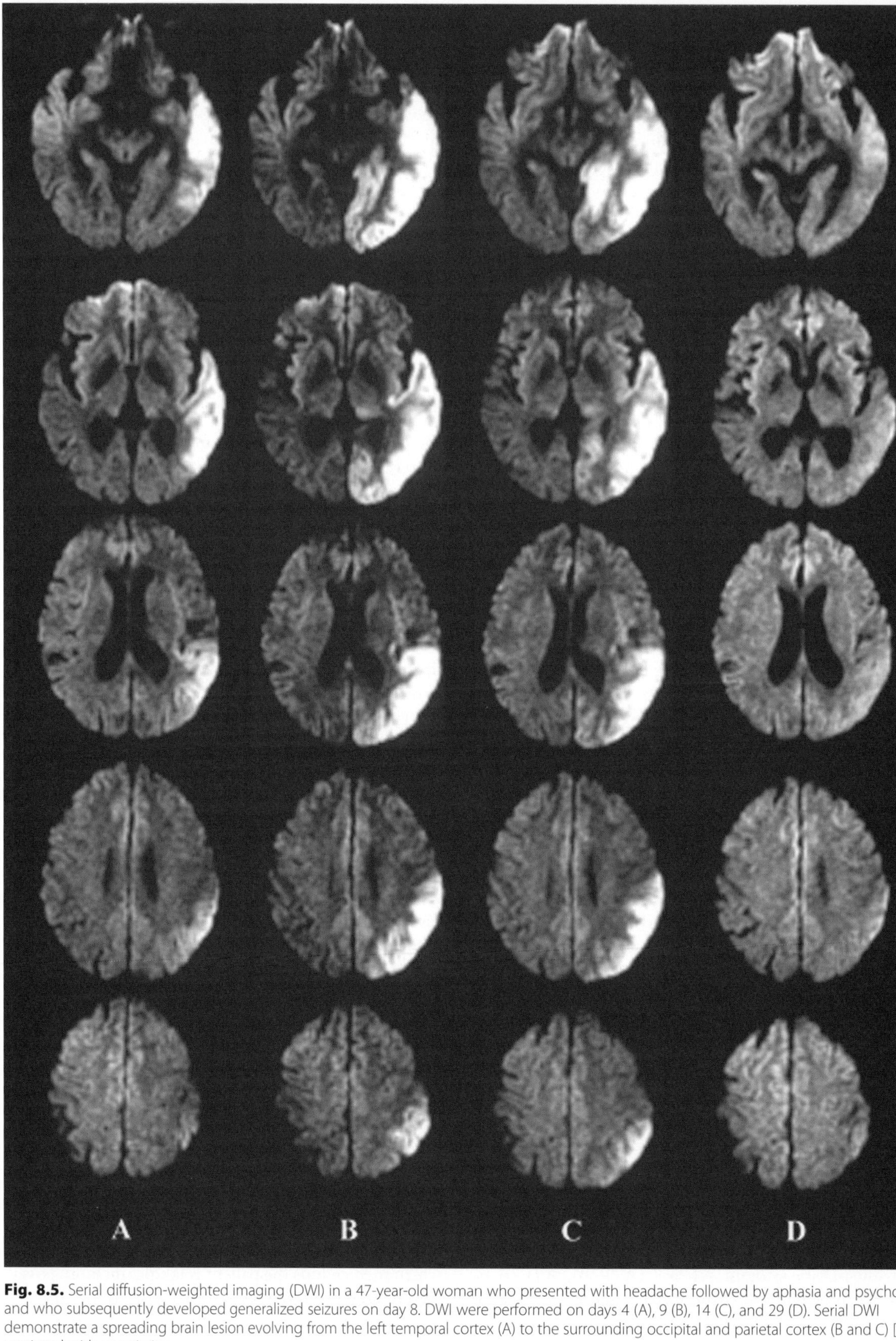

Fig. 8.5. Serial diffusion-weighted imaging (DWI) in a 47-year-old woman who presented with headache followed by aphasia and psychosis and who subsequently developed generalized seizures on day 8. DWI were performed on days 4 (A), 9 (B), 14 (C), and 29 (D). Serial DWI demonstrate a spreading brain lesion evolving from the left temporal cortex (A) to the surrounding occipital and parietal cortex (B and C) [65]; reprinted with permission.

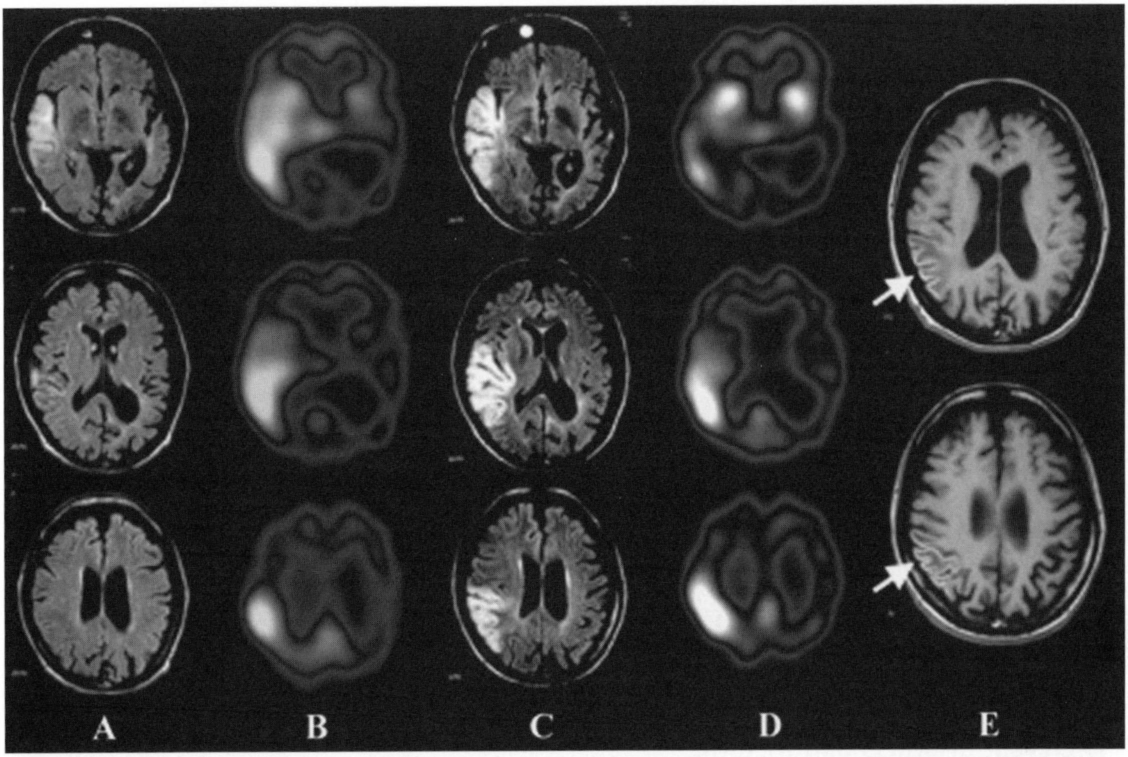

Fig. 8.6. A patient who is experiencing a stroke-like episode at the time of imaging, demonstrating the relationship between the stroke-like lesion on fluid-attenuated inversion recovery (FLAIR) image (A and C) and flow changes on SPECT (B and D) and late cortical changes on T1-weighted image (E). The first FLAIR image performed on day 12 shows high signal intensity in the right anterior temporal lobe (A) while on day 14, SPECT demonstrates focal hyperemia in the right temporoparietal lobe (B). On day 17, the second FLAIR image demonstrates a continuous spread of the brain lesion in the posterior temporal and parietal cortex (C) while on day 28, the second SPECT shows changes in location of the focal hyperperfusion moving toward the parietal cortex (D). A gyriform configuration of T1-weighted high signal intensity compatible with cortical laminar necrosis was identified on MRI obtained on day 52 (arrows, E) [65]; reprinted with permission.

cause both psychosis and headache include L-Dopa and dopamine agonists (such as pramipexole), [72] anticholinergics, corticosteroids, [73] broad-spectrum antibiotics (e.g., quinolone), [74] anti-malaria medication (e.g., mefloquine or chloroquine), [75] and medication used to treat tuberculosis, such as isoniazid. [76] Stimulant medications (e.g., methylphenidate) have also been associated with headache and psychosis in both pediatric [77] and adult [78] patient populations. Both endogenous cortisol production (i.e., Cushing's syndrome), as well as the use of prescription corticosteroid, are associated with a wide range of neuropsychiatric symptoms, including headache and psychosis. [73] It appears that these side effects are dose-dependent, with an increased rate and severity at higher corticosteroid doses. [79]

Substances causing headache and psychosis, both during the intoxication and withdrawal phases, include cocaine, amphetamines/speed, hallucinogens (e.g., LSD, peyote, psilocybin), PCP, anxiolytics/hypnotics (e.g., benzodiazepines and barbiturates), ecstasy, marijuana, and opioids. The time of onset of psychotic symptoms and headache tends to vary depending on the type of substance. For example, cocaine can induce psychotic symptoms and headache over the course of only a few minutes whereas with alcohol, these symptoms tend to occur typically after long-term usage, or during the withdrawal phase. The type of psychotic symptoms can sometimes help differentiate between different substances, i.e., persecutory delusions and tactile hallucinations (e.g., the sensation of bugs crawling under the skin, referred to as *formication*) can be seen with cocaine-induced psychosis whereas predominant visual hallucinations, flashbacks and sympathetic activation would more likely indicate hallucinogen use.

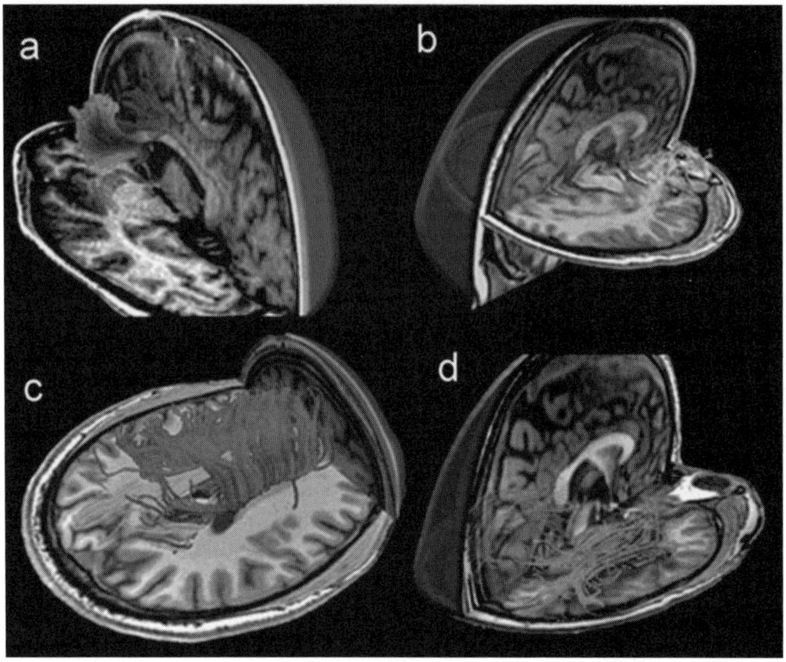

Fig. 8.7. Fiber tractography of commonly damaged tracts in mild traumatic brain injury, including: (a) anterior corona radiata and genu of corpus callosum, (b) uncinate fasciculus, (c) cingulum bundle in green and body of corpus callosum in red, and (d) inferior longitudinal fasciculus [84]; reprinted with permission. See color plate section.

Other relevant disorders and medical conditions

Patients who sustain **traumatic brain injury (TBI)**, especially with a loss of consciousness, are prone to develop a wide range of neuropsychiatric symptoms, including headache and psychosis. [80] Diffuse axonal injury typically occurs when the head is subjected to shear-strain forces, with most lesions emerging at the interface between brain regions that have different tissue densities, such as the junctions between gray and white matter. [81] Diffusion tensor tractography has been used to demonstrate changes in structural connectivity in patients with traumatic axonal injury [82–84] in conjunction with CT and conventional MRI, since the latter two imaging methods are often normal in this patient population. [84] In diffusion tensor imaging (DTI) studies of mild TBI, the most commonly damaged tracts include the frontal association pathways, such as the anterior corona radiata, uncinate fasciculus, superior longitudinal fasciculus, and the anterior corpus callosum (see Fig. 8.7). [84] Some DTI studies have demonstrated that diffuse axonal injury can lead to damage of the thalamic projection fibers which correlate with cognitive deficits following the injury, [85] whereas other studies found that in adults with mild TBI, impaired integrity of frontal and temporal white matter pathways correlates with deficits in specific cognitive domains, including executive attention and memory. [84,86]

Idiopathic intracranial hypertension (IHH, also known as pseudotumor cerebri), is a disorder characterized by increased intracranial pressure (ICP) in the absence of a space occupying lesion and of unknown cause, predominantly seen in women of childbearing age and associated with a history of weight gain. [87] If untreated, IHH may lead to papilledema (i.e., swelling of the optic discs) with visual field deficits, which can ultimately progress to blindness. [88] Isotretinoin (vitamin A) has been associated with an increased occurrence of IHH, and increased rates of IHH have been found in both Behcet's disease [45,89] as well as SLE. [91] The most common symptom of IHH is headache, typically occurring in over 90% of the cases. The headache is characteristically worse in the morning, is generalized and throbbing in nature. [88] The headache can be worsened by activities that increase the intracranial pressure more, such as coughing and sneezing. In addition to headache, some of these patients also experience pulsatile tinnitus (a "whooshing" sensation in one or both ears synchronous with the pulse), generalized weakness, loss of smell, incoordination, and rarely also psychosis. [88, 90, 92]

Both **obstructive** (i.e., with obstruction of the CSF flow) and **non-obstructive hydrocephalus** (i.e., **normal pressure hydrocephalus**) have been associated with headache and psychosis. [93–95] Obstructive hydrocephalus can be caused by congenital abnormalities like the Arnold–Chiari malformation, as well as secondary to processes that affect the CSF flow, including infections, brain tumors, head injury, intracranial hemorrhage (subarachnoid or intraparenchymal) or neurosarcoidosis. [95,96] In cases of obstructive hydrocephalus, the headache can be extremely painful. Patients with normal-pressure hydrocephalus typically present with the classic triad: urinary incontinence, dementia, and gait disturbance. The treatment of hydrocephalus is surgical diversion of CSF. This is accomplished by implanting a shunt to drain CSF from either the intracranial ventricular system or the lumbar subarachnoid space to a distal site, such as the peritoneal or pleural cavity or the venous system, where the CSF can be reabsorbed. The most common shunts typically utilized are ventriculoperitoneal and ventriculoatrial shunts. There is a variable improvement rate after CSF shunting. [97]

Another possibility to be considered in a patient with new-onset psychosis and headache, especially if cognitive deficits and other neurological symptoms are also present, is toxic exposure to **metals** (e.g., mercury or lead) or **organophosphate** poisoning (e.g., in pesticides). [98–101] For severe metal poisoning, chelation therapy may be tried, whereas organophosphate poisoning is usually treated with atropine in conjunction with pralidoxime. Pralidoxime binds to organophosphate-inactivated acetylcholinesterase (a "cholinesterase reactivator").

In rare cases, patients with a demyelinating disorder, such as **multiple sclerosis**, can also present with psychotic symptoms. [102,103] Studies on headache in MS estimate the frequency of headache in MS at approximately 50%. [104] Both the psychosis and headache should be treated with the same medication regimen used in patients with a primary psychotic disorder and a primary headache disorder.

Infectious disease affecting the central nervous system (i.e., the meninges, brain or spinal cord tissue, cerebrospinal fluid, or any combination thereof) can also lead to psychosis and headache. The list of infectious agents that have been reported to sporadically cause psychotic symptoms and headache is long and includes different bacteria, spirochetes such as *Treponema pallidum* (causing neurosyphilis) and *Borrelia burgdorferi* (causing Lyme disease); viruses such as herpes simplex viruses (HSV-1 and -2), Epstein–Barr virus, CMV, influenza, measles, rubella, mumps, polio, enteroviruses such as Coxsackie B4, arboviruses such as Eastern equine encephalitis virus, retroviruses such as the human immunodeficiency virus (HIV) or endogenous human retroviruses, and Borna disease virus; and protozoa such as *T. gondii*. [103] Neurosyphilis involves a syphilitic infection of the central nervous system and is often incorrectly referred to as "tertiary syphilis." [106] Neurosyphilis can occur at any time in the course of the disease, including in the primary stage. Early forms of neurosyphilis primarily affect the meninges, cerebrospinal fluid, and cerebral or spinal cord vasculature whereas the later forms of neurosyphilis primarily affect the brain and spinal cord parenchyma. [106] In the later stages, patients can develop gummas (a space-occupying lesion contiguous with the dura), strokes, psychosis, tabes dorsalis, rapidly progressive dementia with personality changes, and Argyll–Robertson pupils (i.e., bilateral small pupils that constrict when the patient focuses on a near object, but do not constrict when exposed to bright light; see Fig. 8.8a). [106] At times, the medication used to treat or prevent the transmission of an infectious agent can also cause both headache and psychosis, such as isoniazid used to treat tuberculosis. [76]

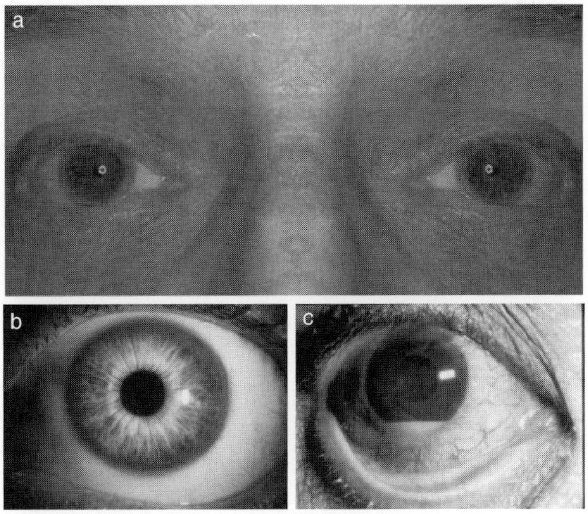

Fig. 8.8. (a) Argyll Robertson pupils (http://www.mrcophth.com/pupils/argyllrobertson.html); (b) Kayser–Fleischer ring (http://dmnemonics.blogspot.com/2011/12/wilsons-diseases.html); (c) Hypopyon and uveitis (http://medicalpicturesinfo.com/hypopyon/). See color plate section.

Rare **metabolic disorders** can also be the cause of both psychosis and headache. One example of this is a urea cycle enzymatic abnormality which is rare hereditary metabolic disorder with a reported incidence of 1/25 000 in the US, and which is usually only reported in children. [107] The serious abnormality or lack of one of the four urea cycle enzymes: carbamyl phosphatase synthetase I, ornithine transcarbamylase, argininosuccinate synthetase, and argininosuccinate lyase can all cause acute hyperammonemia which in adults can be triggered by stress, alcohol or drug use, surgery, infection or delivery in women. [107] The urea cycle enzymatic abnormalities are associated with a wide range of neurologic, psychiatric and gastrointestinal manifestations and the clinical course can vary. Headache is a symptom that frequently arises during the puerperium (~30%–39%), typically manifesting between 3 and 6 days after delivery. [105]

Required work-up of patients with psychosis and headache

Considering the broad differential diagnosis for a patient with psychosis and headache, the work-up should be comprehensive (see Table 8.2). In any patient presenting with psychosis and headache, the physician must take a careful **history**. This includes obtaining details about the psychotic episodes (e.g., type of symptoms, potential triggers, course, psychiatric co-morbidity) and the headache (e.g., type of headache, potential triggers, course); establishing if either of these symptom-clusters appear to be primary or whether they are both likely the result of a separate etiology based on the temporal relationship; medication history (as discussed above, several medication classes such as anti-malarial medication, corticosteroids, and dopamine agonists can all cause psychosis and headache); past medical history (including sexually transmitted diseases/having unprotected sex), and family history (are there any family members with similar symptoms suggestive of a familial inheritance?). Parallel history should also be obtained to evaluate this information for accuracy and completeness. In patients with new-onset memory problems, a **mini-mental state examination** (**MMSE**) or more comprehensive **neuropsychological testing** should be considered.

In addition to this, one has to carry out a comprehensive **physical exam**, which should also include a **mental status exam** to evaluate for psychiatric

Table 8.2. Work-up for patients with headache and psychosis

Diagnostic test	Finding	Associated neuropsychiatric disease
Physical exam	– Oral ulcers – Malar ("butterfly") rash	– Behçet's disease – SLE
Laboratory studies	– TFTs – Thyroid auto-antibodies – Elevated ESR/CRP – ANA and other auto-antibodies – Elevated LFTs – RPR – Elevated serum lead and mercury levels – ACE – Decreased ceruloplasmin	– Thyroid disease – Systemic disease (GCA; SLE; Behçet's disease); infection or inflammatory process – SLE – Wilson's disease – Syphilis – Lead or mercury poisoning – Sarcoidosis – Wilson's disease
Eye exam	– Uveitis; hypopyon – Kayser–Fleischer ring – Argyll–Robertson pupils	– Behçet's disease – Wilson's disease – Syphilis
Fundoscopy MRI	– Papilledema – Bleed or infarct – Tumor – "Slit-like ventricles" – Empty sella sign – Small punctate focal lesions in subcortical white matter – Cortical atrophy – Periventricular white matter changes – Ventricular dilation	– IHH – CVA – Meningioma; glioblastoma multiforme; etc. – IHH – SLE

Table 8.2. (cont.)

Diagnostic test	Finding	Associated neuropsychiatric disease
	– Major infarcts – Gumma's – Tubers – Hamartomas	 – Syphilis – Tuberous sclerosis – NF
DTI	– Diffuse axonal injury/ disrupted axonal integrity – Bleed/infarct	– Traumatic brain injury – CVA
MRSI	– Increased lactate in CNS	– MELAS
PET or PET-CT	– Seizures – Gummas – Tubers, – Hamartomas – Dementia – Malignancy	– Seizure disorder – Syphilis – Tuberous sclerosis – NF – Alzheimer's dementia
Lumbar puncture – CSF analysis	– Opening pressure (can also bring relief) – Protein, glucose, WBCs, RBCs, gram stain, oligoclonal bands, IgG – Identification of neuronal auto-antibodies and antigen – Elevated 14–3–3 protein	– IHH – Bacterial/viral encephalitis /meningitis; MS; Behçet's disease – Limbic encephalitis – Transmissible spongiform encephalopathies (Creutzfeld-Jacob disease)
Temporal artery biopsy	– Vasculitis with giant cells	– GCA
Thyroid – FNA – US – Tc/radioactive iodine uptake thyroid scan	 – Rule out malignancy – Determine whether nodule is cystic, irregular boundaries, calcifications – Thyroid nodule is "hot" or "cold"	 – Thyroid cancer – Benign/malignant thyroid nodule – Hypo/hyperthyroid – Benign/malignant thyroid nodule
EEG	– Seizure activity (e.g., spike and wave discharges)	– Seizure disorder
Genetic testing	– m.3243A>G mutation – ATP7B mutation – CACNL1A4 – HLA type B51	– MELAS – Wilson's disease – Familial migraine – Behçet's disease

symptoms, including psychosis, dementia, and delirium; inspection for oral ulcers (Behçet's disease); eye and fundoscopic examination (e.g., Argyll Robertson pupils in neurosyphilis, Kayser–Fleischer ring in Wilson's disease, uveitis with or without hypopyon in Behçet's disease, or papilledema in IHH); evaluation for rashes (e.g., malar rash in SLE), and so forth. Furthermore, the **neurological exam** can further guide the physician as to whether there is any indication of a specific neurological disease.

Laboratory testing should be broad and could include urine toxicology, urinalysis (protein, protein-creatinine ratio, red blood cells (RBCs), white blood cells (WBCs), cellular casts), CBC with differential, erythrocyte sedimentation rate (ESR) or C-reactive protein (CRP) (e.g., elevated in infections and systemic diseases like GCA, Behçet's disease and SLE), complement, electrolytes, thyroid function tests (TFTs), thyroid auto-antibodies, liver function tests (LFTs), vitamin B12, folic acid (FA), rapid plasma regain (RPR), HIV testing, serum lead and mercury levels, anti-nuclear antibodies (ANA), other auto-antibody tests (e.g., anti-double-stranded DNA (anti-dsDNA), anti-Smith (anti-Sm), anti-RNP antibodies, anti-Ro(SSA), anti-La(SSB), anti-ribosomal P, anti-neurofilament, anti-endothelial cell, antineuronal, and anti-NR2 antibodies – all of which may be present in SLE), antiphospholipid antibodies (present in approximately half of patients with SLE), lupus anticoagulant antibody test, angiotensin converting enzyme (ACE; in patients with suspected neurosarcoidosis), ceruloplasmin level (decreased in patients with Wilson's disease), tumor markers, CSF – standard panel (e.g., glucose, protein, gram stain, IgG, WBCs, RBCs, oligoclonal banding, 14–3–3 protein, which can be elevated in patients with Creutzfeldt-Jacob disease), encephalitis markers, opening pressure (can also alleviate symptoms as in IHH), and neuronal auto-antibodies (e.g., anti-NMDA-R, anti-AMPA-R, anti-GABA-B), and evaluation for inborn errors of metabolism.

In patients who have not had a prior evaluation, **neuroimaging** should always be done. This can involve structural an MRI (e.g., "slit-like ventricles" or empty-sella sign in IHH; gummas in neurosyphilis; tubers in tuberous sclerosis), CT, DTI (e.g., for traumatic brain injury and CVAs), MRSI (e.g., for MELAS), PET and PET-CT (e.g., for tumor screen in patients with suspected limbic encephalitis, seizures, gummas, tubers, and hamartomas like in neurofribromatosis), and SPECT and SPECT-CT (e.g., for MELAS). Repeat neuroimaging should be performed when symptoms do not improve, change, or worsen over time (e.g., a whole-body PET can be repeated in 6 months in a patient with limbic encephalitis typically associated with a tumor and who does not respond to immunosuppressant therapy). **Electroencephalography** (**EEG** – including long-term video-EEG monitoring) should be done in patients with a potential seizure disorder or a neurological condition which is associated with seizures (e.g., limbic encephalitis or tuberous sclerosis). In patients who present with thyroid nodules, in addition to TFTs, physicians should consider **fine needle biopsy** to determine whether a nodule is malignant as well as an **ultrasound** (e.g., to evaluate whether the nodule is cystic, has irregular boundaries, and is calcified) and/or **technetium** or **radioactive iodine imaging of the thyroid** (to determine whether a nodule is "hot" or "cold"). Patients who present with symptoms of giant cell arteritis should be considered for a **temporal artery biopsy**. Finally, **genetic testing** can be done for certain diseases that affect the brain and which can lead to both headache and psychosis (e.g., Wilson's disease, MELAS, and familial migraine).

Treatment considerations in patients with psychosis and headache

The treatment of patients who present with psychosis and headache must be tailored to the specific etiology. When patients suffer from a *primary psychiatric disorder* who suffer from somatic delusions, tactile hallucinations interpreted as headache, or those who suffer from both a psychotic disorder as well as a somatization disorder – when the appropriate psychiatric treatment is implemented to target these symptoms (e.g., by using antipsychotics), both the psychosis and perceived headache should respond to treatment. This can also help further differentiate and confirm whether the experienced headache is indeed a consequence of, or influenced by, the psychotic disorder or whether this may instead represent a co-morbid condition or that both the headache and psychotic symptoms are caused by a separate "organic" neuropathology. Certain medications used for several psychiatric disorders which can present with psychotic symptoms can also be effective for the treatment of some forms of headache. Examples of this include first-line mood stabilizers, such as lithium and divalproic acid, which are both used in the treatment of bipolar disorder as well as for migraine disorder and cluster headache. [108,109] Some researchers have also suggested that migraine disorder is more prevalent in patients who suffer from bipolar disorder. [110] Neuroleptics, especially atypical antipsychotics, have also been increasingly used for severe forms of headache, although at the present time there is no rigorous data supporting this use. [111,112]

When patients suffer from a *primary neurological condition*, the treatment should focus on this condition, since the psychotic symptoms can sometimes respond as well. Examples of these include migraine disorder and seizure disorder (especially temporal lobe epilepsy), which, when treated, can potentially lead to a complete remission of the psychotic co-morbidity.

Finally, when the psychotic symptoms and headache are caused by a *separate etiology* – both of these symptom-clusters can potentially respond if an adequate treatment for the condition is provided. For example, if systemic lupus erythematosis is relatively well-managed (e.g., with glucocorticoids alone or in combination with immunosuppressive medication) both the headache and psychosis can go into complete remission, albeit sometimes only temporarily. [37] If an infectious etiology is identified within a critical time window, adequate treatment can reverse or prevent worsening of the associated neuropsychiatric symptoms. If a patient suffers from Graves' disease, treatment with antithyroid medication, radioiodine, or surgery can completely reverse the associated psychotic symptoms and the headache. Similarly, in cases of hydrocephalus (treatment with a ventriculo-peritoneal shunt for idiopathic intracranial hypertension, treatment with lumbar puncture, acetazolamide, or optic nerve sheath decompression and fenestration or shunting can both lead to significant improvements in the psychotic symptoms and headache. The most dramatic example of a complete reversal of neuropsychiatric symptoms may very well be limbic encephalitis, where patients have neuronal auto-antibodies which target cell surface antigens such as the NMDA-, AMPA-, and $GABA_B$-receptors. In these patients, treatment with immunosuppressant drugs, such as intravenous IgG or Rituximab, can lead to a complete remission of an often dramatic neuropsychiatric presentation which can include psychosis, agitation, headache, seizures, memory and attentional deficits, delirium, autonomic instability, and coma. It underscores the importance of making the correct diagnosis so that the appropriate treatment can be initiated to target the neuropsychiatric condition and the associated neuropsychiatric symptoms.

References

[1] Rosenbaum M. Psychogenic headache. *Dis Nerv Syst* 1947; **8**: 252–6.

[2] Gilman L, Wexberg L. Psychogenic aspects of headache; a symposium. *J Clin Exp Psychopathol* 1949; **10**: 1–26.

[3] Ad Hoc Committee on Classification of Headache. *JAMA* 1962; **179**: 717–18.

[4] Headache Classification Committee of the International Headache Society. Classification and diagnostic criteria for headache disorders, cranial neuralgias and facial pain. *Cephalalgia* 1988; **8**(Suppl. 7): 1–96.

[5] Headache Classification Committee of the International Headache Society. The International Classification of Headache Disorders, 2nd Edition. *Cephalalgia* 2004; **24**(Suppl. 1): 1–160.

[6] American Psychiatric Association. *Diagnostic and Statistical Manual of Mental Disorders* (Revised 4th ed.). 2000. Washington, DC.

[7] Bruyn GW. Migraine equivalents. In FClifford Rose ed. *Handbook of Neurology,* vol 4, *Headache*. Amsterdam: Elsvier Science Publishers, 1986.

[8] Fuller GN, Marshall A, Flint J, Lewis S, Wise RJ. Migraine madness: recurrent psychosis after migraine. *J Neurol Neurosurg Psychiatry* 1993; **56**: 416–18.

[9] Fuller G, Guiloff R. Migrainous olfactory hallucinations. *J Neurol Neurosurg Psychiatry* 1987; **50**: 1688–90.

[10] Kaiser F. Anticipation in migraine with affective psychosis. *Am J Med Genet* 2002; **110**: 62–4.

[11] Schreier HA. Auditory hallucinations in nonpsychotic children with affective syndromes and migraines: report of 13 cases. *J Child Neurol* 1998; **13**: 377–82.

[12] Cotard J. Du délire hypocondriaque dans une forme grave de la melancolie anxieuse. Memoire lu à la Société médico-psychologique dans la Séance du 28 Juin 1880. *Ann Medico-Psychol* 1880; **4**: 168–74.

[13] Cotard J. Du délire des négations. *Arch Neurol (Paris)* 1882; **4**: 152–70.

[14] Pearn J, Gardner-Thorpe C. Jules Cotard (1840–1889): his life and the unique syndrome which bears his name. *Neurology* 2002; **58**: 1400–3.

[15] Bhatia MS, Agrawal P, Malik SC. Cotard syndrome in migraine. *Ind J Med Sci* 1993; **47**: 152–3.

[16] Spranger M, Spranger S, Schwab S, Benninger C, Dichgans M. Familial hemiplegic migraine with cerebellar ataxia and paroxysmal psychosis. *Eur Neurol* 1999; **41**: 150–2.

[17] Ophoff RA, Terwindt GM, Vergouwe MN, *et al.* Familial hemiplegic migraine and episodic ataxia type-2 are caused by mutations in the Ca-channel gene CACNL1A4. *Cell* 1996; **87**: 543–52.

[18] Marmura MJ. Use of dopamine antagonists in treatment of migraine. *Curr Treatm Opt Neurol* 2012; **14**: 27–35.

[19] Ekstein D, Schachter SC. Postictal headache. *Epilepsy Behav* 2010; **19**: 151–5.

[20] Laplante P, Saint JH, Bouvier G. Headache as an epileptic manifestation. *Neurology* 1983; **33**: 1493–5.

[21] Dainese F, Mai R, Francione S, Mainardi F, Zanchin G, Paladin F. Ictal headache: headache as first ictal symptom in focal epilepsy. *Epilepsy Behav* 2011; **22**: 790–2.

[22] Kanner AM. Psychosis of epilepsy: a neurologist's perspective. *Epilepsy Behav* 2000; **1**: 219–27.

[23] Nadkarni S, Arnedo V, Devinsky O. Psychosis in epilepsy patients. *Epilepsia* 2007; **48** Suppl 9: 17–19.

[24] Devinsky O. Postictal psychosis: common, dangerous, and treatable. *Epilepsy Curr* 2008; **8**: 31–4.

[25] Toone BK, Garralda ME, Ron MA. The psychosis of epilepsy and the functional psychosis: a clinical and phenomenological comparison. *Br J Psychiatry* 1982; **141**: 256–61.

[26] Fisher RS, Schachter SC. The postictal state: a neglected entity in the management of epilepsy. *Epilepsy Behav* 2000; **1**: 52–9.

[27] Tadokoro Y, Oshima T, Kanemoto K. Interictal psychoses in comparison with schizophrenia – a prospective study. *Epilepsia* 2007; **48**: 2345–51.

[28] Chemerinski E, Robinson RG. The neuropsychiatry of stroke. *Psychosomatics* 2000; **41**: 5–14.

[29] Almeida OP, Xiao J. Mortality associated with incident mental health disorders after stroke. *Aust N Z J Psychiatry* 2007; **41**: 274–81.

[30] Bourgeois JA, Hilty DM, Chang CH, Wineinger MA, Servis ME. Poststroke neuropsychiatric illness: an integrated approach to diagnosis and management. *Curr Treat Options Neurol* 2004; **6**: 403–20.

[31] Wong VS, Adamczyk P, Dahlin B, Richman DP, Wheelock V. Cerebral venous sinus thrombosis presenting with auditory hallucinations and illusions. *Cogn Behav Neurol* 2011; **24**: 40–2.

[32] Dhasmana DJ, Brockington IF, Roberts A. Post-partum transverse sinus thrombosis presenting as acute psychosis. *Arch Wom Ment Hlth* 2010; **13**: 365–7.

[33] Wasay M, Kojan S, Dai AI, Bobustuc G, Sheikh Z. Headache in Cerebral Venous Thrombosis: incidence, pattern and location in 200 consecutive patients. *J Headache Pain* 2010; **11**: 137–9.

[34] Brockington IF. Cerebral vascular disease as a cause of postpartum psychosis. *Arch Wom Ment Hlth* 2007; **10** (4): 177–8.

[35] Benseler, SM, Silverman ED. Neuropsychiatric involvement in pediatric systemic lupus erythematosus. *Lupus* 2007; **16**(8): 564–71.

[36] Yu HH, Lee JH, Wang LC, Yang YH, Chiang BL. Neuropsychiatric manifestations in pediatric systemic lupus erythematosus: a 20-year study. *Lupus* 2006; **15**: 651–7.

[37] Bertsias GK, Boumpas DT. Pathogenesis, diagnosis and management of neuropsychiatric SLE manifestations. *Nat Rev Rheumatol* 2010; **6**: 358–67.

[38] Brey RL, Holliday SL, Saklad AR, *et al.* Neuropsychiatric syndromes in lupus: prevalence using standardized definitions. *Neurology* 2002; **58**: 1214–20.

[39] Fabiani G, Monteiro de Almeida S, Germiniani FMB, *et al.* Neuro-Behçet: report of three clinically distinct cases. *Arq Neuropsiquiatr* 2001; **59**: 250–4.

[40] Yazici H, Barnes CG. Practical treatment recommendations for pharmacotherapy of Behçet's syndrome. *Drugs* 1991; **42**: 796–804.

[41] Taylor SR, Singh J, Menezo V, Wakefield D, McCluskey P, Lightman S. Behçet disease: visual prognosis and factors influencing the development of visual loss. *Am J Ophthalmol* 2011; **152**: 1059–66.

[42] Yazici H, Fresko I, Yurdakul S. Behcet's syndrome: disease manifestations, management, and advances in treatment. *Nat Clin Pract Rheumatol* 2007; **3**: 148–55.

[43] Al-Araji A, Kidd DP. Neuro-Behçet's disease: epidemiology, clinical characteristics, and management. *Lancet Neurol* 2009; **8**: 192–204.

[44] Kale N, Agaoglu J, Icen M, Yazici I, Tanik O. The presentation of headache in neuro-Behçet's disease: a case-series. *Headache* 2009; **49**: 467–70.

[45] Can E, Kara B, Somer A, Keser M, Salman N, Yalçin I. Neuro-Behçet disease presenting as secondary pseudotumor syndrome: case report. *Eur J Paediatr Neurol* 2006; **10**: 97–9.

[46] Noel N, Hutié M, Wechsler B, *et al.* Pseudotumoural presentation of neuro-Behcet's disease: case series and review of literature. *Rheumatology* (Oxford) 2012 [Epub ahead of print].

[47] Deniz O, Cayköylü, A, Vural G, *et al.* A case study of neuro-psycho-Behçet's syndrome presenting with psychotic attack. *Clin Neurol Neurosurg* 2009; **111**: 877–9.

[48] Bona JR, Fackler SM, Fendley MJ, Nemeroff CB. Neurosarcoidosis as a cause of refractory psychosis: a complicated case report. *Am J Psychiatry* 1998; **155**: 1106–8.

[49] Hoitsma E, Faber CG, Drent M, Sharma OP. Neurosarcoidosis: a clinical dilemma. *Lancet Neurol* 2004; **3**: 397–407.

[50] Nowak DA, Widenka DC. Neurosarcoidosis: a review of its intracranial manifestation. *J Neurol* 2001; **248**: 363–72.

[51] Kale N, Eggenberger E. Diagnosis and management of giant cell arteritis: a review. *Curr Opin Opthalmol* 2010; **21**: 417–22.

[52] Cherry JE, Pearce JM. Unusual variants in the presentation of temporal arteritis. *Postgrad Med J* 1980; **56**: 88–91.

[53] Razavi M, Jones RD, Manzel K, Fattal D, Rizzo M. Steroid-responsive Charles Bonnet syndrome in temporal arteritis. *J Neuropsychiatry Clin Neurosci* 2004; **16**: 505–8.

[54] Vu N, Manolios N, Spencer DG, Howe GB. Charles Bonnet syndrome in giant cell arteritis. *J Clin Rheumatol* 1998; **4**(3): 144–6.

[55] Villa-Forte A. Giant cell arteritis: suspect it, treat it promptly. *Cleve Clin J Med* 2011; **78**: 265–70.

[56] Schadlu AP, Schadlu R, Shepherd JB. 3rd. Charles Bonnet syndrome: a review. *Curr Opin Ophthalmol* 2009; **20**: 219–22.

[57] Roberts CG, Ladenson PW. Hypothyroidism. *Lancet* 2004; **363**: 793–803.

[58] Bunevicius R, Prange AJ Jr. Psychiatric manifestations of Graves' hyperthyroidism: pathophysiology and treatment options. *CNS Drugs* 2006; **20**: 897–909.

[59] Anaissie E, Tohme JF. Reserpine in propranolol-resistant thyroid storm. *Arch Intern Med* 1985; **145**: 2248–9.

[60] Graus F, Saiz A, Dalmau J. Antibodies and neuronal autoimmune disorders of the CNS. *J Neurol* 2010; **257**: 509–17.

[61] Lancaster E, Martinez-Hernandez E, Dalmau J. Encephalitis and antibodies to synaptic and neuronal cell surface proteins. *Neurology* 2011; **77**: 179–89.

[62] Ciafaloni E, Ricci E, Shanske S, *et al.* MELAS: clinical features, biochemistry, and molecular genetics. *Ann Neurol* 1992; **31**: 391–8.

[63] Manwaring N, Jones MM, Wang JJ, *et al.* Population prevalence of the MELAS A3243G mutation. *Mitochondrion* 2007; **7**: 230–3.

[64] Iizuka T, Sakai F, Suzuki N, *et al.* Neuronal hyperexcitability in stroke-like episodes of MELAS syndrome. *Neurology* 2002; **59**: 816–24.

[65] Iizuka T, Sakai F, Kan S, Suzuki N. Slowly progressive spread of the stroke-like lesions in MELAS. *Neurology* 2003; **61**: 1238–44.

[66] Kaufman P, Shungu DC, Sano MC, *et al.* Cerebral lactic acidosis correlates with neurological impairment in MELAS. *Neurology* 2004; **62**: 1297–302.

[67] Ala A, Walker AP, Ashkan K, Dooley JS, Schilsky, ML. Wilson's disease. *Lancet* 2007; **369**: 397–408.

[68] Stremmel W, Meyerrose KW, Niederau C, Hefter H, Kreuzpaintner G, Strohmeyer G. Wilson's disease: clinical presentation, treatment, and survival. *Ann Intern Med* 1991; **115**: 720–6.

[69] Walshe JM. Wilson's disease. The presenting symptoms. *Arch Dis Child* 1962; **37**: 253–6.

[70] Sinha S, Taly AB, Ravishankar S, *et al.* Wilson's disease: cranial MRI observations and clinical correlation. *Neuroradiology* 2006; **48**: 613–21.

[71] Kozic D, Svetel M, Petrovic B, Dragasevic N, Semnic R, Kostic VS. MR imaging of the brain in patients with hepatic form of Wilson's disease. *Eur J Neurol* 2003; **10**: 587–92.

[72] Aiken CB. Pramipexole in psychiatry: a systematic review of the literature. *J Clin Psychiatry* 2007; **68**: 1230–6.

[73] Perantie DC, Brown ES. Corticosteroids, immune suppression, and psychosis. *Curr Psych Rep* 2002; **4**: 171–6.

[74] Tomé AM, Filipe A. Quinolones: review of psychiatric and neurological adverse reactions. *Drug Saf* 2011; **34**: 465–88.

[75] Kukoyi O, Carney CP. Curses, madness, and mefloquine. *Psychosomatics* 2003; **44**: 339–41.

[76] Schrestha S, Alao A. Isoniazid-induced psychosis. *Psychosomatics* 2009; **50**: 640–1.

[77] Klein-Schwartz W. Abuse and toxicity of methylphenidate. *Curr Opin Pediatr* 2002; **14**: 219–23.

[78] Kraemer M, Uekermann J, Wiltfang J, Kis B. Methylphenidate-induced psychosis in adult attention-deficit/hyperactivity disorder: report of 3 new cases and review of the literature. *Clin Neuropharmacol* 2010; **33**: 204–6.

[79] The Boston Collaborative Drug Surveillance Program. Acute adverse reactions to prednisone in relation to dosage. *Clin Pharmacol Ther* 1972; **13**: 694–8.

[80] Halbauer JD, Ashford JW, Zeitzer JM, Adamson MM, Lew HL, Yesavage JA. Neuropsychiatric diagnosis and management of chronic sequelae of war-related mild to moderate traumatic brain injury. *J Rehab Res Dev* 2009; **46**: 757–96.

[81] Li XF, Feng DF. Diffuse axonal injury: novel insights into detection and treatment. *J Clin Neurosci* 2009; **16**: (5) 614–19.

[82] Shenton ME, Hamoda HM, Schneiderman JS, *et al.* A review of magnetic resonance imaging and diffusion tensor imaging findings in mild traumatic brain injury. *Brain Imaging Behav* 2012; **6**: 137–92.

[83] Wang JY, Bakhadirov K, Abdi H, *et al.* Longitudinal changes of structural connectivity in traumatic axonal injury. *Neurology* 2011; **77**: 818–26.

[84] Niogi SN, Mukherjee P. Diffusion tensor imaging of mild traumatic brain injury. *J Head Trauma Rehabil* 2010; **25**: 241–55.

[85] Little DM, Kraus MF, Joseph J, *et al.* Thalamic integrity underlies executive dysfunction in traumatic brain injury. *Neurology* 2010; **74**: 558–64.

[86] Niogi SN, Mukherjee P, Ghajar J, *et al.* Structural dissociation of attentional control and memory in adults with and without mild traumatic brain injury. *Brain* 2008; **131**: 3209–21.

[87] Wall M. Idiopathic intracranial hypertension. *Neurol Clin* 2010; **28**: 593–617.

[88] Binder DK, Horton JC, Lawton MT, McDermott MW. Idiopathic intracranial hypertension. *Neurosurgery* 2004; **54**: 538–51.

[89] Essaadouni L, Jaafari H, Abouzaid CH, Kissani N. Neurological involvement in Behçet's disease: evaluation of 67 patients. *Rev Neurol (Paris)* 2010; **166**: 727–33.

[90] Duggal HS. Idiopathic intracranial hypertension presenting with psychiatric symptoms. *J Neuropsychiatry Clin Neurosci* 2005; **17**: 426–7.

[91] Barahona-Hernando R, Ríos-Blanco JJ, Méndez-Mesón I, *et al.* Idiopathic intracranial hypertension and systemic lupus erythematosus: a case report and review of the literature. *Lupus* 2009; **18**: 1121–3

[92] Restak RM. Pseudotumor cerebri, psychosis, and hypervitaminosis A. *J Nerv Ment Dis* 1972; **155**: 72–5.

[93] Price TR, Tucker GJ. Psychiatric and behavioral manifestations of normal pressure hydrocephalus. A case report and brief review. *J Nerv Ment Dis* 1977; **164**: 51–5.

[94] Yusim A, Anbarasan D, Bernstein C, *et al.* Normal pressure hydrocephalus presenting as Othello syndrome: case presentation and review of the literature. *Am J Psychiatry* 2008; **165**: 1119–25.

[95] Westhout FD, Linskey ME. Obstructive hydrocephalus and progressive psychosis: rare presentations of neurosarcoidosis. *Surg Neurol* 2008; **69**: 288–92.

[96] Franklin D, Westhout MD, Mark E, Linskey MD. Obstructive hydrocephalus and progressive psychosis: rare presentations of neurosarcoidosis. *Surg Neurol* 2008; **69**: 288–92.

[97] Gallia GL, Rigamonti D, Williams MA. The diagnosis and treatment of idiopathic normal pressure hydrocephalus. *Nature Clinical Pract Neurol* 2005; **2**: 375–81.

[98] Kohlmeier RE. Chronic lead poisoning: induced psychosis in an adult? *Am J Forensic Med Pathol* 2002; **23**: 101.

[99] Pelclová D, Lukás E, Urban P, *et al.* Mercury intoxication from skin ointment containing mercuric ammonium chloride. *Int Arch Occup Environ Hlth* 2002; **75**:S54–9.

[100] Levin HS, Rodnitzky RL. Behavioral effects of organophosphate pesticides in man. *Clin Toxicol* 1976; **9**: 391–403.

[101] Damstra T. Environmental chemicals and nervous system dysfunction. *Yale J Biol Med* 1978; **51**: 457–68.

[102] Feinstein A. Neuropsychiatric syndromes associated with multiple sclerosis. *J Neurol* 2007; **254**: II73–6.

[103] Kosmidis MH, Giannakou M, Messinis L, Papathanasopoulos P. Psychotic features associated with multiple sclerosis. *Int Rev Psychiatry* 2010; **22**: 55–66.

[104] Solaro C, Uccelli MM. Management of pain in multiple sclerosis: a pharmacological approach. *Rev Neurol* 2011; **7**: 519–27.

[105] Yolken RH, Torrey EF. Are some cases of psychosis caused by microbial agents? A review of the evidence. *Mol Psychiatry* 2008; **13**: 470–9.

[106] Marra CM. Update on neurosyphilis. *Curr Infect Dis Rep* 2009; **11**: 127–34.

[107] Tonini MC, Bignamini V, Mattioli M. Headache and neuropsychic disorders in the puerperium: a case report with suspected deficiency of urea cycle enzymes. *Neurol Sci* 2011; **32**: S157–9.

[108] Summar ML, Barr F, Dawling S, *et al.* Unmasked adult onset urea cycle disorders in the critical care setting. *Crit Care Clin* 2005; **21**: S1–S8.

[109] Blumenfeld A, Gennings C, Cady R. Pharmacological synergy: the next frontier on therapeutic advancement for migraine. *Headache* 2012 [Epub ahead of print].

[110] Dodick DW, Capobianco DJ. Treatment and management of cluster headache. *Curr Pain Headache Rep* 2001; **5**: 83–91.

[111] Low NC, Du Fort GG, Cervantes P. Prevalence, clinical correlates, and treatment of migraine in bipolar disorder. *Headache* 2003; **43**: 940–9.

[112] Silberstein SD, Peres MF, Hopkins MM, Shechter AL, Young WB, Rozen TD. Olanzapine in the treatment of refractory migraine and chronic daily headache. *Headache* 2002; **42**: 515–18.

[113] Dusitanond P, Young WB. Neuroleptics and migraine. *Cent Nerv Syst Agents Med Chem* 2009; **9**: 63–70.

[114] Keidar Z, Gurman-Balbir A, Gaitini D, Israel O. Fever of unknown origin: the role of 18F-FDG PET/CT. *J Nucl Med* 2008; **49**: 1980–5.

Chapter 9

Chronic daily headache

Robert P. Cowan

Introduction

Chronic daily headache (CDH) is seen in approximately 4% of headache sufferers in the USA, Europe, South America, and Asia. This number has remained consistent over the past 20 years. CDH is the most common presenting headache in headache specialty practices and can be devastating in its effect on patients, their families, and physicians who care for them. At the same time, when treated successfully, the results can be dramatic and rewarding.

CDH is not a diagnosis, but rather describes a condition in which headache is present on a daily or near daily basis for a period of 3 months or more. It is not a discrete headache type and can represent any primary or secondary headache that occurs more than 15 headache days per month. It is not synonymous with chronic migraine (CM), medication overuse headache (MOH), chronic tension-type headache (CTTH) or new daily persistent headache (NDPH). However, each of these is an example of CDH and almost any primary or secondary headache can transform into chronic daily headache. There are several primary headaches in which the initial presentation is chronic and daily, most notably hemicrania Continua and new daily persistent headache.

While the strict definition of CDH specifies discrete parameters of 15 or more days per month for 3 successive months, these reflect the necessities of study design and epidemiologic analysis more than the clinical picture. In practice, a patient with 13 or 14 days of headache per month or persistence for 2½ months should not automatically be excluded from a working diagnosis of CDH. However, once outside these accepted criteria, the index of suspicion for an alternative explanation should increase.

Primary headaches are distinguished from secondary headaches by the absence of an underlying cause. For example, headache in the presence of meningitis, subarachnoid hemorrhage, tumor, or mass would be considered a secondary headache. Therefore, a patient with episodic migraine reporting a change in pattern to daily headache, while using analgesics on a near daily basis, would have both a primary headache disorder (migraine) and a secondary headache disorder (medication overuse headache – MOH).

While chronic headache associated with toxic exposure or medication has been a part of the medical literature for centuries, MOH has become codified in the modern literature over the last 60 years. Peters and Horton report an over-use headache phenomenon in the early 1950s, but it is not until 1982 that Kudrow generalizes the relationship between medication overuse and migraine to include medications other than ergotamine and lays the foundation for the concept of medication overuse headache (Boes [1] 2005). Indeed, the 1988 International Headache Society (IHS) criteria does not include a classification for chronic migraine, but does describe medication overuse. The idea that migraine can become chronic in the absence of medication overuse is a more recent concept.

Currently, CDH is most often associated with medication overuse. Failure to respond to a wide variety of acute and preventive medicines and multiple comorbidities with psychiatric and medical illnesses are more common in CDH than in their episodic counterparts. In 2007, Ferrari, Leone, et al. report that there are significant sociodemographic differences between populations of episodic and chronic migraine. Chronic migraineurs experience earlier onset of headaches, have a great incidence of drug/alcohol abuse in first

The Neuropsychiatry of Headache, ed. Mark W. Green and Philip R. Muskin. Published by Cambridge University Press.

degree relatives, greater incidence of GI disease and use of medication for other medical conditions, and are much more likely to be overusing their headache medications. [2]

Risk factors for CDH can be divided into those that are modifiable and those that are not. From a clinical perspective, this is critical. Factors such as history of episodic migraine, female gender, low socioeconomic status, less education, head and neck trauma and abuse as a child, are not readily modifiable. Factors such as obesity, medication overuse, stress management, sleep apnea, diet (including caffeine), depression (to a degree), and chronobiologic behaviors (sleep, eating, and exercise schedules) when modified are beneficial in converting CDH to an episodic form, particularly when the CDH has transformed from an episodic condition.

Classification and diagnosis

The International Classification of Headache Disorders (ICHD-2) is the standard for codification of headache. It is revised on a regular basis to reflect current data. At this time of writing, a new edition is approaching release. The current ICHD-2 classifications are accessible through the IHS website, Cephalalgia, and a variety of other sources. What follows here is a widely used clinical approach to CDH classification that is entirely consistent with ICHD as presently configured (ICHD II, Revised), but may be more clinically relevant.

When a patient presents with frequent headache, determine whether the headache is primary (not due to an underlying medical condition) or secondary. [3] Part of this process, accomplished through a detailed and careful history, is to distinguish between a headache that is "episodic" and one that is "chronic." CDH can present in different ways. A patient who awakens with a headache every morning that resolves shortly after rising is different from a patient who awakens each morning headache-free but develops a headache as the day progresses. Both have chronic daily headache.

Similarly, a patient who experiences a 10-day headache with her menses and a 5-day headache with ovulation (15 days per month) will likely have a different diagnosis from a patient who experiences headache 3 or 4 days each week (15 days per month). When collecting the history, it is essential to establish a clear natural history (how long the condition has existed and how it has evolved) and the frequency, duration, timing, and severity of each ictus. The standard at this time is set at 15 headache days per month. The ICHD-2 standard includes that this headache should have been present at this frequency or greater for at least 3 months. In practice, the longer a headache has been present and stable, the less likely it is to be secondary, progressive, or sinister. Conversely, the shorter the amount of time a headache has been present, particularly if it is increasing in frequency and/or severity, the more likely a secondary, progressive, or sinister etiology.

Useful questions to ask when obtaining a history on patients presenting with frequent or daily headaches:

- How old were you when you experienced your first headache of any kind?
- When did your headaches become a problem for you?
- Is the headache you are here for today similar or different compared with headaches you have had in the past?
- Have these headaches been increasing in frequency? Duration? Severity?
- Have you noticed a temporal pattern to the headaches (worse in AM, worse on week-ends, clustering for a period and then resolving for a period)?

These questions are just one component of a careful headache history, along with questions about conditions of concern, medication usage, triggers, and lifestyle. These queries separate a chronic daily headache from an episodic headache, and help determine whether that chronic daily headache is superimposed on an episodic primary or secondary headache.

There are secondary headaches that mimic primary CDH. While MOH is by far the most common CDH, missing a primary or secondary CDH other than MOH may have significant consequences. The headaches in this group are rare: medication, post-traumatic, disorders of intracranial pressure, structural, cranial neuralgias, vascular, infectious, and metabolic. It is beyond the scope of this writing to detail the entities within each category, which are well described elsewhere. Consider vasculitides (giant cell arteritis), increased intracranial hypertension, CSF leaks (CSF hypotension) as among the more common.

Another cautionary note with respect to ruling out secondary causes: computerized tomography (CT scan) alone is not an adequate screening tool to rule out secondary causes of CDH. It may fail to detect a variety of vascular, neoplastic and infectious entities and even certain anatomic conditions such as Chiari malformation or acoustic schwannoma. It is not necessary or appropriate to image every patient with chronic headache with MRI. The most valuable diagnostic tool in the patient with chronic daily headache is the history.

Once it has been determined that the patient's headaches are chronic and daily, and secondary headache has been ruled out, the next issue is the duration of the individual attack. When during the day is the headache present? Using ICHD-2 criteria as a guide, the current cut-off for a short-duration vs. long-duration CDH is four hours. The short-duration CDHs include chronic cluster, chronic paroxysmal hemicrania, hypnic headache and chronic trigeminal neuralgia. The frequent long-duration headaches include chronic migraine (CM), transformed migraine (TM), chronic tension-type headache (CTTH), hemicrania continua (HC), and new daily persistent headache (NDPH). Frequent long-duration headache does not distinguish between headaches that are present 24 hours a day, 7 days a week and those that are present for some discrete cluster totaling 15 days or more per month and lasting greater than 4 hours. These data are critical for accurate diagnosis, creating the appropriate treatment plan, and assessing response to treatment.

At this point it can be useful to identify a few "walk-in-the-door" diagnostic pearls for CDH. Like all pearls, they are not pathognomonic, but can be helpful.

- Patient gives you the specific date (and even time) of onset – new daily persistent headache.
- Patient describes continuous unilateral pain with autonomic symptoms – hemicrania continua.
- Patient with history of episodic headaches and now presents with prominent chronic headache that has migrainous features or mixed migrainous and tension-type features – chronic migraine or transformed migraine
- Prominent tension-type features and few or no migrainous features, mild to moderate pain and previous history of similar but episodic headaches – chronic tension-type headaches.
- Patient describes severe unilateral headache behind one eye with autonomic symptoms on that side, often at the same time each night or day – chronic cluster

The classification and nomenclature for these headaches can be confusing. Some CDH is narrowly defined, such as hypnic headache or hemicrania continua. Others have a broad spectrum where syndromes almost merge into one another, as in the various forms of trigeminal autonomic cephalgia (TAC).

This is apparent in the effort to distinguish between migraine that is progressive but purely migrainous, and headaches that begin as episodic migraine but become "something else" as they chronify. The term "transformed migraine" became popular in the early 1990s to describe a headache that may have begun as episodic migraine, but over time took on characteristics suggestive of both migraine and tension-type headache. This progression from episodic migraine into a mixed episodic pattern of migraine and tension and ultimately CDH is generally accepted. Medication overuse and comorbid conditions became apparent during the progression. By the mid 1990s there was wide acceptance of this concept of transformed migraine, best articulated in the Silberstein/Lipton criteria: headache more than 15 days/month with an average duration of more than 4 hours/day, untreated. In addition, they required a previous history of episodic migraine meeting ICHD II criteria, history of increasing frequency but decreasing severity of migrainous symptoms over at least 3 months, and other than duration, the current headache must meet criteria for migraine.

The usual caveats of ruling out secondary or other primary headache applied as well. When the first revision of the ICHD II came out in 2006, the diagnosis of chronic migraine was described as 15 days of headache or more in at least the last 3 months with five attacks meeting criteria for migraine without aura and without evidence of medication overuse. [4] The definition further required that, on eight or more occasions in each of the last 3 months, the headache should meet the ICHD II criteria for migraine without aura.

Transformed migraine currently describes headache occurring 15 or more days per month in a patient with a history of transformation from episodic migraine to chronic headache with migrainous features. Chronic migraine is a subpopulation within transformed migraine in which there is no evidence of medication overuse and at least 8 of the 15 or more headache days meet criteria for migraine without aura.

From a clinical standpoint this is useful. A patient with episodic migraine now experiencing CDH due to medication overuse can realistically expect a return to their episodic migraine baseline (or better) with proper management. A patient with transformed migraine without MOH may have a worse prognosis. The former group will often describe a dull "background" headache that is daily, superimposed on episodic "spikes" that are reminiscent of their previous episodic headaches.

In contrast, identifying chronic tension-type headache is more straightforward, essentially mirroring the criteria for episodic tension-type headache with the exception of frequency and duration (15 or more days per month and duration of hours to continuous, respectively). Other CDH syndromes have had a relatively stable history in the ICHD Classification system. Each of these entities will be discussed in detail later on in this chapter and elsewhere in the text. An additional classification is in wide use and will be elaborated here: identification of CDH in terms of the presence or absence of medication overuse.

This is critical as it may influence the patient's response to treatment, regardless of other CDH diagnoses.

Medication overuse headache (MOH)

MOH is currently the most common cause of CDH in the industrialized countries. MOH is a CDH that has developed in association with increasing use of acute (rescue) medications either in monotherapy or polypharmacy in patients with an underlying headache disorder or a family history of headache disorder. [5] While still controversial, it appears that MOH does not occur in the absence of an underlying primary headache disorder in the patient or family. Studies looking at daily medication use in patients with GI, low back, and rheumatologic pain have not demonstrated the development of CDH with chronic medication use unless they also have a history of primary headache disorder.

While the reasons for the unique response to daily use of acute (rescue) medicines in headache patients is still the subject of much research and speculation, the phenomenon has significant treatment implications. Patients with MOH tend not to respond to preventives (OnobotulinumtoxinA may be an exception), [6] and the rescue medications themselves become increasingly less effective over time. Moreover, the only long-term effective treatment is cessation of the overuse, and if overuse is not identified there will not be a positive outcome.

Epidemiology

For a detailed discussion of the epidemiology of chronic and other headaches, please see Dr. Lipton's chapter in this volume. For CDH, the overall incidence across the USA, Europe and Asia hovers around 4%. [7] Each year, approximately 2.5% of patients with episodic migraine transform to chronic migraine. About half of the CDH patients have TM and approximately one-third of these patients have MOH. In headache clinics in the United States, 50% to 80% of patients present with CDH and 85% of these have TM. Eighty percent of these transformed migraine patients have MOH. [8] Moreover, patients with CDH are approximately three times more disabled than patients with episodic migraine. Between 1% and 2% of this population has MOH. However methodological variability yields a range from 1.3% in a Chinese study to 6% in a study from Brazil. A study in the late 1980s suggests 10% of patients seen at a headache center meet criteria for MOH; however, many headache specialists today report that 60% of the patients they see present with CDH, and most of those have MOH as well. [9] Rapoport and Bigal report a survey of primary care physicians who identified MOH as the third most common cause of headache in their practices. [10] Among adolescents, the prevalence appears to be slightly less for CDH, at 3%, but the incidence of MOH is dramatically greater at more than 50%. [11]

Pathophysiology

The process by which episodic headaches chronify and the pathophysiology of MOH are incompletely understood. A central issue with respect to MOH and its role in chronification is the observation that CDH does not develop in the treatment of other pain syndromes with the same medications that result in chronification for those with headache. This is first noted by Lance in the late 1980s among arthritis patients using daily analgesics. In 2003, Scher reports that about 3% of episodic headache patients chronify each year, and she identifies medication overuse and headache frequency at baseline as most predictive of chronification. [12] In headache centers, the percentage of patients with episodic headaches that become chronic is even higher, at 14%. [13]

This suggests that the predisposition to medication overuse is linked to the pathophysiology of headache, probably on a genetic basis. [14] Headache may have features that are unique in terms of response to medication and perhaps broader treatment strategies as well. Specifically, it appears that the treatment strategies applied to other chronic pain syndromes (CRPS, low back pain, inflammatory syndromes) may not be appropriate in CDH.

There is some suggestion in the literature that MOH is mediated through specific serotonergic pathways. Of particular interest is the 5-HT2A receptor, which has been identified to play a significant role both in migraine prevention and in medication overuse. The 5-HT2A receptor is pro-nociceptive and when up-regulation occurs through medication overuse, this becomes an important step in the process of cortical hyper-excitation and nociceptive facilitation. [15]

Almost 10 years ago, it was demonstrated that chronic exposure to triptans results in a down-regulation of receptors in the trigeminal ganglion and decreased synthesis of serotonin in the dorsal raphe. [16] More recently, central sensitization in MOH is shown to involve cerebral supraspinal structures with an increase in serotonin turnover and is demonstrated in patients overusing medication, regardless of the class. [17] Other studies show genetic links between MOH and CTTH and migraine. [18]

Central sensitization appears to play a major role in distinguishing episodic from chronic headache. [19] There are good animal models for pain, cortical spreading depression, and other mechanisms operating in CHD. [20] Both facilitation of pain processing and decreased pain thresholds are demonstrated in MOH. [21] These electrophysiologic studies are supported and amplified by functional imaging studies that demonstrate increased levels of hypometabolism in patients overusing combination analgesics. [22]

In addition to altered physiology unique to patients with primary headache, it appears that behavioral reinforcement and the behavioral and physical withdrawal symptoms, which are part of normal physiology, play a role in MOH. It is confusing to patients and physicians when medications that initially relieve the headache become less effective when overused. The most common medications in this regard are caffeine, barbiturates and opioids, but other classes, including triptans, analgesics, and muscle relaxants are also implicated in overuse. Even over-the- counter agents have both physical and "psychologic" dependency issues. [23] For example, the main metabolite of carisoprodol is meprobamate, and many popular over-the-counter headache relievers contain caffeine.

While the pathophysiology remains to be fully understood, the phenomenology seems clear. Central sensitization is key, and may result from over-activation of nociceptive pathways. It is possible that there is a direct effect of medication on the brain's ability to inhibit pain, possibly through alterations in the serotonin system. Genetic studies increasingly suggest that there are cellular changes in patients with MOH that are not seen in patients without a predisposition to headache. There is some evidence for structural changes in the periaqueductal gray matter and other brainstem centers [24] and in the cortex. [25] There is also emerging data that the immune system may be involved beyond simple inflammation, [26] as well as endocrine function. [27]

Other risk factors are identified and may provide insight into the process of chronification. Low socio-economic status is shown in several studies to increase the likelihood of chronification. This may reflect decreased access to healthcare, lower education, limited financial resources, or a different stress pattern. Obesity [28] and a history of abuse [29] are associated with greater risk. Head and neck injury are reported to increase risk for CDH, Taken together, these data suggest a significant environmental (and modifiable) contribution to chronification. When combined with genetic and pharmacologic evidence, it appears that CDH in general and MOH specifically reflect a combination of circumstances resulting in chronic pain and increasingly less effective treatment results.

Clinical presentation of CDH and MOH

In general, CDH presents as any head pain that occurs frequently. It can be mild, moderate, or severe. It can be present continuously or at a particular time during the day. It can be short lasting, only seconds, often multiple times throughout the day, or can continue for hours without respite. The distinguishing features of the various CDHs are mentioned above, and are discussed in detail elsewhere in this volume.

MOH, in contrast, has a typical presentation that can be recognized along with other primary headache types. For example, it is common to see both "Chronic migraine" and MOH diagnosed, or "Migraine without aura" and MOH. There are certain characteristics often seen in MOH that are not necessarily part of the underlying primary headache. It can be difficult to diagnose the underlying headache when a patient has MOH. Sometimes this can be accomplished through a careful history of the headache presentation prior to becoming chronic and daily, or before medication use became frequent. Without a careful interview, the underlying headache can be lost in the MOH presentation.

The usual story in MOH is an episodic headache that becomes increasingly frequent over time, requiring a rescue or acute medicine most days. Typically, MOH is not a severe headache. It is mild to moderate, often present on awakening, and somewhat relieved (although usually only partially) by taking a dose of the offending medicine. Often superimposed on this chronic, low-grade headache, patients experience more severe headaches from time to time, and these more severe headaches are becoming unresponsive to rescue medications.

MOH typically has features of both migraine and tension-type headache. Low-grade nausea is often present, particularly if the offending agent has GI issues as a side effect. MOH patients complain of sensitivity to light, sound, or smell in varying degrees, particularly if this is a component of their underlying headache. Cutaneous allodynia is often a prominent feature in MOH, and while present in some patients with episodic headache, it is often more prominent in MOH. In addition to the migrainous features, MOH patients often lose the lateralization of their headaches, but report it during the occasional severe headaches. MOH patients often report neck tightness and stiffness with their daily headaches as well.

Because MOH presents with features of both migraine without aura and tension-type headache, it can easily be mistaken for transformed migraine or chronic tension-type headache. When this presentation is placed in the context of a careful medication history, the diagnosis becomes apparent. It is best to address both the MOH and the underlying primary headache, but sometimes this is not possible until the MOH is treated, revealing the nature of the episodic underlying headache.

When discussing MOH with patients, it is helpful to understand when medication is used. While it is best to treat episodic headache early with the appropriate medication, that becomes increasingly difficult as headache frequency increases. Many headache specialists suggest pre-treating with medication when a patient anticipates a situation that will likely trigger a headache (such as a plane flight, menstrual period, or day in the sun). This may become a problem for patients who slip into anticipatory behaviors and take medication in order to avoid a headache. This may be a fear response and not rational management. It is important to provide patients with guidelines for management of episodic headache in order to prevent the development of MOH.

As primary headaches are usually a chronic condition, there is a bidirectional movement from infrequent headache to low frequency, high frequency and chronic daily headache. The risk of increasing frequency and MOH is always present, but that the trend can be reversed. While the issue of the progressive nature of headache (migraine in particular) is still debated, most experts agree that there is significant reversibility from the CDH state to the episodic state with cessation of medication overuse. [30,31]

Treatment

Treatment strategies depend on the offending agent, frequency of use, underlying primary headache, comorbidities, social, and financial circumstances. It is essential to address each of these elements in order to maximize the likelihood of a good outcome. Introducing a treatment strategy for MOH should not be done abruptly. Patients who enter into treatment for MOH without an appropriate "buy in" period, during which the patient works toward creating a non medication-centered lifestyle, tend to fail. Treatment of MOH can be difficult and is best accomplished in a multi-disciplinary setting where pain psychologist, headache specialist, physical therapist, pharmacist, nutritionist, and nurse educator work together. [32]

The offending agents must be identified. These need not be prescription medicines. Combination over-the-counter analgesics, particularly those containing caffeine, are among the most difficult agents to withdraw. Surprisingly, physicians often fail to query the use of non-prescription and alternative substances. When the agent is an opioid or a barbiturate-containing compound, it is often necessary to move from a short-acting formulation to a long-acting formulation and taper slowly, or to admit the patient and manage withdrawal in the hospital setting. In either circumstance, it is a challenge to manage the pain during this period, so it is critical to have a support system and rescue plan in place before embarking on the withdrawal.

Frequency of use can also be a challenge. Many patients take their medicines "only when necessary" and actually have little concept of their average daily intake. Patients often underestimate (hoping to communicate that things are not that bad) or over-estimate (in hopes that the withdrawal schedule will be more tolerable). For this reason, it is helpful to have patients record their medication intake for at least a few weeks prior to commencing a withdrawal program. For example, if a patient overestimates the amount of daily butalbital being consumed, the conversion to phenobarbital can be greatly overestimated with potentially life-threatening consequences.

One useful strategy is to convert the patient from an "as needed" regimen to a scheduled dosing prior to admission or outpatient tapering. This has the added benefit of demonstrating to the patient the actual role the medication is playing in their headache management and will often uncover additional issues to be addressed. It is also useful to initiate a preventive therapy during the "buy-in" period. There is good evidence for topiramate in chronic migraine, [33] and onobotulinumtoxin A as noted above. Many other preventives used for episodic migraine are also prescribed for CDH, but data are lacking.

The underlying primary headache, when identified, is an important consideration in treating MOH. Remember that a patient with MOH initially suffered an underlying headache type that was not effectively managed. When the offending medications are removed, they will likely revert to the underlying headache frequency and severity. Without a plan for ongoing headache treatment, the patient will likely relapse. [34] One strategy is to begin a preventive medication prior to initiating the withdrawal process. While the preventive is unlikely to be effective until the offending medication is eliminated for some time (depending on the medication), the patient will have achieved an effective dose by the time withdrawal is complete.

A possible exception to the common wisdom that preventives are ineffective for patients in MOH may be onabotulinumtoxin A. Patients with MOH may experience a significant decrease in headache days with onobotulinumtoxin A despite continued over-use of rescue medication. [35] The choice of preventive medication is based on the underlying primary headache, the side effect profile of the preventive, and the comorbidities of the individual patients. There is no one preventive that is felt to be universally superior to any other, but each has advantages in the proper setting.

The last component of the treatment plan focuses on correcting those elements in the patient's life that led to the development of MOH. This begins with education. Many know about "rebound headache," the older but more widely recognized term for MOH. Most do not understand the behaviors that lead to MOH, such as anxiety, stress, physical deconditioning, irregular sleep, and eating behaviors. Unless these are addressed, there is little that can be done to prevent relapse. This is a reason to postpone admission or outpatient withdrawal until the patient has had an opportunity for education and time to implement the changes necessary to avoid relapse.

While overuse of rescue medicines is the immediate antecedent of MOH, it is the increasing frequency of headaches that first leads a patient into overuse. There is evidence that untreated migraine is a progressive disease, and can increase in frequency, duration, and severity. This progression is also affected by changes in internal and external environments, patient behaviors, and comorbid conditions. Moreover, there is strong evidence to suggest that not all overused medications are equivalent in their impact on headache frequency. For example, it appears that NSAIDs and triptans are less likely to cause MOH compared with opioids or barbiturate-containing compounds. There is also increasing evidence that the psychoactive properties of agents can lead to overuse. Given a patient's premorbid psychiatric conditions, there is a tendency to overuse specific medications. Patients with dysphoria are often paired with opioids, while patients with an underlying anxiety disorder are more susceptible to overuse of barbiturate-containing compounds such as butalbital/caffeine/analgesics. Patients with depression may be more likely to overuse caffeine. [36] While this literature is nascent and requires the validation and confirmation of additional study, it suggests a rich area for both research and clinical application.

For the migraineur battling increasing headaches, and for the patient with MOH, it is essential to identify modifiable elements that can reverse, retard, or prevent this progression. Most headache specialists focus on four areas as modifiable and high yielding in patients with CDH and MOH. Three of these areas are related to normal life rituals: sleep patterns, eating habits, and exercise. The fourth is stress management, more difficult to regularize due to the unpredictability of stressors.

Sleep has long been recognized as a restorative process essential to good health. Among migraineurs and other primary headache patients, sleep (either too much or too little) is a frequent trigger. Shift workers, who tend to log the same ratio of sleep time to waking time per 24 hours but vary the timing of sleep, often experience worsening headaches. It is best for those with headaches to maintain a regular sleep cycle and practice good sleep hygiene. Medications that are being overused interfere with this patterned behavior and further complicate the picture. Nonetheless, before patients undertake withdrawal from medications they are overusing, they must regularize their sleep schedule, avoid naps, eating or watching television in bed, and spending time in bed outside of their scheduled sleep time. How well the patient modifies this behavior is often a good indicator for overall success in treating MOH.

Eating behaviors are another critical element in treating MOH. Headache associated with fasting, overeating, or eating specific foods has been a part of the headache literature for hundreds of years. While there is no scientifically validated headache diet, nor are there "universal" food triggers, many patients believe that ingestion of specific foods can trigger a headache. Recent studies have suggested that IgG testing for certain foods may have validity in structuring individual diets. The timing of meals is more widely influencing patients with migraine. While this is difficult to demonstrate in a controlled trial, there is a general perception that those who eat their meals on a regular schedule and remain fairly consistent in their diet do better than those with inconsistent dietary behaviors.

Exercise is the third essential element in modifying the behavior of patients who experience MOH or CDH. Exertion can be problematic as many with chronic pain find that exercise worsens their pain. This is particularly true for migraineurs. There is a vicious cycle involving headache, lack of exercise, declining conditioning, dropping endorphin levels, and increasing headache. Breaking this cycle can be difficult, although necessary to initiate the recovery process and regain health. Aerobic exercise is currently viewed as the most important physical activity to promote for patients with MOH or CDH. Often, they will need to start slowly and consistently build their tolerance to the point where they are getting a minimum of 20 minutes of aerobic exercise daily. Many note that their headache worsens during or after exercise, affording them the opportunity to stop just before they would normally experience the onset of pain. Another useful strategy, depending upon which medications is overused, is to pretreat with a non-steroidal antiinflammatory agent prior to exercise.

Stress management is often a critical component in worsening headaches and in MOH. Every patient who has CDH or MOH should be evaluated by a neuropsychologist or pain psychologist. While not every patient will require an MMPI and formal cognitive testing, some assessment of the patient's coping skills, home and work situation, support and relationships, and history of abuse is critical. This assessment can determine the appropriate behavioral treatments that will help prevent relapse into MOH.

Whether the above strategies are best implemented as an out-patient, [37] or as an in-patient, [38] it is clear that simply stopping the offending medication is not a sole and sufficient solution. [39]

Prognosis

Several outcome studies have evaluated success rates after stopping medication overuse as well as assessing recurrence rates as far out as 4 to 6 years. Additionally, analysis of risk factors for relapse is considered in various settings. Most studies define success as a 50% decrease in headache days per month. Diener *et al.* looks at 17 studies with a combined population of 1101 patients and reports a success rate of 72.4% at 1 to 6 months. These findings are largely consistent with others studies ranging up to 3 years. Longer-term studies are available, out to 6 years revealing a decrease in success rates to the 50% range. It is difficult to interpret these reports, since different centers use different inclusion/exclusion criteria and their approaches to treatment and follow-up vary. [40]

Recently, Manack and colleagues performed an analysis of those patients in the American Migraine Prevalence and Prevention (AMPP) study to characterize which patients are likely to remit from chronic to episodic migraine over a period of three years. [41] In their analysis, only one-quarter of chronic migraineurs remit for 2 years. A higher headache frequency and the presence of allodynia are the best predictors of a negative response. Interestingly, they find that other risk factors for developing chronic migraine are not predictive of remission. These include depression, obesity, and the presence of MOH.

Another observation is that the use of a preventive medication does not predict a better outcome. This finding follows several studies suggesting modest, but statistically significant decrease in headache days with gabapentin, topiramate, and onobotulinumtoxin A. [42]

With respect to relapse risk factors, the results are inconclusive due to procedural variability. However, several groups report that relapse is higher among patients with tension-type headache or mixed tension/migraine headaches. [43] There is controversy about the prognostic importance of the duration of medication overuse. The question of whether overuse of specific medications predicts relapse rates remains unanswered. Clinical experience suggests that triptan overuse has a better outcome after treatment than overuse of opioids or barbiturates, but hard data is scarce. [44]

Continued follow-up is the best predictor of positive outcome after successful treatment of MOH. The fear of a headache brought on by a suspected trigger (impending stress, inability to fall asleep), increases the likelihood of relapse. Therefore, it is important to reinforce the lifestyle changes and rescue strategies that were developed and implemented to treat the patient's MOH.

Conclusions

Whether headache is episodic or chronic, the result of the natural evolution of the disease, or through overuse of medication, the impact on the individual, their family, work and the economy is significant. Through the identification and modification of risk factors, education in lifestyle, treatment strategy and the nature of the disease, as well as the development of improved pharmacologic approaches, the impact of headache can be modified.

The current understanding is that chronic migraine represents a different pathophysiology from episodic migraine. There are enduring changes in the brains of patients with chronic migraine that are not seen, even ictally, in the brains of episodic migraineurs. The process by which chronification occurs is not well understood. Episodic headache is most effectively treated with acute medications. The best indication as a clinical marker of chronification is baseline headache frequency, which should be carefully monitored in episodic headache patients. There are identifiable risk factors, which help define those patients at greatest risk for chronification.

Once a patient has transformed to chronic daily headache, treatment strategies must change from reliance on rescue medication and lifestyle modification to a regimen that provides real-time pain relief while avoiding MOH and shifting the patient's headache frequency back toward the episodic form.

MOH remains the single most common factor in the transformation of episodic headache to chronic headache, and is the default diagnosis when patients present with CDH. [10] The diagnosis is obtained through a careful history and candid interview with the patient, followed by education and the development of a strategy to withdraw the offending medications. Depending upon the medication, dose, and individual patient factors, withdrawal can be complex. In almost every case it is associated with a transient exacerbation of pain. It is a common belief that preventive (and rescue/abortive) medications are ineffective during MOH. This has recently been challenged by data from onobotulinumtoxinA studies suggesting a modest decrease in headache days despite MOH. [45] Most headache specialists initiate preventive medication in anticipation of withdrawal of overused medication. Long-term strategies to revert chronic headache to an episodic occurrence include biobehavioral, lifestyle, and integrative approaches in addition to medication and education.

CDH is a contributor to suffering and economic burden worldwide. Treatment is a time-consuming, often expensive process that rarely offers a linear regression from chronic to episodic headache. As with episodic headache, careful diagnosis, elimination of the possibility of secondary headache (including MOH), and a multidisciplinary team approach to management represent the best hope for improvement for patients and the most rewarding experience for physicians.

Further reading

- Bigal MD, Rapoport AM, Sheftell FD, Tepper SJ, Lipton RB. Trasnsformed migraine and medication overuse in a tertiary headache center – clinical characteristics and treatment outcomes. *Cephalalgia*. 2004; **24**: 483–90.
- Couch JR, Lipton RB, Stewart WF, Scher AI. Head or neck injury increases the risk of chronic daily headache – a population-based study. *Neurology* 2007; **69**: 1169–77.
- Cupini LM, Calabresi P. Medication-overuse headache: pathophysiological insights. *J Headache Pain* 2005; **6**: 199–202.
- Ferrari A, Leone S, Vergoni AV, *et al.* Similarities and differences between chronic migraine and episodic migraine. *Headache* 2007; **47**: 65–72.
- Gaul C, van Doorn C, Webering N, *et al.* Clinical outcome of a headache-specific multidisciplinary treatment program and adherence to treatment recommendations in a tertiary headache center: an observational study. *J Headache Pain* 2011; **12**: 475–83.
- Halker, RB, Hastriter EV, Dodick DW. Chronic daily headache: an evidence-based and systematic approach to a challenging problem. *Neurology* 2011; **76**;S37.
- Moschiano F, D'Amico D, Schieroni F, Bussone G. Neurobiology of chronic migraine. *Neurol Sci* 2003; **24**: S94–6.
- Nicholson RA. Chronic headache: the role of the psychologist. *Curr Pain Headache Rep* 2010; **14**: 47–54.

References

[1] Boes CJ, Capobianco DJ. Chronic migraine and medication-overuse headache through the ages. *Cephalalgia*. 2005; **25**: 378–90.

[2] Bigal ME, Serrano D, Buse D, Scher A, Stewart WF, Lipton RB. Acute migraine medications and evolution

from episodic to chronic migraine: a longitudinal population-based study. *Headache*. 2008; **48**: 1157–68.

[3] Diener, H-C, Katsarava Z, Limmroth Headache attributed to a substance or its withdrawal, in *Handbook of Clinical Neurology*, Vol 97 (3rd series) G Nappi, MA, Moskowitz, eds, *Headache*, Elsevier B.V, 2011

[4] Oleson J, Bousser MF, Diener HC, *et al*. Headache Classification Committee. New appendix criteria open for a broader concept of chronic migraine. *Cephalalgia* 2006; **26**: 742–6.

[5] Cupini LM, Sarchielli P, Calabresi P Medication overuse headache: neurobiological, behavioural and therapeutic aspects. *Pain*. 2010; **150**: 222–4. Epub 2010 May 23,

[6] Dodick DW, Turkel CC, Brin MF, *et al*. Onabotulinumtoxin A for treatment of chronic migraine: pooled results from the double blind, randomized, placebo-controlled phases of the PREEMPT clinical program. *Headache* 2010; **50**: 921–36.

[7] Dowson AJ, Dodick DW, Limmroth V. Medication overuse headache in patients with primary headache disorders: epidemiology, management and pathogenesis. *CNS Drugs* 2005; **19**: 483–97.

[8] Bigal ME, Lipton RB. Excessive acute migraine medication use and migraine progression. *Neurology* 2008; **71**: 1821–8.

[9] Katsarava Z, Buse DC, Manack AN, Lipton, RB. Defining the differences between episodic migraine and chronic migraine. *Curr Pain Headache Rep*, 2011. 15-DOI 10.1007/s11916-011-0233-z

[10] Rapoport AM. Medication overuse headache: awareness, detection and treatment. *CNS Drugs* 2008; **22**;995–1002.

[11] Seshia SS. Chronic daily headaches in children and adolescents. *Curr Pain Headache Rep*, 2011. DOI 10.1007/s11916-011-0228-9

[12] Scher AI, Lipton RB, Stewart W, Risk factors for chronic daily headache. *Curr Pain Headache Rep* 2002; **6**: 486–91.

[13] Bigal ME, Serrano D, Reed M, Lipton RB. Chronic migraine in the population: burden diagnosis and satisfaction with treatment. *Neurology* 2008; **71**: 559–66.

[14] Hershey AD, Burdine D, Kabbouche MA, Powers SW. Genomic expression patterns in medication overuse headaches *Cephalalgia* 2011; **31**: 161–71.

[15] Supornsilpchai V, Legrand SM, Srikiat khachom A, *et al*. Involvement of pro-nociceptive 5-HT2A receptor in the pathogenesis of medication overuse headache. *Headache* 2010; **50**: 85–97.

[16] Meng ID, Dodick D, Ossipov MH, Porreca F. Pathophysiology of medication overuse headache: insights and hypotheses from preclinical studies. *Cephalalgia* 2011; **31**: 851–60.

[17] Ayzenberg I, Obermann M, Nyhuis P, *et al*, Central sensitization of the trigeminal and somatic nociceptive systems in medication overuse headache mainly involves cerebral supraspinal structures. *Cephalalgia* 2006; **26**: 1106–14.

[18] Di Lorenzo C, Sances G, Dilorenzo G, *et al*. The wolframin His611Arg polymorphism influences medication overuse headache. *Neurosci Lett* 2007; **424**: 179–84.

[19] Boes CJ, Black DF, Dodick DW. Pathophysiology and management of transformed migraine and medication overuse headache. *Semin Neurol*, 2006; **226**: 232–41.

[20] Bongsebandhu-phubhakdi S, Srikiatkhachorn A. Pathophysiology of medication overuse headache: implications from animal studies. *Curr Pain Headache Rep*, 2011. DOI 10.1007/s11916-011-1234-y

[21] Curra A, Coppola G, Gorini M, *et al*. Drug-induced changes in cortical inhibition in medication overuse headache. *Cephalalgia* 2011; **31**: 1282–90.

[22] Ferraro S, Grazzi L, Mandelli ML, *et al*. Pain processing in medication overuse headache: a functional magnetic resonance imaging study. *Pain Med* 2012; **13**: 255–62.

[23] Garza I, Schwedt, TJ. Diagnosis and management of chronic daily headache. *Semin Neurol* 2010; **309**: 154–66.

[24] Aurora SK, Kulthia A, Barrodale PM. Mechanism of chronic migraine. *Curr Pain Headache Rep*, 2011. 15–57–63 DOI 10.1007/s11916-010-0165-

[25] Fumal A, Laureys S, DiClement L, *et al*. Orbitofrontal cortex involvement in chronic analgesic-overuse headache evolving from episodic migraine. *Brain* 2006; **129**: 543–50.

[26] Forcelini CM, Danata DC, Luz C, *et al*. Analysis of leukocytes in medication – overuse headache, chronic migraine and episodic migraine. *Headache* 2011: **51**: 1228–38.

[27] Rainero I, Ferrero M, Rubino E, *et al*. Endocrine function is altered in chronic migraine patients with medication overuse. *Headache* 2006; **46**: 597–603.

[28] Bigal ME, Rapoport AM. Obesity and chronic daily headache. *Curr Pain Headache Rep*, 2011. DOI 10.1007/s11916-011-0232-0

[29] Tietjen GE, Brandes JL, Peterlin BL, *et al*. Childhood maltreatment and migraine (part II), Emotional abuse as a risk factor for headache chronification. *Headache* 2010; **50**: 32–41.

[30] Reija G, Granato A, Bratina A, Antonello RM, Zorzon M. Outcome of medication overuse headache after

abrupt in-patient withdrawal. *Cephalalgia*. 2006; **26**: 589–95.

[31] Rizzoli P, Loder EW. Tolerance to the beneficial effects of prophylactic migraine drugs: a systematic review of causes and mechanisms. *Headache* 2011; Se**051**: 1323–35.

[32] Gaul C, Visscher CM, Bhola R, *et al.* Team players against headache: multidisciplinary treatment of primary headaches and medication overuse headache. *Headache Pain* 2011; **12**: 511–19.

[33] Diener HC, Bussone G, Van Oene JC, Lahave M, Schwalen S, Goadsby PJ. TOMPAT-MIG-201 (TOP-CHROME) Study Group. Topiramate reduces headache days in chronic migraine: a randomized, double-blind, placebo-controlled study. *Cephalalgia* 2007; **27**: 814–23.

[34] Bigal ME, Sheftell FD, Tepper SJ Rapoport AM. Discontinuation of medication overuse in headache patients: recovery of therapeutic responsiveness. *Cephalalgia* 2007; **27**: 598.

[35] Gerwin R. Treatment of chronic migraine headache with Onabotulinumtoxin A. *Curr Pain Headache Rep* 2011; **15**: 336–8.

[36] Radat F, Grach C, Swendesen JD, *et al.* Psychiatric comorbidity in the evolution from migraine to medication overuse. *Cephalalgia* 2005; **25**: 519–22.

[37] Krymchantowski AV, Moreira PF. Out-patient detoxification in chronic migraine: comparison of strategies. *Cephalalgia* 2003; **23**: 982–93.

[38] Trucco M, Meineri P, Ruiz L, Gionco M. Medication overuse headache: withdrawal and prophylactic therapeutic regimen *Headache* 2010; **50**: 989–99.

[39] Zeeberg P, Olesen J, Jensen R. Discontinuation of medication overuse in headache patients: recovery of therapeutic responsiveness. *Cephalalgia* 2006; **26**: 1192–8.

[40] Hagen K, Jensen R, Bøe MG, Stovner LJ. Medication overuse headache: a critical review of endpoints in recent follow-up studies. *J Headache Pain* 2010; **11**: 373–7.

[41] Manack A, Buse DC, Serrano D, Turkel CC, Lipton, RB. Rates, predictors, and consequences of remission from chronic migraine to episodic migraine. *Neurology* 2011; **76**: 711–18.

[42] Meskuna CA, Tepper SJ, Rapoport AM, Sheftell FD, Bigal ME. Medications associated with probable medication overuse headache reported in a tertiary care headache center over a 15-year period. *Headache* 2006; **46**: 766–72.

[43] Ashina S, Lyngberg A, Jensen R. Headache characteristics and chronification of migraine and tension-type headache: a population-based study. *Cephalalgia* 2010; **30**: 943–52.

[44] Negro A, Martelletti P. J Chronic migraine plus medication overuse headache: two entities or not. *Headache Pain* 2011; **12**: 593–601.

[45] Aurora SK, Dodick DW, Turkel CC, *et al.* Onabotulinumtoxin A for treatment of chronic migraine: results from the double-blind, randomized placebe controlled phase of the PREEMPT 1 trial. *Cephalalgia* 2010; **30**: 793–803.

Chapter 10

Stress management

Nomita Sonty

Stress management

The rationale for stress management approaches in treating headache disorders is based on the observation that the way individuals cope with everyday stresses can precipitate, exacerbate, or maintain headaches and increase headache-related disability and distress. Individuals learn conditioned perceptual and response styles to stressful events that create habitual patterns of coping. In some instances these coping patterns ameliorate headaches while in others they aggravate them. As stress is dynamic and constantly changing, the demands placed on the individual also change in response. The constant appraisal and reappraisal of these demands is matched by changes in coping, sometimes resulting in the development of avoidant or maladaptive coping mechanisms. This cycle of pain and avoidance, along with catastrophization often acquired through operant conditioning, lays the foundation for anticipatory anxiety associated with headaches. These "conditioned" headaches can themselves become stressors and lead to the chronification of pain. [1] Furthermore, comorbidities such as depression and anxiety interact to increase the complexity of headache presentation and its management, and are often involved in transforming episodic headaches into chronic ones. [2] Research has shown that the contributing role of stress in the onset and maintenance of headache disorders is determined by a number of factors, [3] including physiological, psychological, and environmental. Overall, the unsuccessful behavioral adaptation subsequently impacts the degree of suffering experienced and the quality of life.

As stress is a part of an individual's interaction with the environment, an understanding of generic and individual-specific stressors in triggering headaches is an important part of stress management. Broadly speaking, processes that create an interaction between headaches and stress include: (1) the individual's predisposition and physiologically reactivity to the effects of stress; and (2) an individual's thoughts and beliefs, which influence how one understands and responds to stress. The Transactional Model of Lazarus and Folkman suggests that the cognitive processes involved in the perception of stress include:

(1) **Primary appraisal**, which is the evaluation of the extent of perceived threat, harm, or challenge.
(2) **Secondary appraisal** is the evaluation of how controllable a situation is and what coping resources are available. This process includes acquired beliefs and automatic thoughts that occur in anticipation of pain or in response to it.
(3) **Cognitive and behavioral efforts**, which are needed to meet both the extrinsic and intrinsic demands of the stressors. [4]

Stress is defined as a transaction between an actual or perceived aversive stimuli and the individual's response to it. [5] Therefore, it is a physiological, biochemical, and psychological response to an "unconditioned stimuli" [6] which results in the aggravation of chronic pain conditions including headaches. This chapter reviews the goals of stress management, when to use stress management, and stress management techniques to treat headache disorders. The techniques discussed include relaxation therapy (RT), biofeedback, cognitive behavior therapy (CBT), coping skills and support groups. Two of the evidence-based complementary and alternative medicine (CAM) approaches, yoga and acupuncture, are also discussed as they are often used in comprehensive headache management.

The Neuropsychiatry of Headache, ed. Mark W. Green and Philip R. Muskin. Published by Cambridge University Press.

Table 10.1. US Headache Consortium grading system of nonpharmacological research

Grade A: multiple well-designed randomized clinical trials, which yielded a consistent pattern of findings.
Grade B: some evidence from randomized clinical trials, but scientific support was not optimal.
Grade C: US Headache Consortium committee arrived at a consensus in the absence of relevant randomized controlled trials.

Many of the stress management techniques are borrowed from behavioral medicine, a field in which there is strong emphasis on the development of evidence-based therapies for the treatment of headaches. In an effort to assess the evidence of nonpharmacological approaches available for headache management and make suitable recommendations, the US Headache Consortium developed a grading system based on the quality of research data available (Table 10.1).

The US Headache Consortium consensus report, based on this grading system, notes that individual behavioral therapies including relaxation, biofeedback, and CBT are consistently found to be efficacious in ameliorating headaches, particularly migraines. [7] For migraine headaches, the use of combined therapies consisting of thermal feedback, relaxation therapy, electromyographic biofeedback, and CBT have "Grade A" evidence. There is "Grade B" evidence for the prevention of headaches using combined pharmacotherapy and behavioral therapies. [8,9]

Guidelines for the use of stress management interventions

Stress management approaches are used as a sole treatment, as adjunctive to pharmacological management, or as a replacement to pharmacotherapy. [10] A combination approach of medication and nonpharmacological techniques has been shown to be more effective than any one alone. [11] The efficacy of stress management techniques has been shown to equal pharmacotherapy in some instances. Moreover, stress management techniques do not have the side effects often associated with medications and pharmacological interventions. Such techniques can be relatively cost-effective and have been shown to demonstrate sustained benefit in headache management for up to 7 years. [12]

The US Headache Consortium developed evidence-based and clinically relevant guidelines for the use of behavioral and physical treatments under the following conditions [13]:

(a) When patients prefer nonpharmacological interventions.
(b) When patients are unable to tolerate certain pharmacological treatments.
(c) When there are contraindications for specific pharmacological treatments in the management of the patient.
(d) When patients respond poorly to pharmacological treatments including experiencing significant side effects.
(e) When patients are pregnant, planning pregnancy, or nursing.
(f) When the overuse of analgesics results in rebound headaches.
(g) When patients report significant stress or limited coping skills.

Furthermore, the use of nonpharmacological and stress management approaches is supported for the following [14]:

(a) Patients who are significantly disabled by their headaches.
(b) Patients who have comorbid mood disorders.
(c) Patients who overuse medications.
(d) Patients who prefer to have nonpharmacological headache management.
(e) Patients who have difficulty in identifying and managing stress triggers.

Treatment goals in stress management interventions

Several behavioral treatments have been used for the management of recurrent headaches. The most frequently employed interventions fall into three broad categories: relaxation therapy, biofeedback training (often administered in conjunction with relaxation therapy), and cognitive-behavior (or stress-management) therapy. Behavioral interventions are used also to decrease associated symptoms of sleep disturbance, psychological distress, suffering, and pain-related disability, and to improve overall quality of life. These stress management approaches also focus on improving patients' coping skills by:

(1) Decreasing negative cognitions including catastrophic thinking.
(2) Decreasing a sense of helplessness resulting from chronic, progressive, and unmanageable headaches.
(3) Learning a proactive and preventive approach to managing headaches by identifying and managing stressors, making necessary lifestyle changes, acquiring new coping skills, and generalizing them to other stressors.
(4) Developing a sense of self-efficacy and outcome efficacy.

Behavioral interventions are primarily prophylactic, [15] and their objectives are to decrease the frequency, duration, and intensity of headaches.

Stress management techniques

For purpose of this review, the section on stress management techniques borrows heavily from behavioral medicine.

Relaxation therapy (RT)

Relaxation therapy (RT) is an approach that helps patients gain awareness of their physiological responses and achieve a sense of tranquility [16] by gaining control over their headache-related physiological changes by lowering sympathetic arousal. [16a, 17] When RT was compared with written emotional disclosure (WED) for tension headache management, it was found that RT increased calmness and influenced pain, while WED increased negative mood and had no impact on pain. [18] As predicted, patients who were confident they could prevent and manage their headaches also believed that the factors influencing their headaches were potentially within their control. In addition, self-efficacy scores were positively associated with the use of positive psychological coping strategies to both prevent and manage headache episodes and negatively associated with anxiety. Headache severity, locus-of-control beliefs, and self-efficacy beliefs each explained the variance in headache-related disability.

There are many types of relaxation therapy, but they share some common elements including: deep breathing, progressive muscle relaxation, imagery, and awareness of breathing rate, rhythm, and volume. On average, a relaxation therapy program may consist of 10 to 12 sessions, with some variability in the number of sessions based on the complexity of the headache disorder. Patients are often taught the relaxation technique during treatment sessions and are instructed to practice it at home at least two to three times a day for about 10 to 15 minutes each time. Those patients having difficulty paying attention for this period of time are asked to start with shorter practices and increase the time gradually. Patients may be offered audiotapes or referred to commercially available CDs to assist with relaxation skill acquisition. Once patients master the skill, they also may be taught brief relaxation skills so as to continue to maintain and generalize a state of relaxation. Among the various types of relaxation training, four have been most frequently reported: progressive muscle relaxation, autogenic training, hypnosis and imagery, and meditation.

Progressive muscle relaxation (PMR)

Progressive muscle relaxation (PMR) is designed to teach patients to become aware of how their muscles feel when they are tightened versus relaxed and to label them accordingly. The process includes an introductory phase during which patients are instructed on the procedure, followed by slowly tightening and relaxing 14 muscle groups. The therapist uses a low-pitched monotonous tone when calling out the instructions. Following this step, a deepening procedure is introduced and patients are asked to relax all muscles to a count of 5. Then patients are asked to concentrate on their breath, the cool air as they inhale and the warm air as they exhale. Finally, at the end, an alerting procedure is introduced.

After patients complete PMR, they are asked to rate their experience on a 0 to 10 scale where 0 "no impact" and 10 "the most relaxed." They are also asked to report their pain levels on a 0 to 10 scale where 0 "no pain" and 10 "the worst possible pain." Patients are then given homework and instructed to practice this exercise at least twice a day. Practice allows patients to benefit from the PMR procedure by developing an enhanced sense of self-efficacy. [19]

Autogenic training (AT)

Autogenic training (AT) is a relaxation technique by which a relaxation response is elicited. It involves being seated in a comfortable position and following six exercises to make the body feel warm, heavy, and relaxed. A meta-analysis to evaluate the clinical effectiveness of AT demonstrated that medium-to-large effect sizes (ES) for pre–post comparisons of disease-specific AT effects, with the randomized clinical trials demonstrating larger effect sizes. In this study a comparison of AT with other psychological treatment mostly resulted in no effects or small negative effect sizes. AT effects on mood, cognitive performance, quality of life, and other physiological variables were larger than the main effects. Positive medium range effects of AT and of AT versus control in the meta-analysis were found for tension headache/migraine. [20]

A review of seven studies concluded that the comparative effectiveness of AT over other forms of relaxation did not support the superiority of AT over any other techniques. [21] Contrary to these findings, a prospective study over 8 months on a small sample examined the effects of Schultz-type AT on medication use and headache frequency in patients with migraines, tension headaches, and mixed headaches. Results revealed that, from very early in the AT process, headache frequencies decreased significantly in tension-type and mixed headaches with a delayed response of 3 months in migraine headaches. Decreases in headache frequencies were accompanied by decreases in consumption of migraine medications and analgesics. Despite limitations in this study, the authors concluded that Schultz-type AT is an effective therapeutic approach in the management of headache frequency and medication use. [22]

Biofeedback-assisted AT was studied in female patients with migraine headaches to examine the effect on headache activity, anxiety, and depression. Results of this randomized experimental study demonstrated a greater treatment response rate (defined as ≥ = 50% reduction in headache index) in patients with biofeedback-assisted AT as compared with the monitoring group. The results suggest that the biofeedback-assisted AT is effective for the treatment of migraine; moreover, this effect was mediated by improvement in anxiety. [23]

The efficacy of AT combined with electromyographic biofeedback (EMG) and AT combined with thermal feedback (TEMP) was examined in chronic idiopathic headaches. Findings indicated that treatment groups employing AT + TEMP produced no additional improvements over AT following the 8-week treatment program, or at follow-up over a 12-month period. However, AT + EMG produced significantly greater reductions in headache activity compared with the other treatment groups. Headache activity continued to improve over the follow-up period independent of treatment condition. These authors suggest that EMG biofeedback augments long-term clinical improvements in headache patients who undergo AT therapy. [24]

Hypnosis and imagery

Hypnosis is considered to be a state of heightened focus during which changes in awareness, sensations, and perceptions can occur. There is some controversy about whether or not the hypnotized person is in an altered state of consciousness. Hypnotic pain intervention techniques include alleviation through suggestion, alteration of the pain experience, avoidance/distraction, and awareness of the pain experience. [25] Imagery and visualization are frequently used interchangeably and generally indicate incorporation of visual images. Research has demonstrated that imagery can significantly reduce pain. [26]

Meditation

Meditation has been shown to reduce the frequency and severity of migraine headaches and improve the quality of life of migraineurs. Despite the different types of meditation there are some common elements, such as "self-observation of mental activity, attentional focus training, and cultivating an attitude that highlights process rather than content." [27] Mindfulness meditation emphasizes attentional control by focusing on various stimuli in the moment and in a non-judgmental or analytic manner. The focus of attention can be on internal stimuli such as one's breath, thoughts, and emotions, or on external stimuli such as sights and sounds. Mindfulness meditation is used as a clinical intervention in the form of mindfulness-based stress reduction and mindfulness-based cognitive therapy. Concentration meditation consists of directing attention on some intentional process such as the repetition of a word or phrase (mantra), or the breath. Transcendental meditation is a concentration technique that has demonstrated some benefits with headache disorders. Brain changes during meditation have been documented in numerous EEG and neuro-imaging studies. There is some evidence for meditation effects on endocrine, neurotransmitter, and immune system measures. The role of spiritual meditation in enhancing pain tolerance and decreasing migraine-associated symptoms was examined in a study on 83 migraine sufferers who were trained in one of the following: spiritual meditation, internally focused secular meditation, externally focused secular meditation, or muscle relaxation. Participants practiced for 20 minutes a day for 1 month. Results demonstrated that those who practiced spiritual meditation had greater decreases in the frequency of headaches, anxiety, and negative affect, as well as greater increases in pain tolerance and headache-related self-efficacy. [28]

Biofeedback

Biofeedback is a well-recognized treatment modality in the management of headache disorders and has proven to be more effective than waiting list control group and headache monitoring alone. [29] Biofeedback is defined as "the technique of using equipment (usually electronic) to reveal to human beings some of their internal physiological events, normal and abnormal, in the form of visual and auditory signals in order to teach them to manipulate these otherwise involuntary. . ..signals." [30]

Biofeedback is most useful when provided within the context of a comprehensive treatment plan. It is often used along with different forms of relaxation therapy, CBT, and other complementary and alternative methods. Treatment is initially office based; however, as patients learn to self-regulate, they can be provided with portable biofeedback equipment to practice at home and generalize their skills. These portable devices may be in the form of hand-held thermometers, or GSR or EMG devices. Typical treatment sessions are 50 minutes, once a week for about 8 to 12 weeks.

At a time when cost containment is driving health care, and insurance companies limit coverage, biofeedback may be considered an extremely costly and time-consuming treatment modality. [31] Alternative approaches to the use of biofeedback have been explored. A randomized controlled trial evaluating the efficacy of Internet-based relaxation and biofeedback training found that treatment resulted in significantly greater decrease in headache activity and headache-related disability. This improvement was sustained at follow up in 47% of participants. Medication usage was reduced by 35% in subjects in the treatment group. The authors concluded that the Internet program was more time-efficient and dropout rates were in keeping with other behavioral self-help studies. [32] Using a different model of cost containment, migraine patients were used as lay trainers to work with their fellow migraineurs in a home-based behavioral program. Results at the end of intervention revealed improvement in perceived control, but not in reduction of headache frequency. The same was noted at a 6-month follow-up. [33] The duration of a biofeedback session has been investigated. Earlier studies demonstrated that an adequate feedback response occurs within a few training sessions, and the magnitude of the response does not increase with additional training. [34,35]

Among the many types of biofeedback used for headache management, the two most frequently used are thermal biofeedback and electromyographic (EMG) biofeedback. The other types of biofeedback training less frequently used are cephalic vasomotor biofeedback, electroencephalographic biofeedback (EEG), and galvanic skin response (GSR).

Thermal biofeedback

Thermal biofeedback is a process by which finger temperature is monitored with a thermometer to assess the state of autonomic arousal. Changes in skin temperature are the result of vasoconstriction and vasodilation. Typically, a thermometer or thermistor/temperature probe is placed in contact with skin of the finger; it warms/cools in response to changes in the finger temperature. Training procedures can differ from clinic to clinic but most of them follow some general guidelines. (Table 10.2) [36]

The efficacy of biofeedback in the management of migraines and tension headaches has been well documented. [37,38] A comprehensive review of the efficacy of biofeedback in these two types of headaches was conducted by Nestoriuc and colleagues. [39] From a pool of 150 outcome studies, 94 meeting a strict, pre-defined criteria were selected for two meta-analytic studies. The meta-analytic study on migraine patients demonstrated a medium effect size for all biofeedback interventions (Fig. 10.1) and was seen to be stable over an average follow-up of 17 months. Significant improvement was noted in the frequency of migraine episodes and perceived self-efficacy (Fig. 10.2). Blood-volume–pulse feedback yielded higher effect sizes than peripheral skin temperature feedback and EMG feedback. Biofeedback in conjunction with home training was more effective than therapies without home training. [40] This result was corroborated by another meta-analysis of behavioral techniques used in the management of headaches, which showed that relaxation training resulted in a 35% to 40% reduction in the frequency of headaches. [41]

Table 10.2. General guidelines for thermal feedback training

1.	Establish targets to be achieved within the session.
2.	Determine skills to be acquired via biofeedback.
3.	Choose feedback (auditory, visual, etc.) and modality (EMG, skin temperature, etc.).
4.	Assign homework to generalize skills.
5.	Engage in periodic booster sessions as necessary.

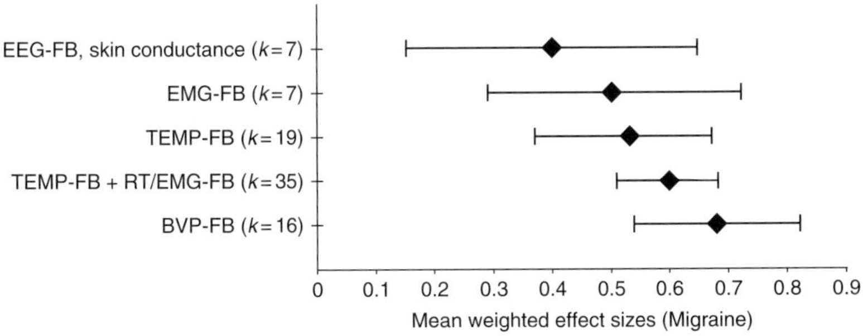

Fig. 10.1. Mean weighted effect sizes for the different feedback modalities in the treatment of migraine. Outcome is measured in headache pain. Mean effect sizes are displayed with their individual 95% confidence intervals (k = number of independent effect sizes). EEG-FB = electroencephalographic feedback, EMG/FB = electromyographic feedback, TEMP-FB = peripheral temperature feedback, RT = relaxation training, BVP-FB = blood-volume–pulse feedback. Printed with permission.

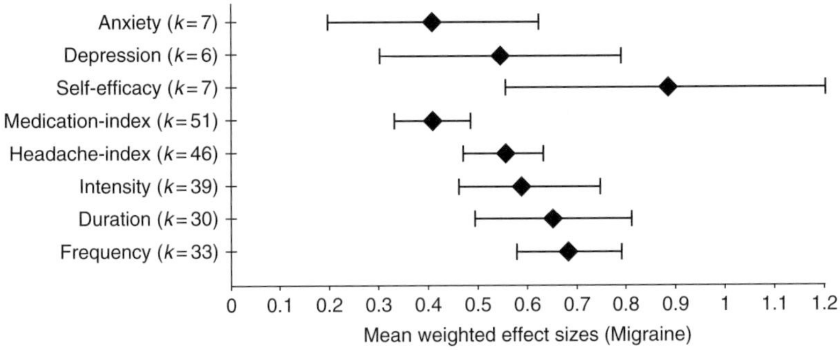

Fig. 10.2. Mean weighted effect sizes for the different outcome variables in the biofeedback treatment of migraine. Outcome is measured in headache pain over all biofeedback modalities. Mean effect sizes are displayed with their individual 95% confidence intervals (k = number of independent effect sizes) [39]. Printed with permission

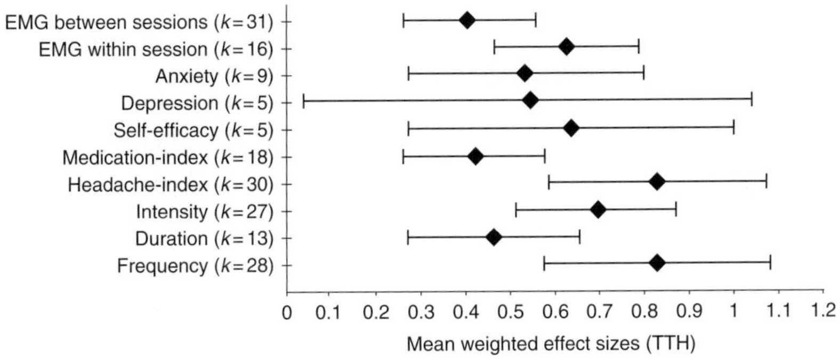

Fig. 10.3. Mean weighted effect sizes for the different outcome variables in EMG-FB for tension-type headache. Outcome is measured in headache pain. Mean effect sizes are displayed with their individual 95% confidence intervals (*k* = number of independent effect sizes). EMG = reduction in muscle tension measured in microvolt through electromyography [39]. Printed with permission.

Electromyograph (EMG) biofeedback

EMG signals are observed through the use of surface electrodes that detect muscle activity from underlying skeletal muscles. These signals, which are seen on a monitor, inform the patient about the amount of activity being detected in that muscle. EMG biofeedback is frequently used in the management of tension headaches. In a meta-analytic study evaluating the efficacy of EMG biofeedback, multidimensional outcomes and treatment moderators of biofeedback were assumed as a treatment for chronic tension-type headache. [29] Nestoriuc and colleagues found a significant medium-to-large effect size that was stable over an average follow-up period of 15 months. Improvements were noted with decreased muscle tension, frequency of headaches, self-efficacy, anxiety, depression, and analgesic medication (Fig. 10.3).

Biofeedback was found to be more effective than headache monitoring, placebo, and relaxation therapies in tension headaches. Combined biofeedback with relaxation training showed the greatest efficacy. Consistent with these findings, the effects of thermal biofeedback, biofeedback plus cognitive therapy, and "pseudomeditation" (body scanning + mental control) on headache pain were examined in a 16-week trial and resulted in a significant reduction in headache-related medication use and in the frequency and intensity of headaches. [42] Examining the effects of different stress management techniques and their effects, Lehrer *et al.* concluded that stress management techniques have specific and varying effects depending on the mechanism that they are targeting, such that EMG biofeedback worked better for tension-type headaches due to the involvement of the muscles, while thermal feedback worked better for migraine headaches due to the involvement of the autonomic system. [43]

Cognitive behavior therapy (CBT)

Cognitive behavior therapy (CBT) has been used as an adjunct in the management of various types of headaches. Its efficacy has varied, depending on the type of headache, such that in episodic migraines and chronic daily headaches CBT has shown prophylactic efficacy, while in cluster headaches it has not been as effective. [44] CBT is based on the assumption that the automatic thoughts, feelings, and behaviors exacerbate, maintain, or decrease symptoms and have a significant impact on pain. This assumption takes into consideration that, through operant learning, thoughts or behaviors that are reinforced increase while those that are ignored decrease. [4] Although it is unclear as to which components of CBT effect change, it is used extensively in pain management, and often used in conjunction with other approaches including biofeedback, relaxation exercises, hypnosis, and mindfulness. Cognitive behavior analysis assessing multiple domains including headache frequency, intensity and duration, medication use, behavioral and stress-related triggers, psychiatric status, and overall interference effects of headaches form the basis of CBT in headache management. [4,44] The development of an internal locus of control and an increased sense of self-efficacy are seen as key mediators to successful headache management. [4] Lipchik and Nash [45] elucidate some of the important self-management strategies used in headache management.

Introducing patients to CBT

(a) *Psycho-education*: In CBT psycho-education consists of explaining the biopsychosocial model of headaches, various triggers, the relationship between stress and arousal, and the concept of self-management. Some headache management programs have patients commit to treatment by signing a behavioral contract, which outlines reasonable expectations in treatment for an optimal outcome. Some patients become more anxious with detailed medical information while others need this information to feel in control. Checking with patients about what they want to know about their headache will help tailor-make the conversation specific to them. Addressing the meaning of chronicity and its impact on course and prognosis will help patients develop realistic expectations and resist engaging in self-blame or catastrophic thinking when they have a flare-up.

(b) *Clinician–patient relationship*: In CBT, the relationship between the patient and treatment provider is a collaborative one. Goals are often established together and agreed upon. It is important to help patients distinguish between wishful thinking and goals so that they can set achievable goals and have success experiences. By successive approximation the targeted goal of headache reduction can be gradually accomplished. Patients are often given homework monitoring headache and stress, maintaining a headache diary, practicing relaxation exercises, and modifying their lifestyle. Acknowledging, approximating, or completing homework is helpful in developing and maintaining new habits.

Addressing cognitions

Discussing the influence of cognitions on headaches and coping will help patients recognize the importance of their role in the maintenance and management of their headaches.

Assessing and enhancing patient's motivation for change

Motivation for change is considered an integral part of self-management of chronic pain including headaches. [46] A framework for assessing a person's readiness for engaging in new adaptive behaviors is proposed by the transtheoretical model. [47] This model suggests that a person's readiness for change can be categorized into one of five stages (Table 10.3).

Knowledge of the patient's motivation allows the clinician to understand the patient's level of commitment or ambivalence toward making the necessary change and to initiate treatment accordingly. Starting intervention at the patient's level of motivation is likely to increase the patient's active participation in treatment as well as increase adherence. [46] It is not unusual for chronic headache sufferers to develop an inflexible cognitive and behavioral style, thus keeping them entrenched in their maladaptive and symptomatic state. These patients can be argumentative, critical, and demanding. The use of motivational interviewing techniques can help clinicians navigate difficult conversations with their patients with empathy and support, and in a non-judgmental manner. [38] Clinicians can enhance treatment adherence by setting appropriate expectations and readiness-based treatment goals and by creating a therapeutic environment that is conducive to helping patients succeed. Empirically-based strategies suggested by Rains and his colleagues maybe helpful in increasing treatment compliance (Table: 10.4). [11].

Table 10.3. Stages of readiness to make change

Stage I:	Precontemplation: not recognizing the need to make change.
Stage II:	Contemplation: recognizing the need to make change but not knowing what to do.
Stage III:	Preparation: understanding the need for change and planning to take action.
Stage IV:	Action: actively involved in managing their headaches.
Stage V:	Maintenance: continuing to use skills automatically to manage headaches even after active treatment may be discontinued.

Skills acquisition

(a) Monitoring headaches, triggers, and identifying patterns
(b) Using a thought record to become aware of catastrophic thinking and replacing it with alternative noncatastrophic thoughts
(c) Using strategies to prevent or ameliorate stress and headaches
(d) Using appropriate medication including timing
(e) Establishing communication skills including assertiveness

Developing self-efficacy

Self-efficacy is the confidence that patients feel in their ability to manage their headaches. Outcome efficacy is the patient's confidence in having a successful outcome. Self-efficacy is a learned behavior that is essential to the

Table 10.4. Empirically based compliance-enhancing strategies

1. **Administrative**
   - Scheduling regular contacts of sufficient duration for complete assessment and rapport-building
   - Recalling missed appointments
   - Clinic orientation
   - Verbal and written recommendations
   - Screen for psychiatric comorbidities
   - Assess and track compliance (multimodal assessment preferred, such as interview, patient monitoring, pill counts, pharmacy records)
   - Encourage participation of key significant others
   - Assess and treat psychiatric comorbidities (e.g,, depression, anxiety)
2. **Psychoeducational**
   - Patient education by provider, staff, computer (prophylactic vs. acute, abortive, overuse consequences)
   - Printed materials for increased retention
   - Involve patient in treatment planning (elicit discussion of barriers [e.g,, cost, side effects])
   - Education on adherence and health behavior change
3. **Behavioral**
   - Simplify regimen
   - Self-monitor compliance
   - Stimulus control (medication reminder systems, cue-dose training)
   - Medication contracts
   - Enhance self-efficacy
   - Reinforcement for successful adherence
4. **Social support**
   - Provider communication/rapport skills (conducive environment, active listening, empathy, adjust language, nonverbal behavior, cultural sensitivity)
   - Collaborative therapeutic alliance (negotiated rather than dictated plan)
   - Spouse/family support

From ref [11]. Printed with permission.

success of any program, as it ensures the continued use of newly acquired skills for management of symptoms. As such, behavioral interventions focusing on self-efficacy can result in sustained improvement in headache self-efficacy and internal locus of control. [48] Higher scores on self-efficacy are associated with more frequent headache monitoring and continued practice of relaxation and stretching exercises. Strategies to acquire self-efficacy behaviors include practicing target behaviors, observing others perform target behaviors without negative consequences, verbally persuading patients to perform the target behavior, and teaching patients strategies to manage anxiety that may occur while acquiring target behaviors. [49] Patients confident in their ability to prevent and manage their headaches also believed that headache triggers were potentially within their control, used more positive psychological coping strategies, and were less anxious. [50]

Coping skills

Coping strategies of chronic headache sufferers include constantly changing cognitive and behavioral efforts to manage stressful events that they appraise as taxing on or exceeding their personal resources. [5] Patients with chronic headaches who use a restricted repertoire of coping strategies may demonstrate inflexibility and dysfunctional coping, while others who use a wider variety of strategies may demonstrate more adaptive coping. Types of coping strategies may include problem versus emotion-focused or cognitive versus behavioral. For example, catastrophizing (cognitive strategy) or avoidance (behavioral strategy) may be seen as examples of dysfunctional coping. Preferential use of these coping strategies can result in associated anxiety and depression. Thus cognitive interventions are aimed at reducing catastrophizing and the resultant avoidance. Some functional and active pain-coping strategies include problem resolution through distraction, reinterpretation or ignoring pain sensations, acceptance, exercise, and task persistence. [51] A study on 144 headache sufferers randomly assigned to one of two treatment groups: cognitive self-hypnosis (CSH) treatment or autogenic training were studied to examine: (1) whether cognitive self-hypnosis training can change appraisal and cognitive coping processes more effectively than a relaxation procedure; and (2) whether these changes in pain appraisal and cognitive coping were related to changes in pain and adjustment in the short and long term. The results indicated that patients were able to successfully change their use of coping strategies and pain appraisals. Cognitive therapy was more effective than relaxation training in changing the use of cognitive coping strategies. However, treatment effects were only related to changes in the use of coping strategies and appraisal processes and their role in pain reduction and better adjustment was inconclusive. [52]

Stress management support groups

Often, patients with conditions like chronic tension headaches or migraines find themselves withdrawing from their social networks because they feel that others may not understand their circumstances of living with pain and unpredictability. For example, cancelling plans at the last minute due to pain or fear of having pain can result in negative reactions from family and friends. This frequently results in social isolation. When stress, social support, and coping were compared in headache and non-headache groups, those with headaches reported having less social support compared with their counterparts, suggesting that interventions aimed at teaching headache sufferers to mobilize social support should be considered as key components of their comprehensive treatment plans. [53] The advantage of stress management support groups is that they provide headache sufferers the opportunity to talk about the impact of their headaches, grieve and obtain support from other people in similar circumstances.

There are many local and national organizations that offer support, each differing in what they offer. Some offer information, while others offer host meetings and yet others bring in experts to discuss the latest treatments available. With the popularity of the internet and the convenience it offers, internet-delivered stress management groups are being offered and are showing promise in treating some disorders including headaches, irritable bowel syndrome, and chronic pain. However, as this is a newer trend, the reported studies have several limitations and caution needs to be exercised in the generalization of their results. [54]

Yoga

Yoga is an ancient Indian, non-religious mind–body way of life that has components of meditation, mindfulness, breathing, and postures. It began as the "science of quieting the mind." [55] Yoga consists of eight stages: Yama, Niyama, Asana, Pratyahara, Dharana, Dhyana and Samadhi. Various forms of Hatha yoga that center on postures are the most commonly practiced in the

USA. Some practices such as Iyengar yoga incorporate props and supports, and may lend themselves more readily to people with neurologic and musculoskeletal disorders. Physiologically, yoga practice is noted to produce changes in heart rate, blood pressure, galvanic skin response, and respiratory rate. Those with headaches use mind–body therapies, including deep breathing, meditation, and yoga more frequently. Few studies document the effectiveness of these techniques in relieving headaches. A randomized clinical trial examining the effectiveness of yoga therapy compared with self-care for migraine was conducted on 72 patients with migraine without aura over a 3-month period. Significant decrease in headache frequency, severity of migraine, pain, anxiety, and medication use in the yoga group compared with the self-care group was reported. [56] Further study of this therapeutic intervention appears to be warranted. More than 50% of adults with migraines/severe headaches reporting CAM use had not discussed it with their health care provider. Correlates of CAM use among adults with migraines/severe headaches included anxiety, joint or low back pain, alcohol use, higher education, and living in the western USA. Only 4.5% of adults with migraines/severe headaches reported using CAM to specifically treat their migraines/severe headaches. [57] In a heterogenous sample of women who participated in a 3-month Iyengar yoga class and who perceived themselves to be emotionally distressed, results showed significant improvements in perceived stress, anxiety, well-being, fatigue, and depression. Those who suffered from headaches also reported marked pain relief. [58]

Acupuncture

Embedded in Chinese medicine is the discipline of acupuncture. It is based on the premise that illness is a "manifestation of an individual's constitutional makeup interacting with his life events." [59] In a randomized control trial of 401 primary care patients with chronic headaches, the effects of acupuncture on medication use, quality of life, resource use and days off sick, and the cost-effectiveness of acupuncture were examined. Patients were randomly assigned to receive up to 12 acupuncture treatments over 3 months or to a control group receiving usual care. Results demonstrated that the intervention group had a lower headache score compared with the controls, had 22 fewer days of headache per year, used 15% less medication, made 25% fewer visits to the doctors, and took 15% fewer days off sick. The study concluded that acupuncture was a cost-effective method to use for headache management with primary care patients suffering from chronic headaches including migraines. Additionally, when acupuncture was compared with topiramate in chronic migraine prophylaxis, results showed that the mean monthly headache days decreased in the acupuncture group and a significantly low adverse event rate of 6% compared with 66% in the topiramate group. [60]

Conclusions

The essence of stress management is to facilitate the physical and psychological adaptation of individuals suffering with headaches. The complexity of headache disorders warrants a comprehensive treatment approach, which addresses the many intrinsic and extrinsic factors that play a role in causation, maintenance and treatment. The transactional model highlights the interaction between the individual and the stressors explaining the individual variance in responses to adverse events. Secondary mood disorders, the conditioned response to pain as well as the development of anticipatory anxiety makes headaches more disabling.

The primary contribution of stress management to the treatment of headaches is its potential for promoting change in order to decrease primary and secondary symptoms. Under the rubric of stress management is an approach and an armamentarium of tools that are available to clinicians that will promote a reduction in symptoms and an improvement in the patient's quality of life. These tools (relaxation therapy, biofeedback, cognitive behavior therapy, coping skills) have been extensively researched, and there is evidence of their importance in headache management.

The emphasis on evidence-based techniques has resulted in the development of a grading system and guidelines for the use of non-pharmacological approaches in headache management. In addition to improve the comparability between clinical trials, the following standards are recommended by the American Headache Society:

(1) The use of a prospective baseline period of at least 1 month
(2) The use of a treatment period of at least 3 months
(3) Continuous monitoring by using a daily headache diary
(4) Use of frequency of attacks per 4 weeks as main efficacy parameter rather than headache index or other measures, and

(5) Use of 50% reduction in attack frequency compared with baseline as the criteria for individual responses.

Despite the understanding that stress in chronic headaches is a significant problem that can be well managed through a variety of adjunctive nonpharmacological treatments, we find that many headache sufferers have limited access to these treatments due to clinician access and reimbursement issues. Increasing physician awareness and making necessary changes in insurance policies will help move this issue forward. In addition, exploring novel approaches to providing stress management are recommended. More robust research on the use of Internet technology to provide biofeedback, relaxation therapies, and psychoeducational activities is needed. An examination of the cost-effectiveness of stress management techniques if offered in a group format, or through programs that involve minimal therapist contact is warranted. Preliminary findings in this area have shown that minimal contact with a therapist, either through limited clinic sessions or via the Internet can be effective. Confirmation of such evidence will result in more options for both clinicians and patients. Such innovation will require changes in policy and practice so as to provide the same high-quality care while safeguarding patient privacy.

Thus, although current research on stress management has proven efficacy using conventional approaches, more well-controlled clinical trials using newer stress management techniques and approaches are needed. In addition, as we move toward patient-centered care, treatment and research will need to consider patient treatment preference on treatment outcome.

References

[1] Vlaeyen JWS, Linton SJ. Fear avoidance and its consequences in chronic musculoskeletal pain: a state of the art. *Pain*. 2000; **85**: 317–32.

[2] Hashizume M. Psychosomatic approach for chronic migraine. *Rinsho Shinkeigaku* 2011; **51**: 1153–5.

[3] Holroyd KA, Labus JS, Carlson B. Moderation and mediation in the psychological and drug treatment of chronic tension-type headache: the role of severity and psychiatric comorbidity. *Pain*. 2009; **143**: 213–22.

[4] Thorn BE. *Cognitive Therapy for Chronic Pain: A Step-By-Step Guide*. New York, Guilford Publications, 2004.

[5] Lazarus RS, Folkman S. *Stress, Appraisal, and Coping*. New York: Springer, 1984.

[6] Flor H, Turk D. *Chronic Pain: An Integrated Biobehavioral Approach*. Seattle, WA: IASP Press, 2011.

[7] Rains JC, Penzien DB, McCrory DC, Gray RN. Behavioral headache treatment: History, review of the empirical literature, and methodological critique. *Headache* 2005; **45**: S92–109.

[8] Silberstein SD. Practice parameter: evidence-based guideline for migraine headache (an evidence-based review). Report of the American Subcommittee of the American Academy of Neurology. *Neurology* 2000; **55**: 754–63.

[9] Holroyd KA, Penzien DB. Psychosocial interventions in the management of recurrent headache disorders. 1: Overview and effectiveness. *Behav Med* 1994; **20**: 53–63.

[10] Holroyd KA, Drew JB. Behavioral approaches to the treatment of migraines. *Semin Neurol* 2006; **26**: 199–207.

[11] Rains JC, Penzien DB, Lipchik GL. Behavioral facilitation of medical treatment for headache – Part II: Theoretical models and behavioral. strategies for improving adherence. *Headache* 2006; **46**: 1395–403.

[12] Blanchard EB. Psychological treatment of benign headache disorders. *J Consult Clin Psychol* 1992; **60**: 537–51.

[13] Campbell JK, Penzien DB, Wall EM. Evidence-based guidelines for migraine headache: behavioral and physical treatments. US Headache Consortium 2000. Available at: http://www.aan.com/professionals/practice/pdfs/gl0089.pdf

[14] Nicholson RA, Buse DC, Andrasik F, Lipon RB. Nonpharmacologic treatments for migraine and tension-type headache: how to choose and when to use. *Curr Treatm in Options Neurol* 2011; **13**: 28–40.

[15] Goslin RE, Gray RN, McCrory DC, Penzien D, Rains J, Hasselblad V. Behavioral and physical treatments for migraine headache. *Tech Rev 2.2.* February 1999.

[16] Holroyd KA, Drew JB. Behavioral approaches to the treatment of migraine. *Semin Neurol.* 2006; **26**: 199–207.

[16a] Arena JG, Blanchard EB. Biofeedback and relaxation therapy for chronic pain disorder. In RJ Gatchell, DC Turk, eds. *Psychological Approaches to Pain Management: A Practitioners Handbook*. The Guilford Press. 1996: 179–228.

[17] Penzien DB, Andrasik F, Frendenberg BM, *et al.* Guidelines for trials of behavioral treatments for recurrent headache, 1st edn: American Headache Society Behavioral Clinical Trials Workgroup. *Headache* 2005; **45**: S110–32.

[18] D'Souza PJ, Lumley MA, Kraft CA, Dooley JA. Relaxation training and written emotional disclosure for tension or migraine headaches: a randomized, controlled trial. *Ann Behav Med*. 2008; **36**: 21–32.

[19] Blanchard, EB, Kim M, Hermann C, Steffek BD. Preliminary results of the effects on headache relief of perception of success among tension headache patients after receiving relaxation. *Headache Quarte.* 1994; **4**: 249–53.

[20] Stetter F, Kupper S. Autogenic training: a meta-analysis of clinical outcome studies. *Appl Psych Bio* 2002; **27**: 45–98.

[21] Kanji N, White AR, Ernst E. Autogenic training for tension type headaches: a systematic review of controlled trials. *Complement Ther Med* 2006; **14**: 144–50.

[22] Zsombok T, Juhasz G, Budavari A, Vitrai J, Bagdy G. Effect of autogenic training on drug consumption in patients with primary headache: an 8-month follow-up study. *Headache* 2003; **43**: 251–7.

[23] Kang EH, Park JE, Chung CS, Yu BH. Effect of biofeedback-assisted autogenic training on headache activity and mood states in Korean female migraine patients. *J Korean Med Sci* 2009; **24**: 936–40.

[24] Cott A, Parkinson W, Fabich M, Bédard M, Marlin R. Long-term efficacy of combined relaxation: biofeedback treatments for chronic headache. *Pain.* 1992; **51**: 49–56.

[25] Appel PR. Clinical hypnosis. In *Alternative Medicine and Rehabilitation. A Guide for Practitioners.* SF Wainapel, A Fast, eds, New York: Demos, 2003.

[26] Fernandez E, Turk DC. The utility of cognitive coping strategies for altering pain perception: A met analysis. *Pain* 1989; **38**: 123–35.

[27] Wahbeh H, Elsas S-M, Oken BS. Mind – body interventions. Applications in neurology. *Neurology* 2008; **70**: 2321–8.

[28] Wachholtz AB, Pargament KI Migraines and meditation: does spirituality matter? *J Behav Med* 2008; **31**: 351–66.

[29] Nestoriuc Y, Rief W, Martin A. Meta-analysis of biofeedback for tension-type headache: efficacy, specificity, and treatment moderators. *J Cons Clin Psychol* 2008; **76**: 379–96.

[30] Basmajian, JV. In Biofeedback: Principles and Practice for Clinicians. 3rd Edition. Basmajian JV (ed.). Williams & Wilkins, 1978;1–4.

[31] Mullally WJ, Hall K, Goldstein R. Efficacy of biofeedback in the treatment of migraine and tension type headaches. *Pain Physician* 2009; **12**: 1005–11.

[32] Devineni T, Blanchard EB. A randomized controlled trial of an Internet-based treatment for chronic headache. *Behav Res Ther* 2005; **43**: 277–92.

[33] Merelle SYM, Sorbi MJ, van Doornen LJ, Passchier J. Lay trainers with migraine for a home-based behavioral training: A 6 month follow up study. *Headache* 2008; **48**: 1311–25.

[34] Kluger M, Tursky B. A strategy for improving finger temperature biofeedback training. *Psychophysiology* 1982; **19**,329 (abstract).

[35] Freedman RR, Ianni P. Self control of digital temperature: Physiological factors and transfer effects. *Psychophysiology* 1983; **20**: 682–9.

[36] Sonty, N. Biofeedback as an adjunct in alternative medicine and rehabilitation. In *Alternative Medicine and Rehabilitation: A Guide for Practitioners.* SF Wainappel, A Fast, eds. New York: Demos, 2003;197–211.

[37] Andrasik F. Biofeedback in headache: an overview of approaches and evidence. *Clevel Clin J Med* 2010; **77**: S72–6.

[38] Buse DC, Andrasik F. Behavior medicine for migraine. *Neurol Clin* 2009; **27**: 445–65.

[39] Nestoriuc Y, Martin A, Rief W, Andrasik F. Biofeedback treatment for headache disorders: a comprehensive efficacy review. *Appl Psych Bio.* 2008; **33**: 125–40.

[40] Nestoriuc Y. and Martin A. Efficacy of biofeedback for migraine: a meta-analysis. *Pain* 2007; **128**: 111–27.

[41] Penzien DB, Rains JC, Andrasik F. Behavioral management of recurrent headache: three decades of experience and empiricism. *Appl Psych Bio* 2002; **27**: 163–81.

[42] Blanchard EB, Appelbaum KA, Radnitz CL, *et al.* A controlled evaluation of thermal biofeedback and thermal biofeedback combined with cognitive therapy in the treatment of vascular headache. 1990;58:216–24.

[43] Lehrer PM, Carr R, Sargunaraj D, Woolfolk RL. Stress management techniques: are they all equivalent, or do they have specific effects? *Biofeedback Self-Regul* 1994; **19**: 353–401.

[44] Lake AE. III Behavioral and nonpharmacologic treatments of headache. *Med Cli North Am* 2001; **85**: 1055–75.

[45] Lipchik GL, Nash JM. Cognitive-behavioral issues in the treatment and management of chronic daily headache. *Curr Pain Headache Rep* 2002; **6**: 473–9.

[46] Nicholson RA, Houle TT, Rhudy JL, Norton PJ. Psychological risk factors in headache. *Headache* 2007; **47**: 413–26.

[47] Prochaska JO, DiClemente CC. Transtheoretical therapy: Toward a more integrative model of change. *Psychother Theory, Res Pract.* 1982; **19**: 276–88.

[48] Seng EK, Holroyd KA. Dynamics of changes in self-efficacy and locus of control expectancies in the behavioral and drug treatment of severe migraine. *Ann Behav Med* 2010; **40**: 235–47.

[49] Bond DS, Durrant L, Digre KB, Baggaley SK, Rubingh C. Impact of a self-help intervention on performance of headache management behaviors: A self-efficacy approach. *Internet J Allied Helth Sci Pract* 2002;Jan (2) 1.

[50] French DJ, Holroyd KA, Pinell C, Malinoski PT, O'Donnell F, Hill KR. Perceived self-efficacy and headache-related disability. *Headache* 2000; **40**: 647–56.

[51] Radat F, Koleck M. Pain and depression: cognitive and behavioural mediators of a frequent association. *Encephale* 2011; **37**: 172–9.

[52] Kuile MM, Spinhoven P, Linssen AC, van Houwelingen HC. Cognitive coping and appraisal processes in the treatment of chronic headaches. *Pain* 1996; **64**: 257–64.

[53] Martin PR, Theunissen C. The role of life event stress, coping and social support in chronic headaches. *Headache* 1993; **33**(6): 301–6.

[54] Andersson G, Ljótsson B, Weise C. Internet-delivered treatment to promote health. *Curr Opin Psychiatry* 2011; **24**: 168–72.

[55] Fishman L. Yoga in medicine. Biofeedback as an adjunct. In *Alternative Medicine and Rehabilitation. A Guide for Practitioners*. SF Wainappel, A Fast, eds. New York: Demos. 2003;139–73.

[56] John PJ, Sharma N, Sharma CM, Kankane A. Effectiveness of yoga therapy in the treatment of migraine without aura: a randomized controlled trial. *Headache* 2007; **47**: 654–61.

[57] Wells RE, Bertisch SM, Buettner C, Phillips RS, McCarthy EP. Complementary and alternative medicine use among adults with migraines/severe headaches. *Headache* 2011; **51**: 1087–97.

[58] Michalsen A, Grossman P, Acil A, *et al.*Rapid stress reduction and anxiolysis among distressed women as a consequence of a three-month intensive yoga program. *Med Sci Monit* 2005; **11**: 555–61.

[59] Kaplan, G. Acupuncture: from Qi to biomedical science. In *Alternative Medicine and Rehabilitation: A Guide for Practitioners*. SF Wainappel, A Fast eds. New York: Demos, 2003.

[60] Vickers AJ, Rees RW, Zollman CE, *et al.* Acupuncture of chronic headache disorders in primary care: randomised controlled trial and economic analysis. *Health Technol Assess* 2004; **8:iii**: 1–35.

Chapter 11

Working with personality and personality disorders in the headache patient

Elizabeth Haase

Introduction

Patients with personality disorders can be difficult people to manage medically. They may distort facts, use maladaptive defenses, and create interpersonal tension. Such patients frustrate physicians by their failure to adhere to agreed-upon regimens and by their seemingly self-destructive health behaviors. They convey their needs poorly through repeated vague complaints that consume time and utilize resources. They can present as clinging and yet be hostile at the same time. Physicians may come to dread their visits, develop guilt-provoking fantasies that such patients will not return, and feel inadequate, helpless, enraged, guilty, or tricked after patient encounters.

Headache patients in particular demonstrate excessive personality dysfunction, the headache often manifesting the patient's interpersonal stress. This is true across divergent cultures such as China, [1] Egypt, [2] and the United States, and across studies using conceptually different tools of personality assessment, including the research-based categorical model of the DSM-III and IV, the patient-derived model of the MMPI, [3] and the temperament-based DAPP. One study, among several, of 100 chronic, non-organic headache patients found 77% to have one or more personality disorders, compared with 24% in the organic headache group. [2] Both these rates are higher than the 10% to 20% prevalence of personality disorder in general population studies. It is highly likely that a headache clinic patient, especially one with chronic, non-organic headache, will have a personality disorder.

Diagnosis

Before discussing the impact of particular personality types on headache, it is necessary to discuss the diagnostic framework that defines personality and personality disorders. The term *personality* refers to habitual and pervasive patterns of thinking, feeling, and acting, based on temperament, the hard-wired aspects of individual emotional response, and character, the non-genetic elements of personality that include abstract thinking, values, ideals, self-concept, fantasies, defenses, and coping styles, and interpersonal patterns. When a particular distortion of personality pervasively and inflexibly causes impairment and distress in a given culture, personality is considered disordered. The current major diagnostic tool for defining personality disorder in the United States, the *Diagnostic and Statistical Manual* (DSM) of the American Psychiatric Association, has been in a state of controversy and flux for several years. A revision, the DSM-V, is planned for release in 2013. The International Diagnostic Code (ICD) of the World Health Organization traditionally follows the DSM system, and is expected to do so in future revisions.

For the past 20 years the DSM has organized personality diagnoses categorically as ten types divided into three clusters, presented in Table 11.1.

The categorical organization of the *DSM-IV* has been marred by high comorbidity with other personality disorders, diagnostic instability over time, arbitrary thresholds for defining illness, and treatment non-specificity. In the coming revision, the DSM-V, four of these diagnoses may be eliminated: schizoid, paranoid, histrionic, and dependent. The diagnosis of personality disorder not otherwise specified (PDO NOS), will be replaced by personality disorder trait specified (PDTS).

Retaining a partially categorical approach, the DSM-V will then additionally rate personality for specific trait domains and level of impairment in two areas, "self-functioning" and interpersonal functioning. This second layer of assessment will describe the personality

The Neuropsychiatry of Headache, ed. Mark W. Green and Philip R. Muskin. Published by Cambridge University Press.

Table 11.1. Personality diagnoses

Personality disorder	Characteristic traits	Fears	Coping style	Physician's experience
Cluster A: odd, eccentric cluster				
Paranoid	Suspicious, wary, easily slighted, holds grudges	Exploitation, harm, deceit, humiliation	Counterattack, Superiority, Secretiveness	Feeling accused, blamed, threatened
Schizoid	Solitary, guarded, emotionless, indifferent to praise or criticism	Intimacy, intrusions into privacy	Insulate self from others, detach, devalue and deny painful realities	Either detachment or wish to break through patient's isolation
Schizotypal	Eccentric, odd, mannered, superstitious	Emotional warmth, violations of privacy	Belief in special powers or magic, Disorganization	Weird and alone feelings, wish to mock/label
Cluster B: dramatic, emotional				
Antisocial	Dishonest, cruel, irresponsible, aggressive, grandiose	Humiliation, betrayal, powerlessness	Seek advantage or gain, exploits, cons, harms	Used, angry, wish to expose and punish
Histrionic	Provocative, melodramatic, impressionistic, suggestible	Loss of love, attention	Seduction, sexualization, attention-seeking	Flattered, aroused, emotionally flooded, wishing to rescue
Borderline	Volatile, angry, impulsive, self-destructive, empty	Abandonment, invalidation	Manipulation, emotional displays, self-destructive acting out with food, sex, violence or drugs	Angry/ guilty, depleted/ heroic, special/ used, acting atypically
Narcissistic	Status-conscious, haughty, envious, entitled,	Loss of face, power, esteem	Demanding, belittling, self-promoting/protecting	Devalued, submissive, hateful
Cluster C: anxious, fearful				
Dependent	Needy, submissive, indecisive,	Neglect, separation, responsibility, anger	Passivity, clinging, regression	Depleted, wish to deny, annoyed
Obsessive-compulsive	Detailed, inflexible, moralistic , cheap, overly serious	Risk, disorder, emotionality	Controlling, intellectualizing, passive resistance	Stubborn, controlling, bored
Avoidant	Hesitant, ashamed, inhibited, avoidant	Disapproval, rejection	Withdraw, escape	Frustrated or impatient, at patient's shame or weakness

characteristics of all patients, whether or not they have a personality disorder. The assessment process is intended to "telescope" the clinician's attention from a global rating of the severity of impairment through increasing degrees of detail and specificity in describing personality psychopathology. [4]

The new *trait domains*, derived largely from the Five Factor Model originated by Cloninger and the 200 item Shedler-Westen Assessment Procedure (SWAP), or SWAP, represent a significant reorganization of personality diagnosis to a *dimensional* conceptualization. Five trait domains (negative affectivity, detachment, antagonism, dis-inhibition vs. compulsivity, and psychoticism) are slotted for inclusion in the revision, as well as facets of these trait groups (for example, impulsivity and rigid perfectionism as sub-facets of compulsivity). Trait evaluation has been shown to improve upon the limitations of categorical diagnosis and upon functional and treatment outcomes, but requires refinement to improve the easy recognition of traits in the clinical context. [5]

Self-functioning includes dimensions of identity and self-directedness. People with a sense of identity that is weak, diffuse, overly conflicted, or splits some behaviors or feelings from awareness suffer a sense of emptiness and have fragmented false exterior selves that change rapidly. They therefore have difficulty with sustained and authentic directed engagement with the world. Interpersonal impairments in the capacities for empathy and intimacy occur from these deficits.

Categorical DSM-IV personality diagnoses are rarely made in primary care settings and there is little research in the area. One British study of general practitioners demonstrates that they identified personality disorder in only 5% of patients with psychiatric illness, despite a 28% prevalence on a formal psychiatric interview. Looking beyond personality disorders, research investigators have attempted to isolate particular personality traits commonly linked to headache. Earlier stereotyping of migraineurs in small studies has not been replicated. Headache patients have been found to have higher rates of both *alexithymia* (trouble labeling emotions verbally or psychologically), and *somatization* (a tendency to experience emotional events through physical distress). [2,3,6] Higher rates of *neuroticism*, a tendency to be worried, irritable, and interpret events negatively, are seen in headache patients. Female migraineurs also have slightly higher rates of *psychoticism*, [7] a term that is most easily defined as the opposite of openness, conscientiousness, and agreeableness: that is, tending to concrete thinking, rigidity, disengagement, and an impersonal, cold, or slightly hostile emotional style.

Certain personality profiles are predictive of the type of headache a patient manifests, with a statistical accuracy of 0.0001 in a chi square analysis. [3] In these studies, migraine patients have showed little personality pathology, although they have consistently scored higher on anxiety and depression and inconsistently higher on hostility, repressed hostility, and alienation from peers. In one non-blinded study, migraineurs with obsessive-compulsive personality disorders were highly likely to develop medication-overuse headaches as well. [6] In contrast, patients with headaches associated with conversion or post-traumatic stress disorder, and those with combination or muscle contraction headaches, had higher rates of personality dysfunction characterized by histrionic and somatizing profiles, the groups separating by degree of neurosis. [12,8]

Medical causes of personality pathology associated with headache

Any acute change in personality over age 35, or over a 1-year period in a child, has a high probability of a biological etiology. The most common personality traits associated with new illness are emotionality, disinhibition, impulsivity, aggressiveness, suspiciousness, or indifference. Personality disorders of this type are currently diagnosed as personality change due to general medical condition and typed according to the dominant emotional change expressed.

Almost any medicine or medical illness can change personality. Medication classes that may present more often with both headache *and* personality change include stimulants, antihypertensives, immunosuppressants, chemotherapeutics, corticosteroids, contraceptives, and high-dose vitamins.

Likely disease sources of a personality change include those that affect the frontal lobes and subcortical structures preferentially. Common examples of the latter include traumatic brain injury, tumors, stroke, subcortical dementias such as AIDS dementia, Huntington's disease, and progressive supra-nuclear palsy, multiple sclerosis, toxins that preferentially attack white matter such as lead, copper, and radiation, vasculitis, and subacute encephalitis, such as Lyme's Disease. More difficult to tease apart from a stable, lifelong personality disorder are gradual changes in personality associated with certain chronic diseases such as alcoholism, epilepsy, thyroid dysfunction, and Parkinson's disease.

Neurobiology of personality relevant to headache

No infant is born with a disordered personality. Personality results when predispositions of temperament are epigenetically codified into typical interpersonal and emotional actions by development and experience. Personality *disorders* result from environmental factors that adversely impact personality, including major single traumas, chronic traumas such as deprivation, neglect, abuse, and abandonment, and child-rearing patterns such as invalidation, communication double binds, and excessive or erratic discipline.

Headache patients, as far as it has been studied, show very few markers of personality dysfunction in childhood. They differentiate from their peers in childhood only in greater personal fearfulness and sensitivity, [9] and perhaps hyperreactivity in infancy. [10] The converse, however, is not true. Patients with personality disorders have multiple neurobiological abnormalities that may predispose them to headaches or may impact upon treatment response.

Patients with *borderline personality* disorder deserve special focus. Etiologically, borderline personality is accompanied by two groups of symptoms to consider independently: significant neurochemical variance from the norm and a typical mode of interpersonal difficulty characterized by interpersonal volatility and the defenses of splitting, projection, and denial. These defenses often arise from family environments that have been either perfectionistic or chaotic, and have interfered with normal attachment physiology by invalidating or neglecting the child's emotional needs and perceptions.

Borderline patients show emotional instability that has been associated with under-activation of the orbital prefrontal cortex (OFC) and hyperactivity of the amygdala in response to emotional challenges, such as memories of abandonment and emotional or angry faces. They are more likely to experience dysphoria with a cholinergic challenge and have abnormalities in the opioid system that include reduced baseline opiates, polymorphism of the mu-opioid receptor, and atypical opioid responses, particularly dissociation. [11]

Borderline patients also show several markers of low central serotonergic function that correlate with impulsivity and aggression. These include reduced responsiveness to fenfluramine challenge; lower platelet paroxetine binding, decreased basal metabolism in the anterior cingulate gyrus (ACG) and orbital prefrontal cortex (OFC). Hippocampal volume is decreased in some. [11] Allelic variation in genes associated with dopamine, serotonin, and MAO-A has also been found in impulsive aggressive patients with borderline and antisocial personalities.

Given this neurobiology, borderline patients are more likely to complain of headache worsening with attachment disruptions and routine stress. They may require extra education about side effects and course of response to help them overcome the innate intensity of their reactions to physical and psychological experience. They may have unusual responses to opioids and are at higher risk of opioid abuse. Their response to serotonergic medications used in headache treatment may be idiosyncratic and inconsistent. The antiepileptic divalproex has perhaps the best data supporting use for both headache and borderline syndromes; carbamazepine and atypical antipsychotics both have efficacy in both conditions. [12]

Schizotypal patients also show considerable neurobiological variation from the norm. Unusual perceptual and somatic experiences are routinely part of their experience and need not be over-read as a psychotic or somatic symptom or side effect. These patients have been found to have cognitive impairments including poor working memory and poor attention and social cue identification that have been correlated with poor rapport and paranoid misreading of personal interactions. Dopaminergic activity is relatively either increased or decreased, and they respond to amphetamines with greater elevations than controls, perhaps correlated with a polymorphism of catechol-O-methyl transferase (COMT) and yield variation in the dopamine buffering system. Imaging studies show reduction in superior temporal gyrus volume and overall ventricular enlargement. They may be particularly sensitive to adverse cognitive side effects of glutaminergic agents such as topiramate and may respond to pro-dopaminergic agents with improved cognition and memory function if such are appropriate. It may also be helpful to repeat education and explanation, reinforced with written or visual aids. [11]

General interpersonal concerns in the headache patient

As the DSM-V revisions suggest, most interpersonal difficulties are not due to personality disorders or pathology *per se*. Understanding common and individual sources of difficulty in collaborating with a patient, rather than the diagnosis of a specific personality disorder, should be an early consideration in every patient that has trouble with the relational aspects of medical care. General concerns that influence a medical encounter include patient reactions to the fear of illness, differing expectations of the social role to be played by patient and physician, the individual's style of attachment, and issues connected to demographic and cultural attitudes towards illness.

Strain and Grossman [13] have outlined *seven psychological fears* that affect patients' responses to physicians. Illness raises the *fear of annihilation*, threatening both physical integrity and activating the accompanying fantasy of protection from destruction by an omnipotent parent. The doctor, often a stranger, demands the patient's implicit trust and full access to the privacy of the body and its intimate experiences, raising early trust issues and *fears of strangers and separation*. Transient paranoia, withdrawal, or anxiety reactions may result. The debilitation of illness requires one to relinquish care to others. For patients who did not have dependable loving caregivers and had to achieve their self-esteem independently, there is an acute *fear of loss of love* and *fear of loss of control* in this dependent state. Needy clinging or dictating care are typical reactions. The invasive procedures of the modern medical office may raise *fears of injury to a body part*, sometimes symbolically processed as a threat to one's potency, both sexual potency and other areas of personal efficacy, or as repetition of physical or sexual abuse. Finally, illness raises *fear of punishment* for transgressions such as eating and smoking. Experiencing a physician's recommendations for treatment as an indictment, patients may feel too attacked or undeserving to participate in efforts to accept help.

Dissonance between doctor and patient can also result from *role discord*. In coming to the doctor, patients place themselves in the sick role, requesting relief from a set of symptoms and an explanation of their cause from an authoritarian figure. The physician aims to diagnose, provide curative treatment or reduce suffering, then empower the patient with the recommendations and medications that allow the patients to resume control. Both parties must play their assigned roles correctly at each stage of the process for the relationship to proceed smoothly.

Both physician and patient must adequately assert authority. Most societies tip this balance to the doctor. The doctor, in order to help the patient become active in his care, must counter this role bias. Physicians can empower and educate the patients regarding their necessary roles. These include providing history, asking questions, reporting side effects, and making decisions about treatment options. Patients who are not heard will soon not be seen either, may act passively about follow-up, or may raise their voices to hostile threats. Conversely, in consumerist societies, the patient may see the doctor as a replaceable commodity and may need counter-balancing reminders of the loss of long-term knowledge and trust in this model.

Patients may show *role abuse* by assuming the sick role to solve non-medical problems. In the extreme, patients with somatization or factitious disorder use symptoms for conscious or unconscious secondary gain. There are common minor abuses as well. If a doctor's visit is the only time that a mother is attended to by her adult children, or if a parent's headaches are the only justification for much-needed household help, a response to routine medical treatment is unlikely.

Role disagreement may also arise. Patients approach caregivers with widely varying expectations regarding the expression of pain and the demand for help based in cultural, intellectual, and medical experience. Their expression of distress may be withheld stoically, exaggerated histrionically, over-psychologized, or expressed in somatic terms. Their cognitive understanding of the etiology of the headache and mechanisms of cure will also have a structure. It may reflect scientific reading, pop-cultural notions of stress effects, mystical or religious systems of thoughts that involve divine punishment, bad karma or evil spirits, or a preoccupation with the toxic effects of a particular environment. For example, a patient who does not accept a treatment plan because of a folk or cultural belief in spirits has violated one of the designated functions of the patient role in coming to a Western medical clinic, to present for care expecting to receive and follow scientifically based medical recommendations.

Role disagreement may also result when doctors and patients have conflicting priorities in their respective roles. For example, the role of doctor as diagnostician may lead to conflict with a patient who may reject routine phlebotomies and repeated tests that have no impact on suffering. Emotional expectations of how needs will be met may also lead to a disagreement about role. Patients' expectations of care range from an assumption of neglect to an entitlement to indulgence, from a belief that the squeaky wheel will get the grease to an anxious preoccupation with following rules to guarantee control over outcome to a paranoid expectation of trickery and abuse. Each of these belief systems dictates particular roles for each party.

Finally, the manner in which a patient will connect to a caregiver and attend to treatment will be powerfully influenced by *attachment style*. [14] Proposed initially by John Bowlby and developed by Mary Ainsworth and others, the attachment system is a biobehavioral system that enhances infant survival by promoting a secure relationship with at least one primary caregiver. Infants have been shown to have at least four basic patterns of attachment: secure attachment, and three insecure attachment styles including inhibited, disinhibited, and disorganized. Self-endangering and indiscriminate styles have also been noted. Bartholomew and Horowitz developed a classification system for adults that includes four styles: secure, dismissing, preoccupied, and fearful. These patterns have been shown to persist throughout life [15] and to be associated with factors associated with outcome in a variety of medical illnesses including chronic pain conditions. Areas investigated to date that correlate with style of attachment include timing of presentation, compliance, number of unexplained symptoms, and adaptation to illness. [16,17]

Patients with *dismissive attachment* downplay the importance of problems and minimize the need for help. As children they learned to do this to keep their bond with an unwilling caregiver who did not like excessive demands. The key to understanding such patients is to keep in mind their paradoxical belief that the fewer their demands, the more care they will get, exactly opposing the physician's impulse to respond to discrete symptoms. These patients will be self-reliant, try not to come in until something is urgent, and use the fewest possible pills. It is easy to collude with the patient's style and inquire less, assume the patient will manage, and go along with the patient's comfortable sense of invincibility. This strategy worsens the problem, as the patient will even further under-report, believing that the first minimization has earned the doctor's approval. Secretly, the patient feels neglected. It is important for the physician to model normal levels of care and emphasize the need to perform all the tests and visits anyone else would get. This message should be repeated every visit, and the doctor should expect it to be a few visits before the patient warms up to these recommendations, as the patient will dismiss and forget the message as well as the care itself until truly sure both are heartfelt.

Fearful attachment occurs when a child depends on a caregiver who is cruel or blatantly neglectful. As adults, such persons mistrust, and have a push–pull, or approach–avoid, style of seeking and fearing help that leads them to demand but to reject. Patients with fearful attachment styles have high rates of symptoms reporting but low primary care costs and fewer visits than average. [18] This patient will respond to help with mistrust and pull away, the opposite of the patient with a dismissive style. It is helpful if the doctor joins the patient's worry that involvement in treatment will lead to danger and pain, and hesitate to do too much, knowing the patient will appreciate sharing his or her anxiety and feel supported in risking next steps. It is also helpful to negotiate with them, demonstrating that both parties are strong, that there will be no violation of their rights in a harmful way, and that the doctor accepts their need to reject care as a self-protective solution.

Patients with *preoccupied attachment* have higher numbers of symptoms, visits and total primary care costs than others. [18] They had caregivers who were inconsistently responsive, this intermittent reinforcement lending a Pavlovian tenacity to their repeated bids for attention. Like the fearful patient, they mistrust, but the external care behavior is diametrically opposite, seeking rather than fearing care. As a result of their operant conditioning, such patients are compulsively hyperactive and hyper-vigilant about getting medical attention. They are terribly insecure about their judgments, as the outcome of their efforts to engage help as children was unpredictable. They report every little symptom and review every instruction repeatedly. They want to know where the doctor went on vacation and what medical school she attended, all activities that reassure them that a relationship is available on demand. They are experienced as clingy, enraging, and childish on the one hand, and gratifying and attentive on the other. Depending on how busy the doctor is that day, these traits will appeal or enrage, engendering the same inconsistency as the patient's original parent. The cheerleader strategy works best here, reducing the patient's fear that the doctor will randomly withdraw but encouraging them to resume the developmental turning away from the parent or doctor towards independent self-care that was stymied and undermined by random withdrawals of support in childhood.

Psychodynamic issues in medical interactions

The medical encounter evokes many aspects of a child/parent relationship. Physicians touch, care for, hurt, and tell their patients what to do. Like children, patients depend on the doctor for functions they normally perform independently. The activation of primitive fears and the parental functions of the physician in the medical encounter lead to *regression*. In regression, patients relinquish more recently matured behavior, returning to earlier coping skills and emotional displays used in interactions with former caregivers. A common example is a child's return to wetting the bed or sucking his thumb after the birth of a sibling. Regression can be both adaptive and maladaptive. For example, a couple's ability to regress from the cares of middle-age to a playful and spontaneous style may facilitate a healthy sexual life, while the tendency to act like a rebellious adolescent with prescriptions can be life-threatening. While the regressive ability of a patient to relinquish control facilitates care, overall, patients' function will be likewise much more child-like in the doctor's office than in the other areas of their lives: less reality-oriented, less stable, and less able to function efficiently in response to the needs of others. In addition, patients expect and recreate patterns of behavior with former caregivers. This phenomenon is known as *transference* because early relationships are transferred into a new situation.

The physician will naturally react emotionally to the behaviors and feelings of the patient. Patients who are needy because they are sensitive to rejection and seek repeated reassurance will elicit rejection by being irritating; patients who complain about what they get out of a sense of deprivation may lead the clinician to feel hopeless and stop offering, repeating the depriving experience. Through these cyclical repetitions, the patient's expectations of interaction become a self-fulfilling prophecy. The *role-responsiveness* emotions of the doctor are known as *counter-transference*, or the reciprocal (counter) response to the transference.

Counter-transference reactions can be helpfully defined as the physician's conscious and unconscious, cognitive and emotional, idiosyncratic and evoked reaction to a given patient. While such responses do often contain emotions that are influenced by the personal situation of the physician (for example, the patient refuses to pay and the doctor was raised in poverty), counter-transference is also profoundly useful information about the emotional actions of the patient.

The counter-transference experience of finding a patient "difficult" is usually the physician's first clue to the presence of a personality disorder. [19] Recognition of the difficult patient or of an underlying personality disorder often starts with a physician's awareness of one of three patterns of unusual subjective response. First, *emotional responses* to such patients tend to be stronger than usual, intruding into professional reasoning. Feelings of wanting to rescue a patient or give special care may alternate rapidly with feelings of hate or betrayal. Physicians may have unusual *fantasies* about a patient in free hours or dream about a patient. The feelings elicited by patients with personality disorders often compel physicians to *atypical behaviors*. Physicians may note urges to order extra tests, perform more invasive low yield procedures on a rejecting patient, or offer free services or drug samples. Such urges almost always reflect a response to emotional needs or pressures from the patient and provide an excellent opportunity to consider how personality dynamics are impacting care.

Recent studies have validated a correlation between the personality style of the patient and the counter-transference that is elicited in the doctor. For example, the narcissistic patient typically causes a doctor to feel dread and resentment towards the patient, to feel devalued and criticized, and to become distracted and avoidant. [20] Eight typical counter-transferences to patients have been described: overwhelmed/disorganized, helpless/inadequate, special/overinvolved, sexualized, disengaged, parental/protective, and criticized/mistreated. Thus one can use one's intuitive emotional response to the patient to learn what kind of personality problem the patient may have in an evidence-based way (see Table 11.1).

General approaches to interpersonal management

The irrational emotional system exerts a profound influence over functions critical to medical care: recall, decision making, persuasion, and information processing among others. While often inaccurate in their judgments, both doctors and patients judge each other's emotions and reveal their liking for each other. [21] In psychotherapy research, the *therapeutic alliance*, a concept highly correlated with feelings of mutual liking and respect between client and therapist, is a better predictor of outcome than the type of treatment delivered. A good alliance in both doctor and therapist treatments is facilitated by unconditional positive regard for the patient, empathy, and a goal-driven collaborative process in which the patient's view is accrued greater significance than that of the professional. [22]

Non-verbal behavior is one way the doctor communicates positive regard. Doctors who sit closer to their patients, lean forward, make more eye contact, read the chart less, and nod and gesture frequently send messages of engagement that yield greater patient satisfaction. Non-verbal behavior is more important even than verbal skill; tone of voice alone has been shown to be predictive of follow-up visits. An anxious or concerned tone combined with positive words and facial expression receives highest patient marks; overtly casual social tones and anger rate most poorly. While impatient nervousness is rated as a sign of physician concern, an impatient dominant style accompanied by low levels of anxiety is linked to being sued. [21]

Patients and doctors read each other even on the basis of small amounts of behavioral information, or "thin slices" of interaction lasting as little as several seconds. [21] Multiple studies show that doctors who have *emotional attunement*, that is, are more skilled at decoding these emotional hints and reciprocate by asking about the patient's concern, get fuller histories, [23] receive higher satisfaction marks, and avoid stalemates generated by emotional concerns. [23] Particularly in situations where chronic illness generates multiple negative affects, hopelessness, helplessness, disappointment and rage, empathic listening becomes a critical therapeutic tool.

Narrative competence is the skill we use as humans to absorb and understand stories told by patients. In contrast to *logicoscientific knowledge*, detached and factual, *narrative knowledge* allows us to understand based on our subjective emotional reactions, memories, associations, creativity, symbolic thought, and cultural experience. The "who, what, when, and how" of a story help the listener sort through the multiple and contradictory possible meanings of different words to understand a single tale. These narrative tasks are essential to getting a whole story and only one story to pursue. [24]

A simple communication strategy to enhance *information gathering* in patients with chronic migraine has recently been supported by phase two of the American Migraine Communication Study (AMCS II). Phase one of this study demonstrates that physicians used closed-ended, short-answer questions to evaluate the key diagnostic criteria of headache frequency and impairment 90% of the time. This closed brief style results in answers different from that those spontaneously reported through open-ended questions in 50% of cases and identification of impairment in only 10% of cases. [25] AMCS II demonstrates that a simple "ask–tell–ask" question sequence significantly improves patient communication and satisfaction. This simple sequence increases the number of visits that address impairment by 80%, narratives about inter-episode functioning by 25%, and raises the satisfaction of both patients and doctors with their visits to 95%. Contrary to physician fears, the length of the visit increases by only 12 seconds on average. [26] The ask–tell–ask sequence is done by *asking* an open-ended question about frequency, *telling* the patient what you have heard, and *asking* if there is any impairment from this, again in an open-ended way.

Obtaining an MMPI or its shorter version, the MCMIII, may also be useful for treatment planning and prognosis. Patients with more depressive personality styles (in contrast to major depressive disorder) and introversion on these scales may have a better prognosis and be better able to use psychotherapy, as they are able to identify sources of distress internally. Research suggests that those with higher scores on the conversion and somatization scales are likely to have a poorer prognosis and are unlikely to benefit from psychological intervention. [3] A specific treatment based on Davenloo's short-term dynamic therapy has preliminary support in headache patients whose style of internalized emotion is expressed somatically. The treatment reduces symptoms and decreases emergency room visits by as much as 75% in those with other psychosomatic disorders. [27]

As interactions become more difficult, the physician's ability to handle his or her own negative emotion becomes increasingly important. Taking time to correctly identify the negative emotions of patient and doctor leads to correction of distorted negative appraisals and active seeking of more information, and is correlated with reduced errors and improved decision making. [28]

Studies of the *malpractice complaints* leading to lawsuits provide another list of rules for managing doctor–patient difficulty. These suggest that the doctor should be careful not to desert, dismiss, or devalue the patient or his symptoms, and should be particularly careful not to dismiss the patient's views. Specific interview techniques that correlate with lower rates of lawsuit include making statements structuring the interview ("I'd like to spend about 10 minutes hearing your side"), encouraging patients to elaborate, checking the patient understands, and using humor. [29,30]

The patient who feels rejected, insulted, or dismissed will become angry. In dealing effectively with an *angry patient*, one is advised to focus exclusively on the incident, commit to keeping cool, and adjust one's body language to a relaxed posture, receptive expression, full eye contact and soft voice. Initially, one should listen respectfully without interrupting or attempting to set limits, and particularly avoiding the temptation to rationalize or defend. Using short simple sentences to paraphrase what the patient expresses, one can then indicate one's commitment to do right by the patient and own the problem. If appropriate, apologize and empathize, and state areas where you agree with the complaint. Pursue the problem until the patient agrees it has been fully understood, and invite the patient to tell you what could help to solve it. While it is unwise to promise a permanent solution, make sure the specific problem is resolved and will not recur before stopping your efforts. [31]

Management of the difficult patient

In navigating the choppy seas of difficult patient interactions, the practitioner is encouraged to reflect deeply on studies and experience telling us that at least half of illness results from behavior and lifestyle. [32] This body of evidence enables us to find the courage and motivation to respond rather than react to the patient's behavioral and psychological style. It is worth the effort, and more importantly, is likely to be the only effort that will work.

General suggestions for working with all difficult patients include:

Consistency: Minimizing changes in plan, medications, schedule, and personnel, making sure all staff respond to a patient with the same information, clarifying the length and time of visits in advance, anticipating and planning for vacations and future events explicitly are all strategies that help difficult patients manage medical care. Consistency is particularly important for dependent and borderline patients.

Clarifying the treatment contract: Explicating the patient's hopes for treatment and explaining the rationale, method, limits, and objectives of treatment can prevent disappointments and misunderstandings to which difficult patients may react dramatically. Paranoid, obsessive-compulsive, and narcissistic patients may especially benefit from this approach.

Sympathetic limit setting: Explaining which behavior or requests will or will not be allowed is the "trump" card of management techniques. It is critical that the physician must neither be manipulated and intimidated nor punitive or rejecting of the patient, as both represent overreactions to the patient's aggression. A confident, balanced, supportive approach allowing some pathological behaviors to go unchallenged while standing firm on others works best. Drug abuse should not be permitted, physical therapy provided, and destruction of property must be prevented while expression of anger is allowed. [33] As personality disordered patients add about 25 minutes of telephone time per clinic hour, most of it for non-emergent urgencies, emergencies, and requests for controlled substances, an explicit program describing how to use the telephone may be helpful. [34]

Specific interventions for difficult personality traits and types

Specific traits found across personality disorders may need intervention informed by an understanding of psychological defenses against unconscious fears. These can be condensed to the following tendencies: suspiciousness, devaluation, neediness, exploitation, inappropriate closeness, and controlled withdrawal.

The *suspicious* patient seeks to make an enemy of the doctor, who is more easily battled than a mysterious illness. Knowing illness is the real fear, one must acknowledge the factual risks of harm to empathize with the patient's vulnerability in placing themselves at risk. The patient's fears are often exaggerated, and should be corrected with information. One should allow the patient to refuse or disagree with care so as not to push them, which will be perceived as a dangerous, coercive, or abusive attack. Avoid blame and punitive finger pointing, which will inflame the patient's fear of further risk from emotionally chaos.

Devaluing patients do so to support self-esteem in situations of vulnerability or humiliation. Critical patients fear they will get bad care because they are worthless. Understanding that the patient feels personally diminished by imperfections in care, one can provide reassurance that you value him or her by stating that you wish to pursue the best options available. If the patient wants more than is actually available, this entitlement can be met with available alternatives elsewhere. Most patients will then feel in control of rejecting an even lesser option.

The requests of needy patients should not be taken too literally. Helping them see their anxiety, make real-world choices, and pursue their fears about outcome is more efficacious. Emphasizing prolonged care, as opposed to gratifying immediate care needs, defuses the tendency to regress without abandoning the patient.

Patients who break boundaries, are *seductive*, or create drama are people who fear loss of love or attention. Staying in the middle ground of logical, warm interaction without becoming too casual or reactive is key to successful management. One can be curious about what that dramatic gesture was intended to achieve, and problem-solve with the patient about more direct or easily recognizable ways to get an appropriate response.

In dealing with patients who *withdraw* through avoiding, controlling, or isolating, one wants to respect their fears of being emotionally overwhelmed while encouraging appropriate participation. Talking them through their distorted concerns helps identify if there is any concrete or real problem they are not able to manage. Demonstrating competence will allow them to relax their need for control and distance.

Finally, it may be helpful to simplify much of what has been discussed by condensing one's view of the patient into one of four difficult patient types, originally described by James Groves, which have proven clinically serviceable over several decades. [35]

Dependent clingers [35] are a common difficult type that can cause the doctor to feel hateful. These patients want an intimate relationship with the doctor more than treatment itself. They present with seemingly insatiable needs paired with an heavily airbrushed image of doctors as inexhaustible mothers with no other duty than to glory in their care through explanation, reassurance, analgesics, or sedatives. After a honeymoon phase in which the doctor typically feels special and powerful, natural weariness will tend to lead to the impatient rejection of a devastated patient. This risk can be diminished by stating as early as possible that the doctor has limits to time, stamina, and scope of ability.

In the headache clinic, pain and chronicity exacerbate clinging traits. The patient, seeking relief of both emotional and physical pain, particularly needs attention, and may then come to the logical but erroneous conclusion that the doctor who provides it is the long-term solution. Therefore, one wants to direct the patient's attention outwards from the clinic to multimodal coping in external life as soon as the first sigh of unclenched breath is heard. A clear statement that the treatment will continue to work can function like a transitional object for the patient to hold on to, while the injunction to imagine the doctor on her shoulder as she works to decrease external stresses that set the treatment back can itself become an on-going companion.

Another type of clinging is affected by the *help-rejecting complainer*. [35] This person also presents with pleas for relief of symptoms, but one detects a ting of smugness as they sabotage or defeat attempts to respond to their complaints. The form of defeat may include misunderstanding instructions, difficulty accepting usual side effects of medications, rejecting consultants, or constantly shifting symptoms once one is addressed. Thus the relationship remains in a stalemate, comfortable for the patient, who prefers a safe balance of closeness and distance, but depressing and frustrating for the doctor. The position of suffering for the patient may serve numerous functions: the garnering of attention, relief from unconscious guilt or anxiety about recovery or success, a compulsion to repeat prior victimization at the hands of a poor caregiver, or a sadistic need to demonstrate the inadequacy of others in order to maintain their own relative self-esteem. The problem in this case is the actions that emerge from the physician's feelings of depression, either an intrusive and forceful attempt to rescue the patient or increasing identification with the patient's helplessness and apathy until finally some real symptom is ignored and a negative consequence results.

In the headache setting, the patient may assume a continuing stalemate with the disease itself. Testimonials of those who have recovered and of a range of modes of recovery may add hope. The notion that headaches may come and go over the life cycle, and that different medicines work at different times, may help the patient develop more flexible means of keeping distance, so that they can give up suffering without fearing loss of contact and care.

The problematic defenses of this patient are manipulation, passive aggressive action, and denial of their own role in relapse. It is helpful to clarify and document carefully what is being offered, and to ask the patient to restate both the offer and which part he or she chooses to accept. Relating to the patient and writing in the chart what the patient is and is not accepting will occasionally augment the patient's attention to his or her own actions. Similarly helpful is to explore how the patient will feel about and handle the likely consequences of, refusal of care. The approach must be balanced, without overblowing alarm scenarios but offering realistic limits for how long their refusal of care is likely to be safe or tolerable to either party. Each of these actions has the added benefit of creating a certain distance without sacrificing the appropriate closeness and compassion of the relationship.

The *self-destructive denier* [35], like the help-rejecting complainer, also sabotages care. There is no complaining, but rather the total absence of responsibility for, and awareness of, one's suffering. These are the patients who remain obese despite sleep apnea, who smoke in their hospital beds after a coronary bypass, or who are repeatedly admitted for variceal bleeding but continue to drink. They appear to glory in their self-destruction. This is because, by their neglect of the problem, they feel both invulnerable to, and triumphant over, the pesky negative future predicted by the worry-wart doctor. Such patients live to preserve invulnerability in the moment, the antithesis of the doctor, who seeks vulnerability in the moment to extend invulnerability into the future. Watching them self-destruct creates rage at one's wasted efforts and dismissed concerns, and leads typically to the wish they would just die now and get it over with. These patients do not want to die. They want to avoid the vulnerability and discomfort of change, and to continue with what pleasures they do have. For these patients, denial is a terminal illness, and they should be treated with the same treatment and comfort measures as any patient with Alzheimer's, stroke, cancer, or other incurable disease that limits the ability for cognitive change. If there are moments of attention to things going south, these can be praised as insight into the illness, and the patient supported in any urges they might have to make an adjustment. Depression should also be assessed.

The final type of generally "hateful" patient is the *entitled demander*. This person often has a narcissistic personality disorder or infantile character, by which is meant someone who has expectations of indulgent care that would be appropriate in a very young child. Typically, such patients make many demands for appointment times, phone calls, special prescriptions, and so forth that are beyond the capabilities of a busy practice. More destructively, they expect their doctors to work more like magicians than physicians, not just evaluating and treating, but also erasing pain and disease. Such patients may be legitimately surprised by the idea of permanent damage, side effects, or mortality risks. It can be tempting to humiliate them with laughter at times, which can create surges of vengeful retaliation for this slight, either through litigation or even more outrageous demands. It is important to remember that such people demand to be important because they fear they are not. Their core sense of self is usually one of terrifying weakness, inadequacy, and fear of neglect. The meeting of each demand provides temporary reassurance against such a view. Bearing this in mind, it is helpful to state clearly to this patient at the beginning of treatment that you value them and appreciate the trust they have placed in you by seeking their care. State that you wish to give them the kind of care that will lead to the best outcome. An important stumbling block here can be the doctor feeling internal shame at not meeting expectations, as if some other doctor might do better, leading to false promises or attempts to provide care beyond one's usual expertise.

Conclusion

Modern approaches to working with the personality of the headache patient are increasingly directed towards trait-based systems of understanding. Alexithymia, somatization, neuroticism, and neurochemical sensitivities are characteristics of headache patients with personality dysfunction that distort the treatment of physical symptoms and make medical interactions more difficult. A careful evaluation of core personality traits, defenses, patient fears, role and attachment patterns, transference–counter-transference feelings, and narrative style of the headache complaint can help the physician develop a thoughtful picture of the patient. This type of evaluation will suggest those modes of medical interaction demonstrated to improve outcome. Following general strategies for open-ended questioning, anger management, interaction with difficult patient types, and avoidance of behaviors associated with conflict and litigation also improve headache patient care. These tools empower the physician to help the patient with the number one cause of all illness, the cause that cannot be measured in the blood or visualized on a scan: the way the patient thinks, feels, and behaves.

References

[1] Wang W, Yang TZ, Zhu HQ, *et al.* Disordered personality traits in primary headaches. *Soc Behav Pers* 2005; **33**: 495–502.

[2] Okasha A, Ismail MK, Khalil AH, *et al.* A psychiatric study of nonorganic chronic headache patients. *Psychosomatics* 1999; **40**: 233–8.

[3] Williams DE, Thompson JK, Haber JD, *et al.* MMPI & Headache: a special focus on differential diagnosis, prediction of treatment outcomes, and patient–treatment matching. *Pain* 1986; **24**: 143–58.

[4] The Personality Disorders Workgroup. Personality and Personality Disorders. 2011.http://www.dsm5.org/ProposedRevisions/Pages/PersonalityandPersonalityDisorders.aspxupdate, (Accessed January 20, 2012)

[5] Skodol A, Bender D. The future of personality disorders in the DSM V. *Am Jl Psych* 2009, **166**: 388–91.

[6] Atasoy HT, Atasoy N, Unal AE. Psychiatric co-morbidity in medication overuse headache patients with pre-existing headache type of episodic tension-type headache. *EJP* 2005; **9**: 285–91.

[7] Brandt J, Celentano D, Stewart W, *et al.* Personality and emotional disorder in a community sample of migraine headache sufferers. *Am Jl Psych* 1990; **147**: 303–8.

[8] Hansen JS, Bendsten L, Jensen R. Predictors of treatment outcome in headache. Patients with the Millon Clinical Multiaxial Inventory III (MCMI-III). *J Headache Pain* 2007; **8**: 28–34.

[9] Waldie KE, Poulton R. Physical and psychological correlates of primary headache in young adulthood: A 26 year longitudinal study. *J Neurol Neurosurg Psychiatry* 2002; **72**: 86–92.

[10] Guidetti V, Ottaviano S, Pagliarini M, Childhood headache risk: warning signs and symptoms in the first six months of life. *Cephalalgia* 1984; **4**: 236–42.

[11] Siever LJ, Weinstein, LN. The neurobiology of personality disorders: implications for psychoanalysis. *J Am Psychoanal Assoc* 2009, **57**: 361–96.

[12] Saper JR, Lake AE. Borderline personality disorder and the chronic headache patient: review and management considerations. *Headache* 2002; **42**: 663–74.

[13] Strain JJ. Psychological reactions to chronic medical illness. *Psychiatric Quarterly* 1979; **51**: 171–83.

[14] Ciechanowski PS. As fundamental as nouns and verbs? Towards an integration of attachment theory in medical training. *Med Ed* 2010; **44**: 122–4

[15] Waters E. Attachment security in infancy and early childhood: a twenty year Longitudinal Study. *Child Dev* 2000; **71**: 684–9.

[16] Thompson D, Ciechanowski PS. Attaching a new understanding to the patient-physician relationship in family practice. *J Am Board Fam Pract* 2003; **16**: 219–26.

[17] Chiechanowski PS, Katon WJ, Russo JE, *et al.* The patient-provider relationship: attachment theory and adherence to treatment in diabetes. *Am J Psych* 2001; **158**: 29–35.

[18] Ciechanowski PS, Sullivan M, Jensen M, *et al.* The relationship of attachment style to depression, catastrophizing and health care utilization in patients with chronic pain. *Pain* 2003; **104**: 627–737.

[19] Schafer S, Nowlis DP. Personality disorders among difficult patients. *Arch Fam Med* 1998; **7**: 126–9.

[20] Betan E, Heim AK, Conklin CZ, Westen D. Countertransference phenomena and personality pathology in clinical practice: an empirical investigation. *Am J Psych* 2005; **162**: 890–8.

[21] Roter DL, Frankel RM, Hall JA, *et al.* The expression of emotion through nonverbal behavior in medical visits. *J Gen Intern Med* 2006; **5**: 28–34.

[22] Norcross JC, Wampold BE. Evidence based therapy relationships: research conclusions and clinical practices, *Psychotherapy* 2001; **48**: 98–102.

[23] Halpern J. Empathy and patient–physician conflicts. *Soc Gen Int Med* 2007; **22**: 696–700.

[24] Charon, R. Narrative medicine: a model for empathy, reflection, profession and trust. *JAMA* 2011; **286**: 1897–902.

[25] Lipton RB, Hahn SR, Cady RK, *et al.* In-office discussions of migraine: results from the American Migraine Communication Study. *J Gen Intern Med* 2008; **23**: 1145–51.

[26] Hahn SR, Lipton RB, Cady FD, *et al.* Healthcare provider-patient communication and migraine assessment: results of the American Migraine Communication Study, Phase II, *Curr Med Res Opin* 2008, **24**: 1711–18.

[27] Abbass A, Lovas D, Purdy A. Direct diagnosis and management of emotional Factors in chronic headache patients. *Cephalalgia* 2008; **28**: 1305–14.

[28] Rao JK, Anderson LA, Inui TS, *et al.* Communication interventions make a difference in conversations between physicians and patients: a review of the evidence. *Med Care* 2007; **45**: 340–9.

[29] Lussier MT, Richard, C. Complaints and legal action: role of doctor-patient communication. *Can Fam Phys* 2005, **51**: 37–42.

[30] Beckma HB, Markakis KM, Suchman AL, *et al.* The doctor-patient relationship and malpractice. *Arch Int Med* 1994, **154**: 1365–70.

[31] Hills L. Defusing the angry patient. *MPM* 2010; **26**: 158–62.

[32] Filipowicz R, Ed. Behaviors: the Actual Leading Causes of Death. *Center for Hlth Stat Study* 2008, **7**: 1–2.

[33] Ferrando SJ, Okoli U. Personality disorders: understanding and managing the difficult patient in neurology practice. *Seminars in Neurology* 2009; **29**: 266–71.

[34] Loder E, Geweke L. Volume and nature of telephone calls in a specialty headache practice. *Headache: J Head Face Pain* 2002; **42**: 883–7.

[35] Groves J. Taking care of the hateful patient. *NEJM* 1978; **298**: 882–7.

Useful links:

Causes of personality change:
http://www.rightdiagnosis.com/symptoms/personality_change/causes.htmA

Chapter 12

Complementary and alternative medicine (CAM) approaches to headache

Maurice Preter and Samuel Lieblich

When I asked the neurologist for a prognosis, he soberly declared, it could get better, it could get worse, it could stay the same. I burst out laughing. He did not see the joke.

Siri Hustvedt, The Shaking Woman or A History of My Nerves [1]

I solve the mind–body problem by stating that there is no such problem. There are, of course, plenty of problems concerning the "mind," and the "body," and all intermediate levels of integration of the nervous system. What I wish to emphasize is that there is no problem of "mind" versus "body," because biologically no such dichotomy can be made. The dichotomy is an artefact; there is no truth in it, and the discussion has no place in science in 1943 . . . The difference between psychology and physiology is merely one of complexity. The simpler bodily processes are studied in physiological departments; the more complex ones that entail the highest levels of neural integration are studied in psychological departments.

Stanley Cobb, Borderlands of Psychiatry (1943) [2]

Introduction

A few general remarks on CAM for the care of the neuropsychiatry patient are necessary, though an in-depth critique of concepts such as "complementary," "alternative" or "conventional" medicine is beyond the scope of this text. It is a truism that the practice of medicine is in constant flux and is subject to scientific as well as to cultural, historic and socio-economic influences. What is conventional now may have been alternative then, massively contested by interested parties supported by an army of scientific experts (e.g., the mid-twentieth century controversy on whether tobacco use causes lung cancer). What is quite alternative in one culture may be conventional in another, such as the practice of the mixed-gender sauna followed by dips in ice-cold water for general wellness and immune support in Northern Europe. Allopathic and CAM practice patterns differ between countries, e.g., in the UK primary care physicians (general practitioners), not specialists, assume most medical care, which at least in theory facilitates (or forces) integration. Neurological consultants have long waiting lists and are rarely involved in the kind of primary neuropsychiatric care currently practiced by many of their US colleagues. China counts about 15 0000 neurologists today, as many as in the USA, but they serve a population approaching five times larger. [3] Consequently, a Chinese neurologist, always based in a tertiary hospital, may see well over 100 patients a day. As psychiatric care is limited, many present with functional symptoms that cannot be addressed in a 2–3-minute patient–physician interaction, and some suffer from undiagnosed and untreated major mental illness. In Germany and Switzerland, more physicians practice some degree of integrated care (allopathic/alternative, and to some extent, neurological/psychiatric) than in the US. Despite these superficial differences, the following applies to biomedicine everywhere.

Despite Cobb's exhortation quoted above, psychiatry and neurology have continued to go their artificially separate ways, [4] leaving both clinical neurology and psychiatry unprepared to care for the complex neuropsychiatric patient, and consequently, often only marginally effective in some cases. [5] This unsatisfying situation is ultimately not being helped by the creation of yet another expert domain to which to refer "non-responders." Non-standard, complementary or "alternative" treatments are not always conceptual

The Neuropsychiatry of Headache, ed. Mark W. Green and Philip R. Muskin. Published by Cambridge University Press.

alternatives to conventional medications: Replacing a standard NSAID with a non-standard (and often non-standardized), frequently self-administered herbal anti-inflammatory as primary therapeutic agent for the chronic disabling head pain of a patient with post-traumatic stress or panic disorder does nothing to address comorbidity and is unlikely to be successful in the long term. Mind–body and manual therapy practitioners are arguably so popular because they respect the suffering person's need for an unrushed, personalized, traditional patient–physician relationship more than most contemporary neurologists, but CAM medications and treatments do not always equal an integrated, patient-rather-than-symptom centered approach. Patients, in ever-increasing numbers interested in pursuing CAM, ought to know that these preparations, whether classified as nutraceuticals, herbs, vitamins, nutrients, or hormones are pharmacoactive substances that are not always safer (e.g., L-tryptophan contamination scandal), nor free of undesired effects (e.g., magnesium), nor cheaper (e.g., SAM-e or quality Omega-3). Navigating the waters between conventional medicine and CAM can be confusing, but to be efficient, professionals involved in the care of the suffering individual, be they neurologists, psychiatrists, psychologists, or others need to acquire a working knowledge of these intricacies. At the same time, the CAM boom notwithstanding, chronic headache patients remain substantially underserved. [5] Many suffer from other chronic, "medically unexplained" (e.g., irritable bowel, backache, genitourinary pain, multiple environmental sensitivities) and psychiatric comorbidities (e.g., panic disorder, depression). Many are psychologically traumatized, often early in life. [6] Frequently, the primary expression of this preverbal, unspeakable suffering is somatic pain. Classified as "medical," many of these patients never come to psychiatrists' attention; rather, they seek (and receive) medical specialty care depending on which body part seems to cause the most distress.

We posit that a truly "alternative," i.e., integrated approach to head pain has to be rooted in contemporary neuroscience perspectives on pain–emotion interactions [7], specifically using current knowledge of:

(1) the migraine–panic interface [8]
(2) the endogenous opioid separation anxiety system [9]
(3) how early life events cause a shift in endogenous opioid reactivity [10]
(4) the inflammation–depression–stress connection [11]
(5) analogies to other "unexplained medical syndromes." [12]

Although awareness of these interdependencies is increasing in the clinical press, [13] integration is far from being achieved. At least since Cobb, neither scientific progress nor patients' needs have been the only driving forces in medicine.

Scope of CAM in headache

In a recent report, half of adults with migraines/severe headaches used CAM in the past 12 months "because conventional treatments were perceived as ineffective or too costly." CAM was most often used adjunctively, frequently without the allopathic physician's knowledge. Mind-body therapies (e.g., meditation, yoga) were used most commonly, ranking just before pharmaceutical herbs and "supplements."[14]

Given space limitations, we list an – idiosyncratic and limited – selection of approaches that appear to be of therapeutic value and to our knowledge, do not expose patients to undue risks. To facilitate comparison, we provide a table at the end of the chapter (Table 12.1). Several established mind-body interventions are covered elsewhere in the book. Allopathic medicine, and perhaps neurology, in particular, tends to be skeptical of alternative approaches. Standard large-scale controlled efficacy studies are rarely available, mainly because there is no economic incentive to carry them out. Those randomized controlled trials (RCTs) that exist are often methodologically problematic, e.g., inadequately blinded and underpowered, and unlikely to successfully compete with industry-funded drug research that has a tendency to report positive more frequently than null results. [15]

While many CAM treatments may have a more favorable risk–benefit profile than standard pharmaceuticals, they should be used just like allopathic drugs, in accordance with patients' wishes (which are increasingly influenced by specialized social networks such as www.patientslikeme.com) and the physician's best judgment, personal experience, and comfort level, while keeping in mind that informed consent is a process, not an event. From clinical experience, for some patients they can be the most effective, low-risk treatments available. Some mind–body and manual therapies take years to learn and are time-intensive; consequently, they tend to be, and should be, therapies to which patients are referred. Because of their pharmacologically based treatment approaches, biomedical physicians may find it relatively easy to accept, become acquainted with, and eventually suggest oral preparations to their CAM interested patients. It is well worth noting that the efficacy of many conventional and CAM treatments alike appears ultimately based on their anti-inflammatory and analgesic properties; this fact should facilitate conceptual integration.

Using Western mind–body dualistic schemata leaves us ill equipped to categorize many CAM approaches. While some treatments conveniently come in pill (or drop) form, it is in many cases impossible to determine whether a treatment is primarily "psychological," "mind-based," or "body-based": mind–body practitioners at any rate, may argue that this distinction is moot.

Lifestyle, exercise, and dietary considerations

Identifying gustatory headache triggers is common practice, although evidence that certain foods actually "cause" migraine remains anecdotal (see [16] for a succinct discussion). Just as basic, but less attended to, lack of regular food and water intake, and of good-quality sleep (including due to shift work and time-zone travel), lack of exercise, of regular social interactions, or of sexual activity can all contribute to or worsen headache. One shared underlying pain-triggering or enhancing mechanism of these dyschronies may be the activation of endogenous inflammatory processes. [17,18]

Given that peripheral inflammation is a risk factor for cerebrovascular and neurogenenerative disease and may increase central pain perception, [19] anti-inflammatory measures should be a priority for the clinician practicing both "headache medicine" and preventative neuropsychiatry. The anti-inflammatory effect of simple cholecalciferol (Vitamin D3) replenishment appears to improve headaches. [20] Special diets, such as the sattvic, strictly non-dairy vegan diet of Vedic India, and certain condiments are recommended by some practitioners as anti-inflammatory. One example is curcumin, a major ingredient in South Asian cuisine studied in numerous clinical trials for its preventive and/or curative effects in animal models of cancer, neurodegeneration and eye diseases. [21]

Oral agents

Magnesium

It is postulated that functional magnesium (Mg^{2+}) deficiency may be pathophysiologically correlated with headache; a number of studies find low levels of Mg^{2+} across headache types, perhaps especially in menstrual migraine. [22] Incidentally, low Mg^{2+} intake and low blood levels are also associated with depression and anxiety in a number of studies. [23] While Mg^{2+} is the fourth most abundant essential mineral in the body and a cofactor for more than 300 metabolic reactions in the body, [24] it is estimated that 75% of Americans do not meet the recommended dietary allowance of magnesium. [24] The evidence for intravenous $MgSO_4$ to treat the acute migraine attack is mixed. Early studies [22] show that response to intravenous magnesium sulfate is inversely correlated with ionized serum Mg^{2+} levels, implying that a functional deficiency may cause migraine. In a small single-blind RCT [25] of 30 patients with moderate to severe migraine attacks, 1 g of intravenous magnesium sulfate is superior to placebo. The same dose provides effective [26] pain reduction in patients with aura, but not in common migraine. There are two other negative RCTs in emergency room settings. [27,28]

There is evidence to support the use of oral magnesium in migraine prophylaxis, variably reducing headache frequency and analgesic use in menstrual migraine, [29] as well as in larger, heterogeneous samples. [30]

Oral magnesium is considered safe below 350 mg of elemental Mg^{2+} daily; higher doses (600 mg) are commonly used in headache prophylaxis. [24] Patients should be cautioned that oral magnesium supplementation can cause diarrhea. Its use is contraindicated in patients with severe renal insufficiency, and in those with neuromuscular disorders. $MgSO_4$ can be used in children and is one of the few oral agents considered safe in women who are pregnant or are trying to conceive.

Feverfew

Feverfew, extracted from the leaves of the ubiquitous weed plant, *Tanacetum parthenium*, is an herbal remedy traditionally used as an antipyretic, anti-inflammatory, and analgesic. Parthenolide has been identified as the main active ingredient and has anti-inflammatory effects possibly explained by its antagonism of the IκB kinase complex. [31] It inhibits prostaglandin synthetase, thereby reducing platelet aggregation. Feverfew inhibits smooth muscle contraction, and may prevent the vascular spasm postulated to be pathophysiologically operant in migraine. It inhibits histamine release from mast cells and is mildly sedative. [31] Several *Tanacetum* varieties contain large amounts of melatonin. Standardized extracts with known quantities of the putatively active compounds are now manufactured; in Canada, one product has received regulatory approval to claim that it prevents migraine headaches. Whether feverfew is an effective preventative remains controversial, probably due to the standardization and methodological issues epidemic in CAM. [32] In positive trials, subjects respond with a decrease in headache frequency of around 2 days per month, but feverfew does not improve headache symptoms or shorten the duration of attacks. [33]

Preliminary data from a recent industry sponsored trial suggest that a proprietary sublingual combination of ginger and feverfew (LipiGesic] may have a role in abortive treatment. [34] It does not limit the second-line administration of a triptan or other conventional acute treatment. Mouth ulceration, nausea and gastrointestinal discomfort are the most frequently reported side effects, which seem to decrease with the use of standardized extractions like MIG-99. [22,31–33]

There are reports of a "post-feverfew syndrome" in prolonged use of raw leaf preparations characterized by rebound migraine, insomnia, anxiety, and pain in joints and muscles. Feverfew is emmenagogic and should not be prescribed to women who are pregnant or breastfeeding. It may cause cross-reactions in those allergic to other plants of the daisy family (like chamomile or ragweed). Its daily use does not limit prescription of other conventional migraine-abortive medications, but because of its antiplatelet activity, co-administration with aspirin, other NSAIDs (which may also interfere with its effectiveness), and anticoagulants is not advisable.

Butterbur

Butterbur is a root extract of the *Petasites hybridus* plant used since antiquity as an analgesic, antipyretic, and spasmolytic. The active ingredients have shown migraine-relevant properties in vitro such as inhibition of COX-1 and COX-2 [35] and blockage of voltage dependent Ca^{2+} channels in vascular smooth muscle.

Several industry-sponsored RCTs, the majority using the proprietary Petadolex at 50 mg or 75 mg BID, demonstrates the safety and efficacy of butterbur as a prophylactic. [22,36,37] It is recommended as a second-line prophylactic agent by the European Federation of Neurological Societies guidelines on the drug treatment of migraine. [38] Petadolex®, Petaforce®, and Tesalin® are all similar standardized extracts containing between 7.5 mg-8.0 mg of petasins in a 50 mg tablet. Butterbur does not appear to significantly inhibit platelet aggregation, making it better suited than feverfew to co-administration with aspirin. Butterbur may potentiate the anticholinergic effects of some drugs and herbal supplements and should not be co-administered with antipsychotics or antihistamines. [39] Unrefined, the plant contains hepatotoxic and carcinogenic pyrrolizidine alkaloids. The extract should contain a minimum of 15% petasins and undergo complete removal of toxic alkaloids ("PA-free"). Reports of adverse events are rare [36] and are limited to benign gastrointestinal symptoms (eructation/"burping"). Butterbur has been recommended for use in children with migraine, [36] but like other herbal preparations, is contraindicated in pregnancy.

Riboflavin

Riboflavin (vitamin B2) is essential to electron transport in oxidative metabolism and at pharmacological doses may relieve oxidative stress due to putative mitochondrial dysfunction in migraine sufferers. [40]

A decrease in headache frequency is seen in an RCT using 400 mg of Riboflavin daily over 4–12 weeks. [41] There is one positive, diary-based open-label study in children with chronic refractory headaches. [42]

Undesired effects are diarrhea, polyuria (both infrequent), and discoloration of urine. There are no significant interactions reported with conventional headache medications or with other nutraceuticals. No safety data exists for high-dose riboflavin in pregnancy.

CoQ10

Another cofactor in mitochondrial oxidative metabolism, Coenzyme Q10 (Ubiquinone) is a potent antioxidant. CoQ10 deficiency has been implicated in numerous disorders, including statin-induced myopathy and childhood migraine where replenishment is prophylactic. [43] It may be effective in adult migraine prophylaxis. [44,45] Undesired effects may include heartburn, agitation, and anxiety at higher doses, and hypotension. Safety of CoQ10 in women who are pregnant or breastfeeding has not been established.

Alpha-lipoic acid

Alpha-lipoic acid is a fatty acid found in many foods such as yeast, spinach, broccoli, potatoes, liver, and kidney. Like riboflavin and CoQ10, it participates in mitochondrial oxygen metabolism. While substantial preclinical interest in its antioxidant, anti-inflammatory, and potentially neuroprotective properties is ongoing, the small clinical literature suffers from methodological problems and remains inconclusive. [[22] for a review] No adverse events have been reported. Alpha-lipoic acid may be beneficial to fetal development, but proper safety data does not exist.

Omega-3 polyunsaturated fatty acids

Clinically relevant omega-3 polyunsaturated fatty acids (PUFAs) are the bioactive lipids eicosapentaenoic acid (EPA) and docosahexaenoic acid (DHA) contained in certain fish and microalgae. They are powerful antiinflammatory substances that attract theoretical and clinical interest in many areas of medicine. [46] While pharmaceutical-grade, quality Omega-3 marine oils are, in our opinion, a highly useful addition to the toolbox of neurologists and psychiatrists, there is to date no published research on PUFAs and headache. Both in published research (e.g., for depression) and in the clinical context, they tend to be under-dosed preventing them from reaching their full therapeutic potential. Since they are still mostly fish-derived, patients need to be aware of quality issues, including potential organochloride and heavy metal contamination. PUFAs prolong bleeding time; they must be stopped several days before any surgical or dental intervention. The EPA component, although it does not cross the blood–brain barrier, is the active mood elevator and can cause hypomania in predisposed individuals. [47]

Ginkgo biloba extract (GBE)

Leaf extracts of the Ginkgo biloba tree (GBE) have been used in traditional Chinese medicine for thousands of years. GBE contains a variety of flavonoid glycosides and terpenoids (ginkgolides, bilobalides) [48] that have antioxidant and anti-inflammatory properties comparable in potency to Vitamin C, E, or glutathione. [49] One gingko terpenoid, Ginkgolide B inhibits platelet activating factor (PAF), a pro-inflammatory and platelet activator [49] that may be released from platelets and leukocytes during acute migraine. [50]

EGb 761, a standardized extract produced in Germany that contains a selection of over 60 components identified in GBE, has been studied in numerous "inflammatory" conditions, including asthma, depression, glaucoma, mild-to-moderate cognitive impairment, and cerebrovascular insufficiency. It is widely used for the latter in European countries and is available in the USA as a nutritional supplement, but for unclear reasons, EGb 761 has never been studied for use in headaches.

The proprietary Migrasoll®, containing 60 mg Ginkgo biloba along with rather minuscule amounts of Co-Q10 and of vitamin B2, may be useful in adult and pediatric migraine prophylaxis based on results of small open-label trials. [50,51] Responders report significantly reduced intra-attack pain, aura duration and aura intensity after 3 months of treatment. [50]

Undesired effects of GBE are rare and may include headache and gastrointestinal disturbances. Subdural hematoma and Stevens–Johnson syndrome have been described. [48] It has not been determined whether or not they were coincidental to Gingko use. A neurotoxin, Ginkgotoxin, known to lower the seizure threshold, is found in small amounts in GBE, and Ginkgo should be used with caution in patients with a history of seizures and those taking other epileptogenic agents used in headache treatment (e.g., tricyclics, chlorpromazine). [48]

Non-pharmacological approaches: body-centered, mind-centered, mind/body-centered and beyond

Some approaches variously classified as psychological, "mind–body," or behavioral, namely biofeedback, cognitive-behavioral therapy, relaxation training, mindfulness and other meditative practices, are discussed under "Stress management" in Chapter 10.

Exercise

While intense physical activity may trigger headaches in some, [52–54] initially raising the specter of a secondary headache, aerobic exercise is commonly recommended to patients with migraine and other types of bodily pain. [55] Regular wellness-promoting physical activity correlates with other psychological, socio-economic and nutritional indices of good health. Physical inertia increases the risk for common headaches in prospective studies. [56] Exercise is a complex behavioral intervention, making it impossible to invoke discrete physiological changes. Nitric oxide [57] and beta-endorphin increases have been postulated as the mechanism of effect. [58] It is worth remembering that headaches often overlap with depression and with panic disorder, both of which respond well to aerobic exercise alone or in combination with other interventions. [59,60]

While the habitual methodological limitations prevail in the literature [61] two recent papers report positive findings. An RCT [62] comparing the efficacy of exercise and topiramate in migraine prophylaxis finds that cycling three times a week has equal efficacy to topiramate and relaxation, without any adverse effects. Significant reductions in the frequency, duration of attacks, and pain intensity are seen after a 10-week exercise program. [63] The authors identify significant differences between responders and non-responders: Patients responding to exercise are fitter at baseline, more competitive, and already less likely to use migraine medication. Stress indices are significantly reduced in patients who exercise regularly and improvements in headache and stress are associated with increased fitness. This argues for the benefits of a broader, patient-, quality-of-life and prevention-centered approach rather than a merely symptomatic one in mind–brain medicine.

Psychotherapeutic approaches

Psychodynamic therapies

Traditional psychotherapies have been in dramatic decline in the past decades, and even before, only a minority of psychoanalytically informed physicians took an interest in the netherworld of mind–body distress. Given the frequent antecedents of traumatic attachment disruptions in patients presenting clinically with an unrelenting headache, [64] integrating into the assessment an understanding of intrapsychic, interpersonal, family, and doctor–patient transference dynamics should be routine. The useful concept of alexithymia, essentially the inability of many chronically overwhelmed and traumatized patients to experience emotional pain as emotional rather than as purely bodily, has fallen by the wayside. While the split in mind–brain medicine continues to be reinforced by the current medical system, the burden of chronic pain to the patient, to society and to the economy (absenteeism, presenteeism, i.e., illness-related loss of productivity while at work) is enormous. Research is sparse, but an interesting argument for using brief psychodynamic psychotherapy interventions in the Emergency Department for unexplained medical symptoms (to wit, head pain and chest pain) is made by Abbas. [65] A small open study of brief psychodynamic psychotherapy in conjunction with drug withdrawal and prophylactic pharmacotherapy finds a statistically greater decrease in headache frequency and medication intake at 12 months, and a much lower relapse rate in the combined treatment group [66] compared with standard treatment alone. A recent overview discusses psychodynamic group therapy approaches to somatoform pain. [67]

Techniques using diverse sensory, non-language-based manipulations to effect change have been summarily called psychosensory therapies. [68] EFT, Havening, and EMDR, all discussed below, originated from a need for brief interventions to relieve acute psychological traumatic stress, but for various reasons seem to be useful in chronic pain and other functional neurological symptoms. Psychosensory therapies promoting mind–body wellness and relaxation include yoga, acupuncture, biofeedback, neuro-feedback, exercise and related activities, music, light, massage, Reiki, aroma therapy, and Rolfing. [68] Research for all these modalities, to the extent it exists is very limited, but these are safe, accessible methods worth knowing about; some will be discussed below.

Hypnosis

Hypnotherapy is not really "CAM." Since Charcot, Bernheim, and the early work of Freud, hypnosis has been central to neuropsychiatric theory and therapeutics. The literature on the analgesic effect of suggestion is comparatively vast, and interest in hypnotherapy is again on the rise. The practice is highly varied, but many contemporary practitioners favor an integrated, eclectic approach based on Ericksonian principles. [69,70] Following trance induction, suggestions may include changing the inner experience from pain to e.g., numbness, reduction in pain, increases in comfort, changes in focus of attention away from pain and increased ability to ignore pain. Post-hypnotic suggestions and encouragement to practice trance auto-induction are commonly used. [70] Hypnosis has been evaluated in a large number of chronic pain conditions, including headache, although the lack of a standardized, properly controlled procedure makes comparisons problematic. Melis [71] found a significant reduction in TTH (tension-type headache) frequency, intensity, and concomitant anxiety, using wait-list controls. In an earlier cross-over study, classic migraine patients aged 6–12 randomized to propranolol, placebo, and self-hypnosis had fewer [5.8] headaches per 3 months in the self-hypnosis group [13] on average in the placebo and 15 in the propranolol groups). [72]. There was an association between decrease in headache frequency and self-hypnosis training, but pain intensity measures were not affected. There are no published studies specifically comparing hypnotic suggestion to more recent standard abortive or prophylactic migraine drugs. However, summarizing methodologically mixed RCTs of hypnotic analgesia for various chronic pain conditions, average effect size across studies was estimated at 0.67, "indicating that the average person treated with hypnosis obtains a greater analgesic response than 75% of individuals who are given standard care or no treatment." [73] Hypnosis does not seem to be superior to progressive muscle relaxation or autogenic training. [73] The general tenor from the literature is that, despite being empirically well supported as efficacious and safe, hypnotic analgesia continues to be greatly underutilized. [73] probably because many contemporary physicians remain un-, or misinformed.

Other techniques potentially helpful for chronic headache patients, such as body-oriented therapy [74] and somatic experiencing, [75] use highly focused attention and aspects of trance and self-hypnosis, but space limitations preclude discussion.

Eye movement desensitization and reprocessing (EMDR)

One mind–body technique originally designed to relieve psychological trauma (which is itself, with panic disorder and depression highly comorbid with chronic headaches) is EMDR. During EMDR, the patient concentrates on a traumatic memory or distressing bodily state, while also focusing on an external stimulus, such as a horizontally moving object or light stimulating saccadic eye movements, or on bilateral tapping. The hypothesis that EMDR may promote interhemispheric connectivity, functionally and anatomically impaired in psychological trauma has not been substantiated. Mostly used for acute and chronic psychological stress, but also obsessive-compulsive disorder, phantom limb pain, specific phobias, and psychogenic seizures, EMDR has also been suggested as an abortive treatment for migraine. In one open-label study, combining EMDR, diaphragmatic breathing, and cranial compression improved or eliminated acute migraine more efficiently and faster than standard abortive medication. During the 1- to-7-day follow-up, 15 out of 26 controls required rescue medication, compared with 9 out of 26 in the treatment group. [76] EMDR has since been studied in small samples of usually acutely traumatized populations with physical pain, such as the South Asian tsunami survivors. Efforts to investigate its effectiveness in headache prophylaxis have been presented in abstract form. [77]

Emotional freedom technique (EFT)

EFT is another poorly understood and under-studied intervention. In a New Age interpretation of traditional chinese medicine (TCM) [78] EFT assumes that traumatic events cause emotional disturbances by interfering with the body's energy field (meridian) system. [79] The therapeutic intervention is light tapping in sequence on acupuncture points on the head, face, upper body, and hands. In TCM, the same acupoints are used to reduce aggressive energy (yang; 阴阳), to "cool heat," i.e., to sedate. Current research is limited to one recent National Health Service (NHS)-supported study comparing EMDR and EFT for psychological trauma, in which both were found to be equally effective in reducing hyperarousal, [79] and one positive, randomized study of internet-administered EFT in fibromyalgia pain. [80] Although so far not formally studied for headache, EFT and other meridian-based, "energy healing" techniques, such as Ronald Ruden MD's Havening, [68] and Tapas acupressure technique (TAT) [81] are easy to learn, widely used CAM treatments of pain, and well worth knowing about.

Alternative medical systems

These can be ancient (and Eastern), such as traditional Chinese medicine (TCM) and Indian Ayurveda, or quite recent (and Western), such as homeopathy. All provide treatment options for chronic pain, including headache. Many good introductory texts are available. [82,83,84]

Chinese medicine

TCM, at least in its modernized version, continues to influence numerous CAM approaches both in modern China and the West. [3] Based on the healing traditions of Taoism (道教), TCM posits that physical and mental health is based on a dynamic, harmonious equilibrium of internal and environmental influences.

These include the two polar, complementary forces, yin and yang (阴阳), the five phases (wu xing; 五行) and qi (气), the vital force that is both matter and energy and flows through the body's dedicated energy channels (jing; 经). Disease is caused by disruption of the balanced state, either in the form of excess, or deficiency. Treatment is aimed at restoring harmony, rather than the identification and eradication of a single pathogen, and consists of pharmaceutical herbs, moxibustion, acupuncture and acupressure, cupping, massage (Tui Na), and physical and mental 'self-cultivation' (yang sheng; 养生), which includes Qigong and Tai Chi. For lack of space, only acupuncture and Tai Chi/Qigong will be mentioned here.

Acupuncture

In contemporary usage the term "acupuncture" describes a family of procedures involving the stimulation of one or several of the hundreds of traditionally described anatomical points along the body's energy channels ("meridians") using hypodermic needles of various thickness and length, sometimes combining them with electrical stimulation (electro-acupuncture), and on occasion, using a laser instead of a needle. These are the same acupoints activated in, e.g., acupressure or cupping (as well as in EFT). The technique most often studied scientifically involves penetrating the skin with thin, solid, metallic needles that are manipulated by hand, or by electrical stimulation.

In Chinese medicine, acupuncture is used in the treatment of numerous neuropsychiatric conditions, from acute delirium to post-stroke spasticity. In Western CAM, it has assumed a particular role in the management of acute and chronic pain. Its "scientific" mechanism of action remains unclear, but involves a possible anti-inflammatory effect, changes to the vascular release of nitric oxide, and modulation of the serotonin, opioid and endocannabinoid systems. [85]

Acupuncture is one of the most frequently employed CAM interventions in headache. [86] Interpretation of available data is problematic. Acupuncture practice varies widely and few Western practitioners have received extensive training in traditional Chinese medicine, which is an 8–12-year curriculum at specialized Chinese institutions. A number of studies found similar efficacy for verum and placebo (sham) acupuncture. [87] "Unspecific," expectancy effects have been invoked, but it has been pointed out that, since we do not have a theory of how needle placement in acupuncture changes physiology, the concept of "sham" is in itself questionable. [88] Others use electroacupuncture which obfuscates the distinction between verum and placebo further because of possible remote effects of the electric current. [89]

Acupuncture compares favorably with prophylactic drugs such as metoprolol in a systematic review. [90] Trials published since have confirmed the conclusions of the Cochrane review. [91,92] Yang *et al.* comparing acupuncture to topiramate finds that it offered similar reductions in headache frequency, but greater increases in social function and significant improvements in headache symptoms with far fewer reported adverse effects (6% compared to 66%) [91]. An accompanying Cochrane review of acupuncture in TTH [93] is dominated by two large studies using "routine-care" (i.e., analgesic use) as the control group [94,95] showing that adding acupuncture reduces the frequency of headaches over the 3 months study period. In an NHS-sponsored study, adding acupuncture to routine care of chronic headache patients yields a cost-effective increase in health-related quality of life measures correlating with the observed reductions in headache severity and frequency; the study does not consider medication cost savings and improved productivity. [96]

Although rarely studied, acupuncture may be effective in acute migraine. Acupuncture compares well head-to-head with subcutaneous sumatriptan as an abortive agent, but is inferior as a rescue medication. [97]

Weintraub [98] describes the use of laser stimulation of He Gu (LI4), an acupoint located near the middle of the second metacarpal to treat acute migraine. In China, LI4 is commonly used in self-administered acupressure for the relief of headache, facial, and dental pain. Also, sham-controlled, intraoral laser application to the maxillary alveolar tender point aborts migraine in 85% of cases. [98]

In experienced hands, acupuncture is a safe therapy with low risk of adverse events. A review of three Chinese trials involving nearly 2000 treatments finds instances of subcutaneous hematoma, bleeding, and needle site pain. [99] Older patients seem to be at greater risk of adverse events. [91,92,94,99] Occasionally, avoidable serious adverse outcomes (hepatitis C, pneumothorax) have been reported.

Tai Chi and Qigong

Tai Chi and Qigong embody the Taoist principle of self-improvement through body–mind practice. Both involve body movements, breathing, and attentional focusing to maintain health and rebalance the qi (气).

Tai Chi, originally a martial art taught at the Shao-Lin and other Buddhist monasteries in classic China evolved into an exercise routine practiced by many Chinese elders in public spaces in China and overseas. Its simplified version includes 24 body positions that appear easy to memorize, but require years of practice to master. A variety of studies demonstrates that tai chi may be a useful treatment for rheumatoid and fibromyalgia pain. [73]

"Internal" Qigong combines focused attention with breathing exercises, while "External" Qigong also includes physical movements, sometimes resembling Tai Chi poses. Some small, positive studies of Qigong in anxiety and depression are reviewed in Brown [100]; Qigong is also effective in a pilot study for fibromyalgia, dramatically reducing both pain and depression measures. Four small studies for various types of chronic pain, including complex regional pain syndrome Type I (reflex sympathetic dystrophy), reviewed in Tan [73] show similar promising results, leading to the conclusion that Qigong is "possibly to probably efficacious for treatment of chronic pain." Thus far, neither Tai Chi nor Qigong have been specifically studied for headache treatment.

Indian medicine

Yoga

Yoga is an ancient spiritual and philosophical system rooted in the religions of the Indian sub-continent. More pragmatically, it is also a mind–body cultivation method as well as a therapeutic modality, and in contemporary India, yoga therapy is one of six officially recognized medical systems, along with allopathy, homeopathy, naturopathy, Ayurvedic medicine, Unani and Siddha. [82]Yoga at its most basic involves stretching exercises, codified postures, deep breathing and meditation. There are many schools of yoga and dozens of traditional postures. Yoga has been shown to improve anxiety and depression and may exert its effect on headache by improvement of comorbid psychological distress. Yoga increases parasympathetic tone and improves sleep, both beneficial in headache. [101] In an RCT of a comprehensive program of yogic techniques (selected asanas, conscious breathing (pranayama), nasal water cleansing (jalaneti) and meditation (kriya) vs. routine care, the yoga program is associated with significant reductions in headache frequency, pain, nausea, anxiety, and medication use. [102] An earlier study comparing yoga with EMG biofeedback finds them similarly effective. [103] A recent meta-analysis of yoga interventions on pain and pain-associated disability shows unequivocal positive effects for back pain, rheumatoid arthritis, dysmenorrhea, and migraine. The generally "moderate" methodological quality of the studies had no impact on the study outcome. Interestingly, short-term interventions yield stronger effects on pain-related disability than longer treatments. [104] Patients who want to try yoga require instruction, supervision, and must practice several hours weekly to maintain therapeutic gain [103,102]; novices are at risk for musculoskeletal injury. Modified yoga is safe in, and may decrease complications of pregnancy. [101] Patients who are pregnant or hypertensive should avoid Bikram and similar hot-room yoga practices.

Homeopathy

Homeopathy is a system of medicine developed by German physician and chemist, Samuel Hahnemann (1755–1843), based on the "law of similars." At its most basic, a homeopathic remedy is said to cure by using infinitesimal dilutions of the purported disease-causing agent in order to stimulate the innate vital healing capacity of the organism and thus "let like be cured by like." To critics questioning how a medicine containing no measurable concentrations of an active agent can affect biological systems, the "memory of water" theory is invoked, which posits that the process of serial dilution transfers disease-relevant information to the solvent. More pragmatically, resemblances between exotic-appearing homeopathic principles and those scientifically accepted are pointed out, e.g., even single-molecule pheromones have long-lasting physiological and behavioral effects, minimal amounts of antigens can trigger hugely amplified immune responses, etc. In the "classical" method of homeopathic prescription the homeopath is guided by the complaint and by idiosyncratic patient features. This highly individualized treatment prevalent in Europe, India, and South America usually arises from a long therapeutic interaction where the patient's symptoms, co-existing conditions and biographical details are discussed. In the USA, where since the 1990s, there has been, a minor homeopathy boom along with the CAM boom, remedies appear to be primarily self-administered (i.e., bought over-the-counter). [84] Around 3.4% of headache patients have tried homeopathic medications. [14] A small number of studies has provided thus far no support for its efficacy over placebo. [16] It should not be neglected that, as a group, people who use homeopathy in a "classic" context (i.e., not simply buying over-the counter remedies in search for more affordable alternatives to standard drugs) are likely to show considerable, long-lasting improvement. [105]

Manual therapies

Chiropractic

Chiropractic is a widely popular, insurance-reimbursed manual method focusing on spinal manipulation that originated in the late nineteenth century in Iowa. Its founder, Daniel David Palmer posited that the body heals itself by "innate intelligence," the operation of which is hindered by spinal subluxations that can be corrected by manipulation. [106] Patients most frequently seek help for musculoskeletal conditions, but also for neurological, gastrointestinal and psychological complaints. [106,107] The chiropractic literature is methodologically fragmented leading systematic reviews to conclude that "[w]ith the possible exception of back pain, chiropractic spinal manipulation has not been shown to be effective for any medical condition," [107], including headache. [16,108] Conversely, a recent review by the Guidelines Committee of the Canadian Chiropractic Association concludes "moderate level" "evidence suggests that chiropractic care, including spinal manipulation, improves migraine and cervicogenic headaches" but is equivocal as to "spinal manipulation as an isolated intervention for patients with tension-type headache." [109] NCCAM lists temporary headaches, tiredness, or discomfort in treated areas as common side effects of chiropractic [110]. There have been rare reports of serious complications such as posterior circulation stroke due to vertebral dissection, although cause and effect are unclear [106,110].

Osteopathy and craniosacral manipulation

Osteopathy is a medical system devised by Andrew Taylor Still in the second half of the nineteenth century in the American Midwest. Osteopaths, like chiropractors, emphasize care of the "whole patient." [111] The four primary precepts posit (1) the body is a unit; (2) the reciprocal relationship of structure to function; (3) the body's self regulatory ability; (4) the inherent ability of the body to defend and heal itself. According to osteopathic theory, imbalances in the musculoskeletal system can affect internal organs via the "somatovisceral reflex", whereas visceral changes can pathologically affect the musculoskeletal system via the "viscerosomatic reflex." [112] In the US, osteopaths are fully licensed to practice allopathic medicine, but distinguish themselves by their particular theory of disease generation and treatment and by use of a manual therapy which is their preserve. [111] While osteopathy focuses on musculoskeletal pain, it is also used in asthma, sinusitis, carpal tunnel syndrome, migraines, and menstrual pain. [111] Treatments can be musculoskeletal, visceral or cranial, the latter manipulating the cranial bones in order to release strains in the dura mater which are thought to cause disease. [113] Commonly, the osteopath will massage cervical soft-tissue using techniques such as "occipital decompression" which is reputed to abort migraines and "myofascial unwinding" which is said to relieve the pain of muscle spasm in the head and neck. [112,114] A single-blind comparison of osteopathic treatments, including cranial osteopathy, plus relaxation vs. relaxation alone finds the combination superior for tension-type headache. [113] In a recent study, osteopathy significantly improves measures of pain, quality of life, and absenteeism in female migraineurs. [115] Adverse events have not been reported in the osteopathic literature on headache.

Reiki

Reiki, while it has a "manual" aspect and is therefore mentioned here for simple convenience, is more correctly classified as an energy healing/Biofield therapy (for a review [116]). The term derives from the Japanese words *rei* (universal) and *ki* (vital energy). The practice was developed by Mikao Usui, a Japanese spiritual healer living in the early twentieth century.

Reiki practitioners place their hands on the patient in approximately 15 different hand positions. In this way they claim to collect "universal energy" (ki or qi) which flows from them to the patient and facilitates a healing response. [117] The technique is highly variegated, with some practitioners' hands contacting the patient, and others' just above the patient, while some practitioners claim to be able to "send" Reiki to distant patients with appropriate training. [117] Some people report it effective when self-applied. [118] The 2007 National Health Interview Survey reported that around 1.2 million adults and 161 0000 children had used energy healing methods like reiki in the previous year. [119] While Reiki practitioners report efficacy in a range of diseases, the treatment has been subjected to only six RCTs and three systematic reviews listed on pubmed. In a recent review, nine of twelve trials have positive findings, but none are methodologically sound. [120] Control groups have received sham Reiki administered by untrained actors [121] or have met with a Reiki master who administered distance-Reiki to some subjects and not others, whilst supposedly maintaining subject blinding. [122] One study of 100 patients with fibromyalgia concludes that neither Reiki nor therapeutic touch, against which it was controlled, had a significant effect on pain. [121] Conversely, a wait list controlled study of 20 elderly patients receiving Reiki for general well-being reports significant improvement in pain, including neck pain, depression, and anxiety. [123]

Electromagnetic stimulation

The idea that the application of magnetic currents may be therapeutic is ancient. Interest in various types of surface electrical and magnetic stimulation has been intense from the eighteenth century, but scientific study of alternate modalities slowed down in the 1930s with the introduction of the highly efficacious electroconvulsive therapy. ECT involves transcranial electrical stimulation at significantly higher intensities than the techniques mentioned here.

Renewed interest in low-intensity superficial brain stimulation through magnetic or electric currents was sparked by the observation that transcranial magnetic stimulation (TMS) may be therapeutic for a number of neuropsychiatric conditions, including pain.

TMS originated as a functional brain mapping method and has been commercially available since 1985. Magnetic coils are applied to areas on the skull surface that correspond to functional cortical areas. Research on TMS is comparatively vast and of higher methodological quality compared to other electrotherapies. Multiple techniques (single pulse vs. more commonly used repetitive stimulation) have been studied. Much work has been done in depression and given the high co-morbidity, rTMS should be useful in chronic pain conditions, such as fibromyalgia and headache. There are no large-scale studies convincingly showing that rTMS benefits neuropsychiatric conditions and pain. [124] An industry-funded RCT shows that single-pulse TMS self-administered to the occiput with a battery-powered device may abort classic migraine headaches. [125] Both active and sham treatment involved the application of electrodes to the occiput. Primary outcome was absence of pain at 2 hours post-intervention, but 75% of patients in the verum group had either "no pain" or "mild pain" before the intervention (compared to 67% in the sham group). Therapeutic gain was calculated as 17%. Given the substantial cost of neurostimulators, a head-to-head comparison between such a device and simple, properly applied, essentially no-cost acupressure to, e.g., Feng Chi (GB 20) between the occipital insertions of the sternocleidomastoid and trapezius muscles might be instructive.

In addition to TMS, the therapeutic potential of non-invasive electrical stimulation of the brain (ESB) in neuropsychiatry continues to attract interest, but evidence for its effectiveness remains sparse. A company-sponsored literature review of the popular Fisher-Wallace cranial electrotherapy stimulation (CES) device shows a moderate effect size compounded from a number of methodologically limited studies of sleep disorders and depression. [126] A recent systemic review of all currently used techniques (rTMS, CES and direct current stimulation, tDCS) finds a possible, "beneficial short-term effect of single-dose high-frequency rTMS applied to the motor cortex [...] not conclusively exceed[ing] the threshold of minimal clinical significance" (i.e., 15%.). [127] The small number of CES and tDCS studies provide no evidence for any effect superior to sham.

Hypothalamic deep brain stimulation (DBS), and less risky, occipital nerve stimulation have been proposed for refractory cluster headache; occipital nerve stimulation was also suggested for intractable migraines, but the authors of a recent review caution that refractory migraine patients "may experience huge improvements when the co-existing psychiatric disorder is properly treated." [128] In late 2011, Saint Jude Medical received regulatory approval in Europe for an implantable occipital nerve stimulator for the treatment of "intractable migraines." Intractable was defined as at least 15 migraines causing at least moderate disability and not responding to three or more preventive drugs, but it is unclear from an integrated neuropsychiatric perspective whether these "refractory patients" had indeed exhausted all treatment options before undergoing a costly, invasive procedure.

Table 12.1. Comparison of some CAM approaches

Agent	Special utility	Dose	Safety			
			Interactions	Side-effects	Precautions/ Contraindications	Pregnancy and breastfeeding
Feverfew		100 mg daily [22]	NSAIDs, Anticoagulants	Mouth ulcerations, Nausea, gastrointestinal discomfort Post-feverfew syndrome (rebound migraine, insomnia, anxiety, muscle and joint pain)	Pediatric Daisy family allergy	Not safe (emmenagogic)
Butterbur	Pediatric [36]	50–75mg bd [22]	Anti-cholinergics [39]	Burping (rare)	Butterbur may increase liver enzyme levels	Insufficient safety data
Magnesium	Menstrual [29] Magnesium deficiency [22] Migraine w/aura [26]	350mg-600mg daily [24] Monitor serum level			Renal insufficiency Neuromuscular disorder	Safe [22]
Riboflavin	Pediatric [42]	400mg daily in divided doses daily [41]		Diarrhea Nausea Polyuria Benign discoloration of urine.	None	Insufficient safety data at headache doses
Co-Q10	Possibly useful in children with demonstrable CoQ10 deficiency [43]	150–300mg daily (Max. 12 mg/kg/day)		Heartburn Headache Rash Agitation and anxiety (high doses) Hypotension Reduced CVS risk		Insufficient safety data
α-lipoic acid	None	600mg daily [129] 300 mg daily with topiramate[130]				Insufficient safety data
Omega-3				"Fish burps"	Potential heavy metal and organic solvent contamination Prolonged bleeding time	Beneficial on theoretical grounds but insufficient safety data
Homeopathy			n/a	n/a		
Ginkgo	Migraine with aura [49–51]		60 –120 mg daily [49–51]	AEDs NSAIDs Anti-coagulants Epileptogenic medications [48] Headache gastrointestinal discomfort	Epilepsy Bleeding diathesis	Insufficient safety data

				bleeding complications dermatitis [48]. Bilateral subdural hematoma and Stevens-Johnson syndrome in two case reports [48] Lowers seizure threshold [48]		
Acupuncture		10 sessions carried out twice weekly [22]	n/a	Headache [86]	Subcutaneous hematoma Bleeding Needle site pain [99]	Safe in expert hands but activation of some meridians is emmenagogic
Vegan, sattvic and other traditional diets	Probable Neurovascular prevention, anti-inflammatory				Risk of unbalanced diet Vit. B12 deficiency	
Yoga		Min. 4 training sessions 1–5 hours/wk practice [102,103]	n/a	n/a	Bikram yoga contraindicated in some patients	Safe in modified form
Exercise		Unclear in migraine 2–12 mins./day resistance exercise in cervicogenic [131]	n/a	n/a	n/a	Safe in modified form
Chiropractic		Variable		Headache Neck pain Headache Tiredness Localized discomfort Rare reports of serious complications such as stroke, although cause and effect are unclear[106]		
Osteopathy		Variable				
Reiki		Variable 1 session/ wk for 8 weeks [123]				Safe

References

[1] Hustvedt S. *The Shaking Woman, or a History of my Nerves*. 1st edn. New York: Henry Holt, 2010. 213 p.p.

[2] Cobb S. *Borderlands of Psychiatry*. Cambridge, MA: Harvard University Press, 1943.

[3] Wang XP, Zhang WF, Huang HY, Preter M. Neurology in the People's Republic of China – an update. *Eur Neurol* 2010; **64**: 320–4.

[4] Preter M, Bursztajn HJ. Crisis and opportunity – The DSM-V and its neurology quandary. *Asian J Psychiatry* 2009; **2**: 143-.

[5] Jones A. High rate of unmet treatment needs occurs in patients with episodic migraine. *Neurol Rev* 2011; **19**, 17.

[6] Tietjen GE, Brandes JL, Peterlin BL, *et al.* Childhood maltreatment and migraine (part I). Prevalence and adult revictimization: a multicenter headache clinic survey. *Headache* 2010; **50**: 20–31.

[7] Eisenberger NI, Lieberman MD. Why rejection hurts: a common neural alarm system for physical and social pain. *Trends Cogn Sci* 2004; **8**: 294–300.

[8] Breslau N, Schultz LR, Stewart WF, Lipton R, Welch KM. Headache types and panic disorder: directionality and specificity. *Neurology* 2001; **56**: 350–4.

[9] Panksepp J, Watt D. Why does depression hurt? Ancestral primary-process separation-distress (PANIC/GRIEF) and diminished brain reward (SEEKING) processes in the genesis of depressive affect. *Psychiatry* 2011; **74**: 5–13.

[10] Preter M, Lee SH, Petkova E, Vannucci M, Kim S, Klein DF. Controlled cross-over study in normal subjects of naloxone-preceding-lactate infusions; respiratory and subjective responses: relationship to endogenous opioid system, suffocation false alarm theory and childhood parental loss. *Psychol Med* 2011; **41**: 385–93.

[11] Rooks C, Veledar E, Goldberg J, Bremner JD, Vaccarino V. Early trauma and inflammation: role of familial factors in a study of twins. *Psychosomatic Med.* 2012; **74**: 146–52.

[12] Hotopf M, Wilson-Jones C, Mayou R, Wadsworth M, Wessely S. Childhood predictors of adult medically unexplained hospitalisations. Results from a national birth cohort study. *Br J Psychiatry* 2000; **176**: 273–80.

[13] Jones A. Adverse childhood experiences are associated with risk for migraine later in life. *Neurol Rev.* 2011; **19**: 24–9.

[14] Wells RE, Bertisch SM, Buettner C, Phillips RS, McCarthy EP. Complementary and alternative medicine use among adults with migraines/severe headaches. *Headache* 2011; **51**: 1087–97.

[15] Kjaergard LL, Als-Nielsen B. Association between competing interests and authors' conclusions: epidemiological study of randomised clinical trials published in the BMJ. *BMJ.* 2002; **325**: 249.

[16] Nicholson Ra, Buse DC, Andrasik F, Lipton RB. Nonpharmacologic treatments for migraine and tension-type headache: how to choose and when to use. *Curr Treatm Opt in Neurol.* 2011; **13**: 28–40.

[17] Morris A, Coverson D, Fike L, *et al.* Sleep quality and duration are associated with higher levels of inflammatory biomarkers: the META-Health Study. *Circulation* 2010; **122**: A17806.

[18] Rubin DA, Hackney AC. Inflammatory cytokines and metabolic risk factors during growth and maturation: influence of physical activity. *Med Sport Sci* 2010; **55**: 43–55.

[19] Wu L-J, Toyoda H, Zhao M-G, *et al.* Upregulation of forebrain NMDA NR2B receptors contributes to behavioral sensitization after inflammation. *J Neurosci.* 2005; **25**: 11107–16.

[20] Knutsen KV, Brekke M, Gjelstad S, Lagerløv P. Vitamin D status in patients with musculoskeletal pain, fatigue and headache: a cross-sectional descriptive study in a multi-ethnic general practice in Norway. *Scand J. Primary Helth Care.* 2010; **28**: 166–71.

[21] Ritch R. Natural compounds: evidence for a protective role in eye disease. *Canad J. Ophthalmol.* 2007; **42**(3): 425–38.

[22] Sun-Edelstein C, Mauskop A. Alternative headache treatments: nutraceuticals, behavioral, and physical treatments. Headache Currents. *Headache.* 2011: 469–83.

[23] Stradford D, Vickar G, Berger C, Cass H. *Flying Publisher Guide to Complementary and Alternative Medicine Treatments in Psychiatry*: Flying Publisher, 2012.

[24] Guerrera MP, Volpe SL, Mao JJ. Therapeutic uses of magnesium. *Am Fam Phys.* 2009; **80**: 157–62.

[25] Demirkaya S, Vural O, Dora B, Topcuoglu MA. Efficacy of intravenous magnesium sulfate in the treatment of acute migraine attacks. *Headache* 2001; **41**: 171–7.

[26] Bigal ME, Bordini CA, Tepper SJ, Speciali JG. Intravenous magnesium sulphate in the acute treatment of migraine without aura and migraine with aura. A randomized, double-blind, placebo-controlled study. *Cephalalgia* 2002; **22**: 345–53.

[27] Cete Y, Dora B, Ertan C, Ozdemir C, Oktay C. A randomized prospective placebo-controlled study of intravenous magnesium sulphate vs. metoclopramide in the management of acute migraine attacks in the Emergency Department. *Cephalalgia* 2005; **25**: 199–204.

[28] Corbo J, Esses D, Bijur PE, Iannaccone R, Gallagher EJ. Randomized clinical trial of intravenous magnesium sulfate as an adjunctive medication for emergency department treatment of migraine headache. *Ann Emerg Med* 2001; **38**: 621–7.

[29] Facchinetti F, Sances G, Borella P, Genazzani AR, Nappi G. Magnesium prophylaxis of menstrual migraine: effects on intracellular magnesium. *Headache* 1991; **31**: 298–301.

[30] Peikert A, Wilimzig C, Köhne-Volland R. Prophylaxis of migraine with oral magnesium: results for a prospective, multi-center, placebo-controlled and double-blind randomized study. *cephalalgia* 1996; **16**: 257.

[31] Pareek A, Suthar M, Rathore GS, Bansal V. Feverfew (*Tanacetum parthenium* L.): a systematic review. *Pharmacognosy Rev*. 2011; **5**: 103–10.

[32] Pittler MH, Ernst E. Feverfew for preventing migraine. *Cochrane Database Syst Rev* 2009, pp. 1–13.

[33] Diener HC, Pfaffenrath V, Schnitker J, Friede M, Henneicke-von Zepelin H-H. Efficacy and safety of 6.25 mg t.i.d. feverfew CO_2-extract (MIG-99) in migraine prevention-a randomized, double-blind, multicentre, placebo-controlled study. *Cephalalgia* 2005; **25**: 1031–41.

[34] Cady RK, Goldstein J, Nett R, Mitchell R, Beach ME, Browning R. A double-blind placebo-controlled pilot study of sublingual feverfew and ginger (LipiGesic™ M) in the treatment of migraine. *Headache* 2011; **51**: 1078–86.

[35] Fiebich BL, Grozdeva M, Hess S, *et al.* Petasites hybridus extracts in vitro inhibit COX-2 and PGE2 release by direct interaction with the enzyme and by preventing p42/44 MAP kinase activation in rat primary microglial cells. *Planta Med*. 2005; **71**: 12–19.

[36] Danesch U, Rittinghausen R. Safety of a patented special butterbur root extract for migraine prevention. *Headache* 2003; **43**: 76–8.

[37] Lipton R, Gobel H, Einhaupl K, Wilks K, Mauskop A. Petasites hybridus root (butterbur) is an effective preventive treatment for migraine. *Neurology* 2004; **63**: 2240–4.

[38] Evers S, Afra J, Frese A, *et al.* EFNS guideline on the drug treatment of migraine – revised report of an EFNS task force. *Eur J. Neurol* 2009; **16**: 968–81.

[39] Giles M, Ulbricht C, Khalsa KPS, Kirkwood CD, Park C, Basch E. Butterbur: an evidence-based systematic review by the natural standard research collaboration. *J Herbal Pharmacother*. 2005; **5**: 119–43.

[40] Sparaco M, Feleppa M, Lipton RB, Rapoport AM, Bigal ME. Mitochondrial dysfunction and migraine: evidence and hypotheses. *Cephalalgia* 2006; **26**: 361–72.

[41] Schoenen J, Jacquy J, Lenaerts M. Effectiveness of high-dose riboflavin in migraine prophylaxis A randomized controlled trial. *Neurology* 1998; **50**: 466.

[42] Condò M, Posar A, Arbizzani A, Parmeggiani A. Riboflavin prophylaxis in pediatric and adolescent migraine. *Jo Headache Pain* 2009; **10**: 361–5.

[43] Hershey AD, Powers SW, Vockell A-LB, *et al.* Coenzyme Q10 deficiency and response to supplementation in pediatric and adolescent migraine. *Headache*, 2007; **47**: 73–80.

[44] Sándor PS, Di Clemente L, Coppola G, *et al.* Efficacy of coenzyme Q10 in migraine prophylaxis: a randomized controlled trial. *Neurology* 2005; **64**: 713–15.

[45] Rozen TD, Oshinsky ML, Gebeline CA, *et al.* Open label trial of coenzyme Q10 as a migraine preventive. *Cephalalgia* 2002; **22**: 137–41.

[46] Simopoulos AP. Omega-3 fatty acids in inflammation and autoimmune diseases. *J Am Coll Nutr* 2002; **21**: 495–505.

[47] Sublette ME, Ellis SP, Geant AL, Mann JJ. Meta-analysis of the effects of eicosapentaenoic acid (EPA) in clinical trials in depression. *J Clini Psychiatry* 2011; **72**(12): 1577–84.

[48] Miller LG. Herbal medicinals. *Arch Intern Med* 1998; **158**: 2200–11.

[49] Maclennan KM, Darlington CL, Smith PF. The CNS effects of Ginkgo biloba extracts and ginkgolide B. *Progr Neurobiol*. 2002; **67**: 235–57.

[50] D'Andrea G, Bussone G, Allais G, *et al.* Efficacy of Ginkgolide B in the prophylaxis of migraine with aura. *Neurol Scie*. 2009; **30** : S121–4.

[51] Usai S, Grazzi L, Bussone G. Gingkolide B as migraine preventive treatment in young age: results at 1-year follow-up. *Neurol* 2011; **32**: S197–9.

[52] Nadelson C. Sport and exercise-induced migraines. *Curr Sports Med Rep* 2006; **5**: 29.

[53] Razavi M. Hemiplegic migraine induced by exertion. *Arch Neurol*. 2000; **57**: 1363.

[54] Pascual J. Cough, exertional, and sexual headaches. *Neurology*. 1996; **46**: 1520.

[55] Tepper SJ, Tepper DE. *The Cleveland Clinic Manual of Headache Therapy* Springer Verlag 2011.

[56] Varkey E, Hagen K, Zwart J-A, Linde M. Physical activity and headache: results from the Nord-Trøndelag Health Study (HUNT). *Cephalalgia* 2008; **28**: 1292–7.

[57] Narin SO, Pinar L, Erbas D, Oztürk V, Idiman F. The effects of exercise and exercise-related changes in blood nitric oxide level on migraine headache. *Clin Rehabil* 2003; **17**: 624–30.

[58] Köseoglu E, Akboyraz A, Soyuer A, Ersoy AÖ. Aerobic exercise and plasma beta endorphin levels in patients with migrainous headache without aura. *Cephalalgia* 2003: 972–6.

[59] Broocks A, Bandelow B, Pekrun G, *et al.* Comparison of aerobic exercise, clomipramine, and placebo in the treatment of panic disorder. *Am J Psychiatry* 1998; **155**: 603–9.

[60] Kruisdijk FR, Hendriksen IJ, Tak EC, Beekman AT, Hopman-Rock M. Effect of running therapy on depression (EFFORT-D). Design of a randomised controlled trial in adult patients [ISRCTN 1894]. *BMC Publ Helth* 2012; **12**(1): 50.

[61] Busch V, Gaul C. Exercise in migraine therapy – is there any evidence for efficacy? A critical review. *Headache* 2008; **48**: 890–9.

[62] Varkey E, Cider A, Carlsson J, Linde M. Exercise as migraine prophylaxis: A randomized study using relaxation and topiramate as controls. *Cephalalgia* 2011; **31**: 1428–38.

[63] Darabaneanu S, Overath CH, Rubin D, *et al.* Aerobic exercise as a therapy option for migraine: a pilot study. *Int J. Sports Med* 2011;**32**: 455–60.

[64] Scher AI, Stewart WF, Buse D, Krantz DS, Lipton RB. Major life changes before and after the onset of chronic daily headache: a population-based study. *Cephalalgia* 2008; **28**(8): 868–76.

[65] Abbass A, Kisely S, Kroenke K. Short-term psychodynamic psychotherapy for somatic disorders. Systematic review and meta-analysis of clinical trials. *Psychother Psychosomat* 2009;**78**: 265–74.

[66] Altieri M, Di Giambattista R, Di Clemente L, *et al.* Combined pharmacological and short-term psychodynamic psychotherapy for probable medication overuse headache: a pilot study. *Cephalalgia* 2009; **29**: 293–9.

[67] Nickel R, Ademmer K, Egle UT. Manualized psychodynamic-interactional group therapy for the treatment of somatoform pain disorders. *Bull Menninger Clinic* 2010; **74**: 219–37.

[68] Ruden RA. *When the Past is Always Present: Emotional Traumatization, Causes, and Cures.* New York, NY: Routledge, 2010.

[69] Tiers M. *Integrative Hypnosis: A Comprehensive Course in Change.* CreateSpace; 2010.

[70] Dillworth T, Jensen MP. The role of suggestions in hypnosis for chronic pain: a review of the literature. *Open Pain Jo.* 2010;**3**: 39–51.

[71] Melis PM, Rooimans W, Spierings EL, Hoogduin CA. Treatment of chronic tension-type headache with hypnotherapy: a single-blind time controlled study. *Headache* 1991; **31**: 686–9.

[72] Olness K, MacDonald JT, Uden DL. Comparison of self-hypnosis and propranolol in the treatment of juvenile classic migraine. *Pediatrics* 1987; **79**: 593–7.

[73] Tan G, Craine MH, Bair MJ, *et al.* Efficacy of selected complementary and alternative medicine interventions for chronic pain. *J Rehab Res Deve* 2007; **44**(2): 195–222.

[74] Kozlowska K, Khan R. A developmental, body-oriented intervention for children and adolescents with medically unexplained chronic pain. *Clin Child Psychol Psychiatry* 2011; **16**(4): 575–98.

[75] Available from: http://www.traumahealing.com/somatic-experiencing/index.html.

[76] Marcus S. Phase 1 of integrated EMDR. *An Abortive Treatment for Migraine Headaches.* 2008.

[77] Konuk E, Epözdemir H, Hacıömeroğlu Atçeken S, Aydın, YE, Yurtsever A. EMDR treatment of migraine. *J EMDR Pract Res* 2011; **5**; 166–76.

[78] Craig G. *Emotional Freedom Techniques: The Manual*: The Sea Ranch, California; 1999.

[79] Karatzias T, Power K, Brown K, *et al.* A controlled comparison of the effectiveness and efficiency of two psychological therapies for posttraumatic stress disorder: eye movement desensitization and reprocessing vs. emotional freedom techniques. *J. Nerv Mental Dis* 2011; **199**: 372–8.

[80] Brattberg G. Self-administered EFT (Emotional freedom techniques) in individuals with fibromyalgia: a randomized trial. *Integr Med* 2008; **7**: 30–5.

[81] http://www.tatlife.com/.

[82] Svoboda R. *Ayurveda: Life, Health and Longevity.* London, New York: Arkana, 1992.

[83] Kaptchuk TJ. *The Web that Has no Weaver: Understanding Chinese Medicine.* Rev. edn. Chicago, Ill: Contemporary Books, 2000.

[84] Chapman E. Homeopathy. In MIW, eintranb, ed. *Medical Guides to Complementary and Alternative Medicine: Alternative and Complementary Treatment in Neurologic Illness* Churchill Livingstone; 2001.

[85] Lin JG, Chen WL. Acupuncture analgesia: a review of its mechanisms of actions. *Am J. Chinese Med* 2008; **36**: 635–45.

[86] Rossi P, Di Lorenzo G, Malpezzi MG, *et al.* Prevalence, pattern and predictors of use of complementary and alternative medicine (CAM) in migraine patients attending a headache clinic in Italy. *Cephalalgia* 2005; **25**: 493–506.

[87] von Peter S, Ting W, Scrivani S, *et al.* Survey on the use of complementary and alternative medicine among patients with headache syndromes. *Cephalalgia* 2002; **22**: 395–400.

[88] Moffet HH. Sham acupuncture may be as efficacious as true acupuncture: a systematic review of clinical trials. *J Altern Complement Med* 2009; **15**: 213–16.

[89] Li Y, Zheng H, Witt CM, *et al.* Acupuncture for migraine prophylaxis: a randomized controlled trial. CMAJ : *Canad Med Associ Jo* 2012; **184**: 401–10.

[90] Linde K, Allais G, Brinkhaus B, Manheimer E, Vickers A, White AR. Acupuncture for migraine prophylaxis. *Cochrane Database Syst Rev* 2009, p. 1–104.

[91] Yang C-P, Chang M-H, Liu P-E, *et al.* Acupuncture versus topiramate in chronic migraine prophylaxis: a randomized clinical trial. *Cephalalgia* 2011; **31**: 1510–21.

[92] Wang L-P, Zhang X-Z, Guo J, *et al.* Efficacy of acupuncture for migraine prophylaxis: a single-blinded, double-dummy, randomized controlled trial. *Pain* 2011; **152**: 1864–71.

[93] Linde K, Allais G, Brinkhaus B, Manheimer E, Vickers A, White AR. Acupuncture for tension-type headache. *Cochrane Database Syst rev* (Online)2009, p. 1–51.

[94] Jena S, Witt C, Brinkhaus B, Wegscheider K, Willich S. Acupuncture in patients with headache. *Cephalalgia* 2008; **28**: 969–79.

[95] Melchart D, Streng A, Hoppe A, *et al.* Acupuncture in patients with tension-type headache: randomised controlled trial. *BMJ* (*Clin rese edn*). 2005; **331**: 376–82.

[96] Wonderling D, Vickers AJ, Grieve R, McCarney R. Cost effectiveness analysis of a randomised trial of acupuncture for chronic headache in primary care. *BMJ* (*Clin rese edn*). 2004; **328**: 747.

[97] Melchart D, Thormaehlen J, Hager S, Liao J, Linde K, Weidenhammer W. Acupuncture versus placebo versus sumatriptan for early treatment of migraine attacks: a randomized controlled trial. *J. Intern Med* 2003; **253**: 181–8.

[98] Weintraub M. Laser biostimulation. In: MI W, ed. *Medical Guides to Complementary and Alternative Medicine: Alternative and Complementary Treatment in Neurologic Illness.* Churchill Livingstone; 2001.

[99] Zhao L, Zhang F-w, Li Y, *et al.* Adverse events associated with acupuncture: three multicentre randomized controlled trials of 1968 cases in China. *Trials* 2011; **12**: 87.

[100] Brown R, Gerbarg PL, Muskin PR. *How to Use Herbs, Nutrients, and Yoga in Mental Health Care* w. W. Norton & Company; 2009.

[101] Field T. Yoga clinical research review. *Complement therap Clini Pract.* 2011; **17**: 1–8.

[102] John PJ, Sharma N, Sharma CM, Kankane A. Effectiveness of yoga therapy in the treatment of migraine without aura: a randomized controlled trial. *Headache* 2007; **47**: 654–61.

[103] Sethi BB, Trivedi JK, Anand R. A comparative study of relative effectiveness of biofeedback and shavasana (yoga) in tension headache. *Ind J. Psychiatry* 1981; **23**: 109–14.

[104] Bussing A, Ostermann T, Ludtke R, Michalsen A. Effects of yoga interventions on pain and pain-associated disability: a meta-analysis. *Journal Pain* 2012; **13**(1): 1–9.

[105] Witt CM, Ludtke R, Mengler N, Willich SN. How healthy are chronically ill patients after eight years of homeopathic treatment? – results from a long term observational study. *BMC Publ Helth* 2008; **8**: 413.

[106] Bronfort G, Pickar J, Meeker W, Khalsa P. Chiropractic: an Introduction. National Center for Complementary and Alternative Medicine, 2007 [updated October 2010; cited 2012 01/18/2012]; Available from: http://nccam.nih.gov/health/chiropractic/introduction.htm.

[107] Ernst E. Chiropractic: a critical evaluation. *J Pain Symptom Managem* 2008; **35**(5): 544–62.

[108] Posadzki P, Ernst E. Spinal manipulations for tension-type headaches: a systematic review of randomized controlled trials. *Complement Ther Med* 2012; **20**: 232–9.

[109] Bryans R, Descarreaux M, Duranleau M, *et al.* Evidence-based guidelines for the chiropractic treatment of adults with headache. *J Manipulative Physiol Ther* 2011; **34**: 274–89.

[110] http://nccam.nih.gov/health/chiropractic/introduction.htm.

[111] AOA. Available from: http://www.osteopathic.org/Pages/default.aspx.

[112] Cole S, Reed J. When to consider osteopathic manipulation. *J Fam Pract* 2010;59:E5-E8.

[113] Anderson RE, Seniscal C. A comparison of selected osteopathic treatment and relaxation for tension-type headaches. *Headache* 2006; **46**: 1273–80.

[114] Keays AC, Neher JO, Safranek S. Is osteopathic manipulation effective for headaches? *J Fam Pract* 2008; **57**: 190–1.

[115] Voigt K, Liebnitzky J, Burmeister U, *et al.* Efficacy of osteopathic manipulative treatment of female patients with migraine: results of a randomized controlled trial. *J Altern Complement Med* 2011; **17**(3): 225–30. Epub 2011/03/10.

[116] Jain S, Mills PJ. Biofield therapies: helpful or full of hype? A best evidence synthesis. *Int J Behav Med* 2010; **17**: 1–16.

[117] Miles P, Yount GL, Moquin BE, Khalsa P. Reiki: An Introduction. National Center for Complementary

and Alternative Medicine; 2009 [updated August 2009; cited 2012 01/17/2012]; Available from: http://nccam.nih.gov/health/reiki/.

[118] Brathovde A. A pilot study: Reiki for self-care of nurses and healthcare providers. *Holist Nurs Pract* 2006; **20**(2): 95–101.

[119] http://www.centerforreikiresearch.org.

[120] vanderVaart S, Gijsen VM, de Wildt SN, Koren G. A systematic review of the therapeutic effects of Reiki. *J Altern Complement Med* 2009; **15**: 1157–69.

[121] Assefi N, Bogart A, Goldberg J, Buchwald D. Reiki for the treatment of fibromyalgia: a randomized controlled trial. *J Altern Complement Med.* 2008; **14**: 1115–22.

[122] Bowden D, Goddard L, Gruzelier J. A randomised controlled single-blind trial of the effects of Reiki and positive imagery on well-being and salivary cortisol. *Brain Res Bull* 2010; **81**: 66–72.

[123] Richeson NE, Spross JA, Lutz K, Peng C. Effects of Reiki on anxiety, depression, pain, and physiological factors in community-dwelling older adults. *Res Gerontol Nurs* 2010; **3**: 187–99.

[124] Wassermann EM, Zimmermann T. Transcranial magnetic brain stimulation: therapeutic promises and scientific gaps. *Pharmacology Therap* 2012; **133**: 98–107.

[125] Lipton RB, Dodick DW, Silberstein SD, *et al.* Single-pulse transcranial magnetic stimulation for acute treatment of migraine with aura: a randomised, double-blind, parallel-group, sham-controlled trial. *Lancet Neurol* 2010; **9**: 373–80.

[126] Smith R. *Cranial Electrotherapy Stimulation. Its First Fifty Years, Plus Three.* A Monograph. Washington, DC 2006.

[127] O'Connell NE, Wand BM, Marston L, Spencer S, Desouza LH. Non-invasive brain stimulation techniques for chronic pain. *Cochrane Database Syst Rev* 2010(**9**):CD008208.

[128] Leone M, Cecchini AP, Franzini A, Bussone G. Neuromodulation in drug-resistant primary headaches: what have we learned? *Neurol Sci* 2011; **32** : S23–6.

[129] Magis D, Ambrosini A, Sándor P, Jacquy J, Laloux P, Schoenen J. A randomized double-blind placebo-controlled trial of thioctic acid in migraine prophylaxis. *Headache* 2007; **47**: 52–7.

[130] Ali AM, Awad TG, Al-Adl NM. Efficacy of combined topiramate/thioctic acid therapy in migraine prophylaxis. *Saudi Pharmaceut J.* 2010; **18**: 239–43.

[131] Andersen LL, Mortensen OS, Zebis MK, Jensen RH, Poulsen OM. Effect of brief daily exercise on headache among adults-secondary analysis of a randomized controlled trial. *Scand J Work, Environm Helth* 2011; **37**: 547–50.

Chapter 13

Somatoform disorders and headache

Filza Hussain, Peter A. Shapiro, and Philip R. Muskin

Introduction

Headache is one of the most common complaints in the general population, causing significant distress and impairment in quality of life. As is the case for some other high-prevalence pain symptoms, such as those involving the joints, chest, abdomen, and back, headache is a complaint that remains poorly understood. [1]

The International Headache Society classification includes the category of "headaches secondary to psychiatric disorders," which in turn includes headaches due to somatization disorder and due to psychotic disorder. [2][Table 13.1] This classification presents several challenges: some headaches do not fit neatly into any one category, there are other somatoform disorders not included in the IHS classification that may present with headaches and there are also times when a patient's unexplained pain symptoms are not accompanied by an overt psychiatric illness.

This chapter reviews the phenomenon of somatization as a ubiquitous process and the so-called somatoform disorders. It is our goal to assist the clinician to appropriately characterize headaches due to psychiatric disorders and hence find the most helpful treatment approach.

Somatization as a process

Somatization refers to the conscious experience of an abnormal somatic sensation or changes in bodily function, in the absence of, or out of proportion to, a somatic stimulus or lesion accounting for that sensation or change. Somatization occurs ubiquitously in people with no psychiatric diagnosis as well as in patients with various psychiatric disorders. Common somatic symptoms that may occur as a result of somatization include pain, weakness, nausea, fatigue, and shortness of breath. Two theories of the process by which somatization occur are: (1) psychodynamic and (2) somatic amplification. These theories are not mutually exclusive.

Psychodynamic theories of somatization

Early psychoanalytic theory of neurotic symptom formation posited that some wishes, drives, and impulses are recognized in the unconscious mind as unacceptable. This provokes unconscious anxiety, and the wishes are repressed from reaching consciousness. When the repression of the wish is not successful, the resulting conflict is expressed in symbolic form as a deviation from normal function that may be perceived as troublesome or impairing function, i.e., a neurotic symptom. Examples include parapraxes, slips of the tongue, phobias, inexplicable forgetting, and some somatic symptoms. As is the case for other neurotic symptoms, a somatic symptom arising as a consequence of unconscious psychic conflict might be understood as a representation of the conflict; that is, it may include elements of both the original wish and the defense against the wish. For example, a young woman who has the impulse to verbally attack her boyfriend over a perceived slight, but is also fearful of the loss of the relationship if she attacks him, might develop the sensation of burning tongue pain and difficulty speaking. With the development of the symptom, she inhibits the interpersonal attack, protecting the relationship (and perhaps even eliciting the caretaking attention of her boyfriend thereby reassuring herself about the relationship), while at the same time symbolically expressing her "acid-tongued" impulse. For some patients with acute conversion disorder, it is indeed possible to identify and interpret the psychological conflict "behind" the symptom, with subsequent relief of the symptom. In empirically based case series, however, many medically unexplained somatic symptoms are not readily understood or treated in this way. [3] A more modern

The Neuropsychiatry of Headache, ed. Mark W. Green and Philip R. Muskin. Published by Cambridge University Press.

Table 13.1. IHS classification

Primary	Secondary
Migraine	Headache attributed to:
Tension-type headache	Head and/or neck trauma
Cluster headache and other trigeminal	Cranial or cervical vascular disorder
Autonomic cephalalgias	Non-vascular intracranial disorder
Other primary headaches	Substance or its withdrawal Infection Disorder of homeostasis Disorder of cranium, neck, eyes, ears, nose, sinuses Teeth, mouth or other facial or cranial structures Psychiatric disorder
	1. Headache secondary to somatization disorder 2. Headache secondary to psychotic disorder

psychodynamic model of mental function focuses on the relationship of the self with other people of emotional significance to the self, i.e., so-called object relationships, and the representation of object relationships within the mind. According to object relations theory, an individual's sense of self derives from the internalized (that is, stored in memory, both consciously and unconsciously) representations of innumerable past object relationship experiences. A person's behavior and/or conscious experience of the self at a given moment may be a "re-playing" of a previous object relationship experience, embodying the representation of either the self or the object. Acting toward your child just like your parent used to act toward you as a child is a common example; the self has taken on the characteristics of the internalized representation of the parental object. In mourning, when the mourner, yearning for the lost loved one, begins to experience symptoms similar to those thought by the mourner to have been experienced by the deceased object we can see a similar, common example. The widower whose wife died of a brain tumor complains of headache in the area of the head where his late wife's tumor was located. He keeps the lost object alive by replicating her experience.

It is important to understand that these experiences of the self and of somatic symptoms are not under one's volitional, conscious control, but may be a function, at least in part, of potentially modifiable psychological traits. When psychological stress overwhelms psychological coping capacity, somatic symptoms may develop. The ability to use language, metaphor, and symbol formation to articulate and communicate feeling states comprises one aspect of psychological coping skill. Some investigators have noted that symptoms occurring under stress can develop without any specific symbolic meaning, particularly when such skills are absent or have been compromised. The term "alexithymia," i.e., "no words for feelings," refers to the characteristic of having a relatively impoverished concept of, and language for, the experience and expression of emotions. Alexithymia appears to be associated with an increased prevalence of medically unexplained somatic symptoms. Variation in the level of conscious emotional awareness is inversely correlated with predisposition to experience somatic symptoms. Emotion processing in higher cortical centers is associated with both conscious emotional awareness and neural traffic regulating activity in mid-brain structures in the thalamus and limbic system. Thus difficulty in processing emotion in "emotional" terms may be related to dysregulation of sensation and of efferent neural control of somatic processes through autonomic, cranial, and skeletal nerves and neuroendocrine pathways. This dysregulation may result in medically unexplained symptoms and in a heightened risk for development of a number of somatic disorders. [4] The degree to which emotional awareness and alexithymia can be modified, and the results of such modification on cortical function, mid-brain function, somatic symptoms, and the development of somatic disease remain to be established.

Somatic amplification theory

A second, complementary theory about somatization phenomena is based on the notion of somatic amplification, the tendency to experience normal somatic sensations as especially intrusive, intense, noxious, or disturbing. [5] It is a cognitive bias in interpreting sensations that reach consciousness. [6]

Somatosensory amplification has three core elements: (1) Increased attention to normal bodily sensations or physiologic processes such as awareness of one's heartbeat or feelings of fatigue; (2) Predisposition to focus and concentrate on infrequent or weak bodily sensations; and (3) reacting to sensations with cognitions and affect in a manner that makes them more alarming. [6,7]

The tendency to somatic amplification can be thought of as both a state and a trait. As a state, it depends on a variety of factors including external circumstances, perceived stress, and mood; in unfavorable conditions, some individuals may have heightened sensitivity to minute changes in sensations and to consider them distressing, while the same individuals may be able to ignore the same sensations when they are not stressed. Conversely, even highly salient somatic sensations may be screened out of conscious awareness under circumstances that demand highly focused attention to the environment, e.g., soldiers not experiencing pain from serious injuries while in combat. The degree to which an individual tends to amplify somatic sensation is also a trait, an enduring perceptual style, and may be either "hard-wired" at birth or developed in childhood through early experiences. "High-amplification" individuals tend to be unable to "tune out" background somatic sensory information no matter what the external circumstances, leading to distress and illness behaviors. Psychodynamic and somatic amplification theories can be utilized to understand somatization experiences occurring in persons without mental illnesses, and also in the various somatoform disorders.

Somatoform disorders

Classification

Current psychiatric nosology, as laid out in the American Psychiatric Association *Diagnostic and Statistical Manual (DSM) of Psychiatric Disorders*, 4th edn with Text Revision [DSM IV-TR] describes seven different types of Somatoform disorders [Table 13.2].

The current DSM scheme is being revised, with several changes proposed for the DSM-5. These changes include renaming the category as "somatic symptom disorders" and bundling somatization disorder, undifferentiated somatoform disorder, and pain disorder under "complex somatic symptom disorder." The cognitive distortions and unintentionally produced somatic symptoms are shared core features of all such patients. The group also proposes modifiying the name "convosion disorder" to "conversion disorder (functional neurological symptom disorder)." Factitous disorder will be included in the somatic symptom disorders category. [8] This chapter will adhere to the current DSM IV-TR classification, and we include factitious disorders and malingering, as they also involve medically unexplained symptoms.

Table 13.2. DSM IV TR somatoform disorders

Somatization disorder	Onset before age 30, extends over a period of years, and is characterized by a combination of pain, gastrointestinal, sexual, and neurologic symptoms.
Undifferentiated Somatoform disorder	Unexplained physical complaints of at least 6 months duration that are below the threshold for a diagnosis of somatization disorder
Somatoform pain disorder	Pain that causes distress or impairment in functioning and in which psychological factors are judged to play a role
Conversion disorder	A loss or change in sensory or motor function that is suggestive of a physical disorder but is caused by psychological factors
Hypochondriasis	Preoccupation with and conviction of having a serious disease, even after appropriate medical evaluation and reassurance of good health
Body dysmorphic disorder	Preoccupation with an imagined or exaggerated defect in physical appearance
Somatoform disorder NOS	Symptoms that do not meet full criteria for a single somatoform disorder

Conversion disorder

Definition and clinical features

Conversion disorder involves the abrupt onset of voluntary motor or sensory deficits that suggest a neurological or general medical condition, without corroborating evidence from history, physical examination, or laboratory data that suggest the presence of a somatic lesion. History should reveal that the psychological stresses are temporally related to the onset of the somatic symptoms. Conversion disorder should only be diagnosed after appropriate history, physical examination, and corollary investigation has taken place, and when the occurrence of a relevant psychological stressor can be temporally linked to the onset of the symptom. Research from the 1960s suggests a high rate of patients with medically unexplained symptoms being misdiagnosed as conversion disorder. [9] A 2005 review [10] reports a decrease in diagnosing medically unexplained neurological symptoms as conversion disorder from 29% in the 1950s and 17% in the 1960s to a consistent 4% in every decade thereafter. This is thought likely to be secondary to improvements in imaging techniques.

Symptom production in conversion disorder is based on the patient's concept of the condition. Medically naïve patients may have implausible presentations. It is important to remember that conversion symptoms can co-exist with true neurological illnesses, for example, non-epileptic seizures in patients with epilepsy. [11]

Conversion symptoms can be viewed as examples of the classical psychodynamically mediated process of somatization, in which the somatic symptom represents an unconscious conflict in symbolic form. However, the DSM-IV criteria do not endorse this theoretical construct, although they do require that psychological factors be associated with the conversion symptoms and correlate temporally with the onset or exacerbation of the symptom. The presence of "la belle indifference," the patient's lack of distress despite symptoms, was at one time considered a key feature of conversion disorder, but empirical data do not support this association and "indifference" to the symptom is no longer a criterion for the diagnosis. [3]

Classically, conversion refers to disorders of special senses and voluntary motor function, e.g. blindness, deafness, or paralysis. Unilateral symptoms on the left side were once thought to be common, but there is insufficient evidence to support this claim. Some authors have included pain, including headache [12] in the spectrum of conversion symptoms, while others, including the DSM-IV, separate pain from conversion. Patients with headaches may have anesthesia or parasthesias.

The course of conversion disorder is variable. Individual episodes can be sudden in onset with quick resolution, though recurrence over time is common. [13] Most patients show a rapid response to treatment, or spontaneous remission, while others go on to a chronic course.

Epidemiology

The DSM-IV reports prevalence rates in general population samples varying from 11/100 000 to 500/100 000. Conversion symptom rates range from 1% to 14% in general medical and surgical inpatients. [13] Other research suggests a rate of 0.3% in the general population, and rates of 1%–14.5% in samples of medical and neurological inpatients. [14]

Psychologically unsophisticated people from rural settings, who may have a poor understanding of medical concepts, are more likely to have conversion symptoms. Typical age of onset is adolescence and early adulthood, but cases also occur in children and older adults. Women are affected more frequently than men, with reported ratios varying from 2:1 to 10:1. [13]

Headache and conversion disorder

There are no direct data on the prevalence of headache as the principal feature or an accompanying symptom in conversion disorder. A recent large prospective study by Stone *et al.* [15] looked at the frequency with which the initial diagnosis of medically unexplained symptoms changes in neurological patients on further follow-up. Twenty-six percent of patients received an initial diagnosis of headache. Almost half of these patients had "other" headache as a diagnosis, rather than migraine or tension-type headache. Eighteen percent of the sample had previously been given a diagnosis of conversion disorder, but the relationship between the headache and conversion disorder diagnoses was not clarified. In a sample of patients with non-epileptic seizures, 61% of the sample suffered from headaches, suggesting a high prevalence of headaches in patients with a previously known conversion disorder. [16]

Clinical features of headache in conversion

Little has been written about headache as a cardinal presentation of conversion. In DSM-IV-TR, such a presentation would most likely be classified as pain disorder or as an unspecified somatoform disorder. However, associated complaints of head numbness, tingling, or paresthesias might fall under the rubric of conversion.

Treatment

Approaches to treatment of conversion derive from the theoretical model used to understand it. A first step is to validate the patient's experience of symptoms as real, while highlighting that no neurological disorder is present as indicated by the history and physical examination. Careful history-taking that includes attention to the personal, family, social history, and the patient's own ideas about the nature, origin, and meaning of the symptom may enable the clinician to formulate the relationship between a specific psychosocial stressor and the symptom. It may be worthwhile to offer this formulation to the patient. This is most likely to be helpful for symptoms of very recent onset, and may lead to dramatic symptom relief. Patients often reject such formulations, and offering them in a tactless manner may actually harm the therapeutic alliance. Suggesting that the symptoms tend to improve spontaneously over a few hours to days and that improvement can be aided through exercise, physical therapy, or rest, is a more tactful approach. This will provide the patient with a tactful and face-saving route to symptom resolution. In parallel with the prescription of physical therapy, intervention aimed at the psychosocial stressor can be carried out without explicitly linking this intervention to the origin of the symptoms. It is also important to identify and treat co-occurring psychiatric conditions. [17]

Example

A 17-year-old high school student was brought to the emergency room by his parents with abrupt onset of headache and difficulty phonating. Examination was negative. The patient had previously expressed anxiety about an upcoming oral examination for which he felt unprepared. His parents expressed concern about the effect of his missing an exam on his grades and college applications. The patient was informed that he would be admitted for rest and a speech therapy consultation and that it was expected that his symptoms would likely improve within 24 hours. While in the hospital, a psychiatric consultant spoke with him about his exam preparation and anxiety dealing with his parents about college planning, suggested breathing and relaxation exercises to reduce stress, offered further counseling for his anxiety, and counseled his parents about balancing their expectations for their son's academic performance. He recovered, missed a day of school, and made up his exam without incident 2 days after it was originally scheduled.

A recent review [17] found no evidence that reached level 1 quality for the efficacy of any treatment of conversion disorder. Most evidence is at level 4, including clinical anecdotes, case series, and case reports. Although there is some increase in our knowledge of the neurobiological basis of conversion through fMRI studies, [18] not enough is known to derive a rationale for any specific psychopharmacological treatment, and clinical trials of pharmacotherapy have reported inconclusive results. [17] Meanwhile, psychotherapy continues to be the mainstay of treatment. One could say that Freud, as a treatment of conversion disorder, invented psychodynamic psychotherapy. More than 100 years after Freud there are no reported systematic or comparative studies of this approach. In a series of ten cases of conversion disorder treated with 12 weeks of psychodynamic psychotherapy, the response rate was 70%. [19] A Cochrane review of hypnotherapy for treatment of conversion disorder, noting lack of power calculation and other methodological shortcomings, concluded that the benefits of hypnotherapy and other psychosocial interventions are not established. [20]

Abreaction can result from an interview conducted in a pharmacologically induced relaxed state with the help of benzodiazepines or barbiturates. The patient is relaxed, more suggestible, and more amenable to exploration of psychological and social events preceding the conversion symptoms. A recent meta-analysis noted that, although the evidence base for this treatment is weak, core features of the technique are amenable to randomization and more studies are needed in this area as a treatment for conversion. [21] General treatment principles hold true for the neurologist who suspects a conversion headache. Exploring other aspects of the patient's history including social stressors and life circumstances could explain the context of conversion. A timely referral to psychiatry can be helpful, although the patient may be resistant to the idea that his or her symptoms are psychiatric in origin.

Pain disorder

Definition and clinical features

The DSM-IV-TR defines pain disorder as pain in one or more sites, not accounted for by a medical or neurological condition, with psychological factors playing an important role in the onset, severity, exacerbation, or maintenance of the pain, and subjective distress and/or impairment in function. Pain disorder and conversion disorder differ primarily in that the primary symptom in pain disorder is pain rather than symptoms in organs of special sense or voluntary motor function. The challenge with this diagnosis is to ascertain that this pain is not better accounted for by another psychiatric disorder such as a mood disorder or somatization disorder, and that the patient is not feigning symptoms. Symptoms generally begin abruptly and increase in severity over weeks or months. The prognosis is variable and pain disorder is often chronic and completely disabling. Pain is often localized in a distribution that is psychologically meaningful to the patient, but does not conform to neuroanatomical or pathophysiological models for pain arising from peripheral lesions. [12]

Chronic pain can predispose patients to depression, anxiety, and substance abuse. They frequently have sleep problems and are also at a higher risk for suicide. They spend an inordinate amount of resources in an attempt to seek cure, increasing their risk for iatrogenic injury. [13]

Epidemiology

A 1998 review of pain literature indicates point prevalence rates of chronic pain of between 2% and 40% in a population of adults between 18–75 years of age. This wide range is partially explained by the differences in diagnostic criteria used, duration of studies, and cultural groups sampled. [22] Using a standardized diagnostic interview in 4181 German patients between the ages of 18–65, Frolich *et al.* [23] found pain to be an extremely common phenomenon, with 22% of all men and 34% of all women having experienced clinically significant medically unexplained pain at least once in the past year. According to the DSM IV-TR, pain disorder is diagnosed twice as frequently in women as in men, with peak age of onset in the fourth to fifth decade of life, perhaps due to lowering of the pain threshold with age.

Headache and pain disorder

Frolich *et al.* note that excessive headache is the most frequent painful condition, affecting 12.7% of the sample, with a female to male ratio of 2:1 (16.7% v. 8.2%). [23] Compared with pain disorder patients, non-pain disorder patients tend to localize pain more, give more detailed sensory descriptions, and link their pain more clearly to situations that increase or decrease the pain. [24]

Treatment

Pain disorder tends to be a chronic condition, and pain disorder patients are high utilizers of medical care. Treatment literature often does not distinguish pain disorder treatment, in particular, from other non-malignant chronic pain syndromes. The goals of treatment are to reduce the patient's experience of pain and to optimize the patient's ability to maintain function despite pain. Decreasing health care utilization can also be a secondary goal of treatment. The biopsychosocial approach is helpful in conceptualizing pain disorder and planning a multi-modal approach to treatment. This approach recognizes that pain is a complex experience that can be conceptualized at the levels of physiology, individual thoughts and emotions, and sociocultural influences. [25] Medications used for pain management are only partially helpful and should be used in conjunction with other therapeutic modalities such as biofeedback, behavioral medicine techniques, and psychotherapy, such as CBT.

Opioids

Opioids act on endogenous opioid receptors to reduce the sensory and affective components of pain. Although helpful in the acute setting, the development of tolerance, physiologic dependence, and aberrant drug-related behaviors limits their use. The American Academy of Pain Medicine and the American Pain Society have established guidelines for opioid use in pain treatment. [26,27] In treating non-cancer chronic pain with opioids, the pain should be of moderate to severe intensity lasting for more than 3 months. It should also cause significant functional disability, with insufficient relief from other treatments. [28]

Opiate addiction in pain patients

The overall point prevalence of opioid addiction in chronic pain patients is 3.27%, and, in a subset with no previous history of substance use, the prevalence is only 0.19%. [29] The risk of creating addiction certainly exists but can be minimized by educating patients, treating underlying causes of pain, and designating one provider as the prescribing physician. The "universal precaution for prescription of opioids" as suggested by Gourlay *et al.* enumerates ten key points highlighting good clinical practice and includes an appropriate diagnosis and differential, psychological assessment of the patient to screen for substance abuse problems, forming an alliance with the patient and delineating rules of treatment and frequent re-assessment to monitor efficacy. Careful and adequate documentation is both a medicolegal requirement and in the best interest of the patient and the physician. [30]

Another approach to treatment of pain disorder is multi-modal, comprehensive pain rehabilitation, with a cognitive-behavioral psychotherapy approach to help patients to cope better with their pain and depend less on opioids. Cognitive-behavioral individual and group psychotherapy approaches target patients' catastrophic beliefs about their pain experience, and are used along with graduated exercise and physical therapy to reduce pain symptoms and increase functional status.

Antidepressants

A review of the use of antidepressants in chronic pain finds the analgesic effect of antidepressants to be independent of their antidepressant effect. [31]

Antidepressants seem to act on the neuroregulatory mechanisms associated with pain perceptions and transmission. Tricyclic antidepressants have been used effectively for treatment of migraine as well as facial pain syndromes. [31] A meta-analysis of randomized controlled trials concludes that tricyclic antidepressants are effective for all headache syndromes and their effectiveness seems to increase over time, although their use is limited by side effects. [32] A typical analgesic dose regimen would be amitriptyline, 10–50 mg once daily at bedtime. Adverse effects such as orthostatic hypotension, cardiac conduction disturbances, drowsiness, and anticholinergic effects such as constipation may limit amitriptyline use.

Smitherman *et al.* report that the evidence supporting use of the selective serotonin re-uptake inhibitors as headache prophylaxis is poor; their use should be reserved for treating comorbid depression in a patient who also has a headache disorder. [33] Selective serotonin/norepinephrine reuptake inhibitors [SNRIs] may produce better analgesic effects compared with SSRIs. Small, randomized trials of venlafaxine indicate efficacy both for migraine and tension-type headache. [34] Duloxetine blocks serotonin and norepinephrine reuptake and is somewhat effective in other chronic pain syndromes, such as fibromyalgia and neuropathic pain. There are data supporting a modest effect of duloxetine for headache, osteoarthritic pain, and pain secondary to Parkinson's disease; however, the data is from single-blinded or open-label trials that require further corroboration with larger randomized studies. [35] Duloxetine has not yet been directly compared with other antidepressants or anticonvulsants for the treatment of somatoform pain syndromes.

Anticonvulsants

Anticonvulsants are used as prophylactics in migraine treatments. Though the evidence for using sodium valproate and topiramate for migraine prophylaxis is robust, the evidence for their efficacy in the use of other chronic headaches is lacking, as most studies are small open-label trials. [36] (See Chapter 2.)

Complementary and Alternative Methods

The National Institute of Health's National Center for Complementary and Alternative Medicine defines complementary and alternative medicine (CAM) as "a group of diverse medical and health care systems, practices, and products that are not generally considered part of conventional medicine." [37]

CAM practices are becoming more widespread and are most commonly used to treat musculoskeletal problems, including back and neck pain, joint pain, and arthritis [38]. There are not much data describing the use of CAM by adults with migraines/severe headaches. Only 4.5% of adults with migraines/severe headaches report using CAM to specifically treat their migraines/severe headaches. [39] The most common treatments are mind–body therapies (deep breathing exercises, meditation, and yoga). Chronic tension-type headache patients prefer physical training and relaxation training over acupuncture for improvement of symptoms and report subjective well-being. [40] The absence of evidence from controlled trials precludes specific recommendations for CAM treatment for pain disorder with headache.

Somatization disorder and undifferentiated somatoform disorder

According to the DSM-IV-TR, somatization disorder is an illness arising before age 30, characterized by multiple somatic complaints involving several different organ systems and causing subjective distress and functional impairment or medical help-seeking behavior, for which no adequate medical explanation can be found, i.e., even if a somatic lesion or disease process is present, the symptoms are not fully accounted for by that lesion or disease process. In its current iteration, a diagnosis of somatization disorder requires a history of at least four pain symptoms, two gastrointestinal symptoms, one sexual symptom, and one pseudo-neurological symptom that is medically unexplained.

Undifferentiated somatoform disorder is diagnosed in individuals who have unexplained physical complaints such as fatigue, loss of appetite, or urinary complaints lasting at least 6 months, but below the threshold needed for a diagnosis of somatization disorder.

Epidemiology

The lifetime prevalence ranges from 0.2%–2.0% in women to less than 0.2% in men. [13] No studies for undifferentiated somatoform disorders exist, but it has been estimated that 4%–11% of the population have multiple medically unexplained symptoms consistent with a sub-syndromal form of somatization disorder. [41]

Headache and somatization disorder

In a retrospective chart review of 8479 patients presenting to an emergency headache center in Paris, only 1% of these patients are given a diagnosis of headache secondary to psychiatric disorder and, of those, 70% were women. [42] Somatization disorder and undifferentiated somatoform disorder represent 1% and 3% of these patients, respectively. [42] In a review of the psychiatric charts of this subpopulation, 6% of the patients are given the diagnosis of somatization disorder. [42]

In a unique study attempting to reclassify medically unexplained symptoms, the authors report that the study sample could be statistically divided into five different groups according to number and type of symptom cluster. [43] For example, Group 1 consists only of those with complaints of back pain; Groups 2–4 have single symptom complaints such as chronic fatigue or gastrointestinal symptoms; Group 5 have multiple complaints similar to what we know to be somatization disorder. Women are more common than men in Groups 2–5. Recurrent headache is a common complaint in Group 5 (74.8%). Given the similarity of Group 5 to somatization disorder, one may infer that headaches may be quite common in somatization disorder. The lack of sensitivity of the current classification system leads to the reported low prevalence rates of somatization headaches. [43]

Clinical features

The typical patient with somatization disorder is a young woman who is a vague historian with multiple bodily complaints. She presents with headaches that do not conform to a typical headache diagnostic category, and with a medical chart notable for many unexplained medical symptoms. The diagnosis of somatization disorder is strongly suggested by the presence in the past medical history and review of systems of multiple symptoms and problems in many organ systems, with inconclusive or negative work-ups. Of note, patients may not accurately report that their previous evaluations failed to identify a specific illness. For example, a patient may state that she had surgery for appendicitis, but omit to report that the surgical pathology examination revealed a normal appendix. Comorbid psychiatric disorders such as depression, dysthymia, panic disorder, other anxiety spectrum disorders, and personality disorders are also common. The designation of somatization in headache patients is problematic because many headache patients experience numerous somatic symptoms and there is no objective manner to determine whether they are "unexplained." Somatic symptom counts may be a surrogate marker for somatoform disorder. Kroenke *et al.* suggest that a threshold of 7 symptoms on the 15-item checklist of the PRIME-MD Patient Questionaire should trigger screening for somatoform disorder, with a positive predictive value of 25%. [44]

Treatment

Core principles of treatment are similar to other somatoform disorders. The doctor should be supportive to the patient; empathic in acknowledging the patient's suffering, and non-judgmental. Communication between all treating physicians (neurologist treating headache and the referring internist treating other physical maladies) is key in order to avoid excessive diagnostic investigations, polypharmacy, and other invasive procedures. Both to minimize risk of iatrogenic injury and to help reduce the patient's preoccupation with symptoms, invasive procedures and treatments should only be undertaken when objective evidence from the physical examination and non-invasive laboratory tests indicate an abnormality. Regularly scheduled frequent follow-up appointments that are not symptom-driven are also helpful to the patient and reduce health care utilization by reducing ER visits and hospitalization. The appropriate goal of treatment for patients with somatization disorder is improvement in functioning, rather than symptom relief or "cure." [45] Medications have not been useful in treating somatization disorder and the most evidence exists for CBT as an effective management strategy. [17]

Other somatoform disorders

Hypochondriasis

Hypochondriasis is characterized by preoccupation with the fear of having a serious illness, based on the individual's misinterpretation of innocuous bodily symptoms that persist despite medical reassurance. [13] The obsessional nature of these fears have led to the suggestion that in DSM-5 hypochondriasis should be included among the anxiety disorders rather than be labeled a somatoform disorder; however, it appears likely that the proposed diagnosis of illness anxiety disorder will remain in the somatic symptom disorders. [8]

Epidemiology

General population and primary care studies estimate the prevalence of hypochondriasis to be between 0.02% and 8.5%, with the population prevalence increasing to as much as 10.7% when abridged criteria are used. Onset can occur at any age, but is most common in adulthood. Hypochondriasis is equally common in men and women. [46]

Clinical features

The core feature is fear that one has a disease and hence increased vigilance towards bodily sensations, and sensory amplification is common. The individual may be preoccupied with a particular bodily function. The perception of the heartbeat and its variability may be perceived as an ominous sign of disease, a trivial abnormal physical state such as a cough can be misinterpreted and a vague physical sensation such as numbness, or a diagnosis such as cancer may become the focus of this preoccupation. Patients with hypochondriasis have a high risk of psychiatric comorbidity with the most common diagnoses being mood and anxiety disorders. High medical utilization by patients is common, increasing risk for iatrogenic injury. The hypochondriacal preoccupation becomes the patient's core identity, impairing function and relationships. [13]

Patients seeking a neurologist with headache symptoms and hypochondriasis most likely will present with altered sensation or vague indescribable symptoms, which they believe to be harbingers of severe illness, e.g., a brain tumor. The clinical course is poorly understood but, in general, acute onset, brief duration, mild symptoms, absence of secondary gain, presence of a comorbid general medical condition, and absence of psychiatric comorbidity are positive prognostic factors. [13]

Treatment

Psychopharmacology

Case reports exist about the use of antipsychotics, antidepressants, benzodiazepines, and even electroconvulsive therapy to treat hypochondriacal preoccupations. In a RCTof 112 patients assigned to paroxetine (Paxil), CBT, or placebo both CBT and Paxil are better than placebo in reducing symptoms. The trial was not adequately powered to compare the active treatments with one another. [47] An exploratory study indicates that patients with hypochondriasis consider CBT more acceptable and more effective than medication. [48]

Psychotherapy

Similar to other somatoform disorders, there is good evidence in support of CBT for treatment of hypochondriasis. CBT challenges the cognitive distortions about illness and aims to modify behaviors of avoidance and reassurance seeking. In a Cochrane review of psychotherapies for hypochondriasis, CBT, exposure plus response prevention, and behavioral stress management approaches are effective in reducing symptoms of hypochondriasis; however, the studies are small in size, different therapies are not compared, and the size of effect is unknown. [49]

Somatoform disorders not otherwise specified

This diagnosis is included for coding disorders with somatoform symptoms that do not meet the criteria for any of the specific somatoform disorders. Some patients with headache as their predominant symptom might be classified as having somatoform disorder not otherwise specified, but most should receive a diagnosis of pain disorder.

Deception syndromes: factitious disorder and malingering factitious disorder

The DSM describes factitious disorder as the intentional production of symptoms in order to assume the sick role. Although factitious disorder is not a somatoform disorder, it should always be considered in the differential for patients with medically unexplained symptoms. There are two subtypes: (1) pychological, in which patients feign memory loss, hallucinations, or worsening mood symptoms; and (2) physical, in which patients primarily feign physical symptoms such as pain, or falsify or fabricate objective findings such as fevers, hematuria, or rash. Individuals with factitious disorder tend to be unreliable historians who provide vague but often elaborate and unbelievable histories. Eventually, these patients are "found out" by the medical team; the ensuing confrontation may lead to resolution of the symptoms or to a precipitous discharge followed by presentation for care at a different medical center. The term "Munchhausen syndrome" is sometimes used synonymously with factitious disorder, or used more specifically to refer to persons who seem to spend all of their time in serial presentations of factitious illness at different hospitals, often traveling to distant cities. These patients often are unable to maintain long-term employment and stable family relationships. Patients with factitious disorder are consciously aware that they are intentionally fabricating symptoms, but generally have difficulty articulating a reason to desire the sick role. External incentives, such as avoiding military conscription or receiving financial damages, are not present.

Epidemiology

According to the DSM, there is limited information on the prevalence of factitious disorder. Standard epidemiological techniques are constrained by the fact that factitious disorder always involves deception and sometimes peregrination as well, and so it often may not be recognized. On the other hand, the chronic form of the disorder may be over-reported because the same individual may present to different physicians at different hospitals, often using pseudonyms. In large general hospitals, factitious disorder is diagnosed in about 1% of patients who undergo mental health consultation. [13] The prevalence appears to be greater in highly specialized treatment settings.

In a review of 45 reports of factitious disorder in a neurological setting comprising 90 cases with neurological presentations of factitious disorder, a wide range of neurological presentations are included, [50] the most common being functional motor symptoms/ simulated strokes, and seizures/blackouts. Although pain is an inclusion symptom, no reports of factitious headaches were found. [50]

Headaches and factitious disorder

There are only case reports of factitious headache. In a few of these cases headache was not the primary complaint, but rather a supporting symptom of factitious subarachnoid hemorrhage or meningitis. Solomon described the case of a man with factitious headache; however, a careful review of the case report reveals that there may have been an element of malingering as the man had, "read up all he could on headache" and wanted to see a headache specialist to "trump up" insurance claims. [51]

Treatment

No specific treatment exists for factitious disorder. The general principles of management include search for evidence of fabrication of symptoms and confrontation of the patient with the factitious nature of the illness when such evidence is available. This is accompanied by a reformulation of the problem as a psychiatric problem for which treatment is offered if the patient will accept it, treatment of self-induced medical or surgical conditions, protecting the patient from self harm and iatrogenic injury, and attempting to limit the patient's care to one primary care physician and to one hospital. Most patients do not accept the offer of psychiatric treatment, and only a minority acknowledges the factitious nature of the illness, even on confrontation. The confrontation frequently results in elimination or reduction of the factious illness presentation, at least temporarily. [52]

Munchausen's syndrome is generally regarded as irremediable. [53] Due to their assumed identities and peregrination, it is challenging to engage patients in psychological treatment. Only a few reports exist in the literature using inpatient behavioral techniques for treatment. In one case, successful treatment was achieved by means of a structured, dynamic, behavior modification program lasting 3 years. [54] The level of evidence is poor and applicability to the headache population unknown.

Malingering

According to the DSM-IV-TR, malingering is a form of deception and symptom production that is motivated by "secondary gains" such as financial compensation, disability claims, evading criminal prosecution, etc. Malingering is categorized as a "condition of interest" rather than as a psychiatric disorder *per se*. The DSM states that a "strong suspicion" of malingering is warranted when at least two of the following four circumstances are present in a patient with medically unexplained symptoms: (1) medicolegal context of presentation; (2) marked discrepancy between claimed stress or disability and objective findings; (3) lack of cooperation in diagnostic process and in compliance with treatment regimen; and (4) presence of antisocial personality disorder. This model has been criticized as vague, moralistic, and not validated. [55]

Despite the growth of literature on the subject, the framework in the DSM for evaluating suspected malingering has not changed in 30 years. Berry and Nelson propose that a revised diagnostic scheme be based on empirically based criteria for detecting false symptom reports using validated tools. [56]

Prevalence

The DSM does not provide an estimated prevalence of malingering. In a review of detection of exaggerated pain-related disability, Fishbain *et al.* report that malingering exists in 1.25%–10.4% of disability claims secondary to chronic pain. Given the poor quality of studies reported, Fishbain also cautions against the reliability of these prevalence figures. [57] There are reports of prevalence rates of malingering in 20%–50% in chronic pain patients with financial motives, depending on the clinical method and rating scales used for detection of malingering. [58] Of this subset of patients, 26.3% report chronic headache. [58]

Management

Little has been written about the management of malingering. The general principles include refusal to provide the secondary gain sought by the patient and confrontation of the patient with evidence that the symptoms are malingered when such evidence is available. Confrontation may help in directing the patient to seek care for comorbid psychiatric illness, but as the "patient's" intention is to deceive the physician rather than to form a therapeutic alliance, the likelihood of successful referral is low. Documenting evidence of malingering is key in communicating with other providers who treat the same patient.

Approach to the patient

Screening

Given the high comorbidity of headache and psychiatric disorders, clinicians evaluating headache patients should be alert for the presence of a psychiatric disorder, including somatoform disorders. Psychiatric tools, such as the PRIME-MD, utilize a short self-report questionnaire followed up with semi-structured interview questions. Answers in the affirmative to somatic complaints can serve as an effective screening measure. More detailed structured interviews for psychiatric diagnosis such as the Mini-International Neuropsychiatric Inventory (MINI) provide more information but require more time to administer and may be better reserved for selected patients. [59]

Common principles of management

The basic principles of management are similar for all somatoform disorders and the most important goal is to care for the patient rather than cure the patient. The headache patient with a somatoform disorder is more likely to seek neurological care than psychiatric care, and the neurologist's stance in the management of these symptoms is crucial. In a classic study, Smith and colleagues conducted psychiatric evaluations of a large series of patients with multiple medically unexplained symptoms. [45] Patients are randomized to control and intervention groups. In the control condition, the patient's primary physician receives a brief letter from the study staff simply thanking him or her for permitting the study team to meet with the patient. In the intervention condition, the patient's physician receives a letter from the study staff giving the diagnosis of somatization disorder (when appropriate) and outlining principles of management including: scheduling appointments on a regular basis rather than driven by symptoms; physical examination at every visit; inquiry into other aspects of the patient's life and functioning at every visit; acknowledgment of the symptoms as a real problem for the patient along with encouragement about improving function as best as possible despite symptoms; and conservative treatment with avoidance of invasive procedures unless dictated by objective findings. At 2-year follow-up, subjects assigned to the intervention group, compared with those in the comparison group, have decreased health care utilization, fewer emergency room visits, fewer hospitalization days, and decreased health care costs, with no decrement in objective measures of health status. In a subsequent review, Kroenke and colleagues find this pattern of outcomes, improved functional status rather than decreased psychological distress or somatic symptoms, and decreased health care utilization and costs. This is replicated in three of the four additional trials. [17] Successful management requires that the patients believe they are being taken seriously and that the physician does not underestimate the patients' distress. Feedback to patients must be provided in a supportive non-judgmental way. The process of helping patients recognize links between physical symptoms and psychological factors, with reattribution of symptoms to psychological stress, can generally occur only gradually, if at all. [60] When patients feel that the relationship with their physician is secure, it may be possible to introduce cognitive-behavioral therapy approaches to improve function and self-management.

Cognitive behavioral therapy

Reviews of the treatment of somatoform disorders [17] and of medically unexplained symptoms [61] both conclude that cognitive behavioral therapy is the treatment with the best-established evidence for effectiveness. Cognitive-behavioral treatments include a focus on behavior modification as well as an emphasis on modifying maladaptive patterns of thinking. The goal is to increase the patient's self-efficacy and thus improve clinical outcomes. The core elements for management of somatoform disorders and headaches include: (1) patient education; (2) collaborative approach; (3) self-monitoring; (4) problem-solving; (5) cognitive restructuring; (6) behavioral assignments and action plans; and (7) breathing and relaxation training.

Patient education

Patients can be educated about their diagnosis, using the bio-psycho-social model as a framework. Explaining a patient's genetic predisposition based on history and the role of stressors in the environment in symptom trigger and exacerbation should be attempted. Aiding the individual to learn about cognitive distortions and restructuring is also important.

Patient–provider partnership and collaborative care

A collaborative care approach relies heavily on joint decision making about treatment, recognizing that the everyday responsibilities of chronic illness fall mostly on the patient. This approach empowers the patient with concrete problem solving and coping skills by optimizing medication adherence, identifying and responding to triggers, making and maintaining lifestyle changes, coping with affective distress associated with chronic illness, and improving stress management. This is all done in the service of improving functioning and limiting disability. [1]

Self-monitoring

Self-monitoring is a well-known concept in headache management. Headache logs are recommended for assessing episode frequency, intensity, and other associated symptoms. The log enables the patient to identify triggers and to monitor self-management efforts. With regular review and feedback by the provider, self-monitoring contributes to self-awareness and review of progress. [1]

Problem solving

Self-monitoring also helps in identifying problems patients have in illness management. A therapist can then work with the patient to come up with techniques to improve decision making and adapt behaviors to fit varying circumstances. Building on identified triggers for symptoms, the patients can identify past maladaptive responses and generate alternative solutions. [1]

Behavioral assignments/action plans

Homework is an integral component of CBT. Patients are not only expected to work on materials required for the next session such as mood, headache and symptom logs, but also to put together information and skills learned in previous sessions to build action plans. An example might be, "When I have a feeling of tingling and fullness in my scalp, rather than going to the ER, or taking extra Ativan, I will first go for a 15-minute walk." Building action plans helps to consolidate newly acquired skills and puts them in context for the patient.

Cognitive restructuring

Cognitive distortions include irrational and unfounded modes of thinking. These include catastrophizing, overgeneralization, dismissing the positive, exaggerating the negative, and all-or-nothing thinking. A headache patient might think, "My head feels numb. I must have bad blood circulation to the brain." He catastrophically attributes his sensation of numbness to vascular disease, without evidence and without considering alternative hypotheses or the evidence that would support or refute his ideas. Once patients have learned to label these distortions, the next step is to challenge and learn to change these maladaptive ways of thinking. The patient described above, might progress to the thought. "My head feels numb; in the past I jumped to the conclusion that I had bad circulation and was dying, but now I can see that this happens when I am nervous, and it does not mean I am having a stroke. Practicing relaxation skills now might help the sensation go away." Cognitive restructuring teaches patients to change their reaction to situations by counteracting stress-generating distorted thoughts by identifying and challenging the accuracy of the underlying inaccurate beliefs. [1]

Relaxation and breathing retraining

Relaxation and breathing retraining are typically used in conjunction with cognitive therapies to teach patients control over physiological responses and lower sympathetic arousal. Abdominal breathing, progressive muscle relaxation, and biofeedback are common techniques. [1]

Summary and conclusions

Headaches can present as a symptom of somatoform disorders and deception syndromes. Such headaches can be a diagnostic and management challenge. Comorbidity is common with other psychiatric disorders, frequently with depression and anxiety. Management strategies for symptom control cut across the various disorders and emphasize support and empathy towards the patient, good communication between different providers, protecting the patient from undue testing and procedures, treating comorbid psychiatric disorders, and utilizing CBT for symptom control. Medications, especially narcotics, should be used sparingly.

References

[1] Lipchik GL, Smitherman TA, Donald B. Penzien DB, Holroyd KA. Basic principles and techniques of cognitive-behavioral therapies for comorbid psychiatric symptoms among headache patients. *Headache* 2006; **46** :S119–32.

[2] The International Headache Society. http://ihsclassification.org/en/02_klassifikation/03_teil2/12.00.00_psychiatric.html (Accessed May 28th 2012).

[3] Ford CV, Folks DG. Conversion disorder: an overview *Psychosomatics* 1985; **26**: 371–83.

[4] Lane RD. Neural substrates of implicit and explicit emotional processes: a unifying framework for psychosomatic medicine. *Psychosom Med.* 2008; **70**: 214–31.

[5] Barsky AJ, Goodson JD, Lane RS, Cleary PD The amplification of somatic symptoms *Psychosom Medi* 1988 **50**: 510–19.

[6] Nakao M, Barsky AJ. Clinical application of somatosensory amplification in psychosomatic medicine. *Biopsychosoc Med* 2007 **9**; 1: 17.

[7] Duddu V, Isaac MK, Chaturvedi SK. Somatization, somatosensory amplification, attribution styles and illness behavior: a review. *Int Rev of Psychiatry* 2006 **18**:1 25–33.

[8] American Psychiatric Association DSM -5 Development. http://www.dsm5.org/ProposedRevision/Pages/SomaticSymptomDisorders.aspx (Accessed May 29 2012).

[9] Slater E: Diagnosis of hysteria. *BMJ* 1965; **1**: 1395–9.

[10] Stone J, Smyth R, Carson A, *et al.* Systematic review of misdiagnosis of conversion symptoms and "hysteria." *BMJ* 2005 29; **331**: 989.

[11] Lazare A. Current concepts in psychiatry. Conversion symptoms. *N Engl J Med* 1981 **24**;305:745–8.

[12] Engel GL. "Psychogenic" pain and the pain-prone patient. *Am J Med* 1959; **26**: 899–918.

[13] *Diagnostic and Statistical Manual of Mental Disorders*, 4th edn Text Revision. APA, 2000.

[14] Toone BK. Disorders of hysterical conversion, In C Bass, ed. *Somatization: Physical Symptoms and Psychological Illness*. Boston, MA: Blackwell Scientific, 1990, pp 207–34.

[15] Stone J, Carson A, Duncan R, *et al.* Symptoms 'unexplained by organic disease' in 1144 new neurology out-patients: how often does the diagnosis change at follow-up? *Brain*. 2009; **132**: 2878–88.

[16] Ettinger AB, Devinsky O, Weisbrot DM, Goyal A, Shashikumar S Headaches and other pain symptoms among patients with psychogenic non-epileptic seizures. *Seizures* 1999; **8**: 424–6.

[17] Kroenke K. Efficacy of treatment for somatoform disorders: a review of randomized controlled trials. *Psychosom Med* 2007; **69**: 881–8.

[18] Stone J, Zeman A, Simonotto E, *et al.* FMRI in patients with motor conversion symptoms and controls with simulated weakness. *Psychosom Med* 2007; **69**: 961–9.

[19] Hinson VK, Weinstein S, Bernard B, Leurgans SE, Goetz CG Single-blind clinical trial of psychotherapy for treatment of psychogenic movement disorders. *Parkinsonism Rel Disord* 2006; **12**: 177–80.

[20] Ruddy R House A. Psychosocial interventions for conversion disorder. *Cochrane Database Syst Revi* 2005 **19**;CD005331.

[21] Poole NA, Wuerz A, Agrawal N. Abreaction for conversion disorder: systematic review with meta-analysis. *Br J Psychiatry* 2010; **197**: 91–5.

[22] Verhaak PF, Kerssens JJ, Dekker J, Sorbi MJ, Bensing JM Prevalence of chronic benign pain disorder among adults: a review of the literature *Pain* 1998; **77**: 231–9.

[23] Fröhlich C, Jacobi F, Wittchen HU. DSM-IV pain disorder in the general population. An exploration of the structure and threshold of medically unexplained pain symptoms. *Europ Arch Clin Psychiatry* 2006; **256**: 187–96.

[24] Adler R, Zamboni P, Hofer T, Hemmeler W. How not to miss a somatic needle in a haystack of chronic pain. *Journal of Psychosom Res* 1997 **42**: 499–505.

[25] Roditi D, Robinson ME. The role of psychological interventions in the management of patients with chronic pain. *Psychol Res Behav Managem* 2011; **4**: 41–9.

[26] American Academy of Pain Medicine http://www.painmed.org/ (Accessed May 27, 2012).

[27] American Pain Society http://www.ampainsoc.org/resources/clinician.htm (Accessed May 27, 2012).

[28] Passik SD, Weinreb HJ. Managing chronic nonmalignant pain: Overcoming obstacles to the use of opioids. *Adv Ther* 2000; **17**: 70–83.

[29] Fishbain DA, Cole B, Lewis J, Rosomoff HL, Rosomoff RS What percentage of chronic nonmalignant pain patients exposed to chronic opioid analgesic therapy develop abuse/addiction and/or aberrant drug-related behaviors? A structured evidence-based review *Pain Med* 2008; **9**: 444–59.

[30] Gourlay DL, Heit HA, Almahrezi A. Universal precautions in pain medicine: a rational approach to the treatment of chronic pain. *Pain Med* 2005; **6**: 107–12.

[31] McCleane G. Antidepressants as analgesics. *CNS Drugs* 2008; **22**: 139–56.

[32] Jackson JL, Shimeall W, Sessums L, *et al.* Tricyclic antidepressants and headaches: systematic review and meta-analysis. *BMJ* 2010; **20**: c5222.

[33] Smitherman TA, Walters AB, Maizels M, Penzien DB The use of antidepressants for headache prophylaxis *CNS Neurosci therape* 2011; **17**: 462–9.

[34] Adelman LC, Adelman JU, Von Seggern R, Mannix LK Venlafaxine extended release (XR) for the prophylaxis of migraine and tension-type headache: A retrospective study in a clinical setting. *Headache* 2000; **40**: 572–80.

[35] Bellingham GA, Peng PW Duloxetine: a review of its pharmacology and use in chronic pain management. *Reg Anesth Pain Medi* 2010; **35**: 294–303.

[36] D'Amico D. Antiepileptic drugs in the prophylaxis of migraine, chronic headache forms and cluster headache: a review of their efficacy and tolerability. *Neurol Scie* 2007; **28**: S188–97.

[37] National Center for Complementary and Alternative Medicine Bethesda (MD): National Institutes of Health; 2011 updated 2011 Jun 20; cited 2010 Dec 20.

[38] Barnes PM, Bloom B, Nahin RL Complementary and alternative medicine use among adults and children: United States, 2007. *Nat Hlth Stati Rep* 2008; **10**: 1–23.

[39] Wells RE, Bertisch SM, Buettner C, Phillips RS, McCarthy EP Complementary and alternative medicine use among adults with migraines/severe headaches *Headache*, 2011; **51**: 1087–97.

[40] Söderberg EI, Carlsson JY, Stener-Victorin E, Dahlöf C Subjective well-being in patients with chronic tension-type headache: effect of acupuncture, physical training, and relaxation training. *Clin J Pain* 2011; **27**: 448–56.

[41] Escobar JI, Manu P, Matthews D, Lane T, Swartz M, Canino G Medically unexplained physical symptoms, somatization disorder and abridged somatization: studies with the Diagnostic Interview Schedule. *Psychiatric Dev* 1989; **7**(3):235–45.

[42] Radat F, Milowska D, Valade D. Headaches secondary to psychiatric disorders (HSPD): a retrospective study of 87 patients *Headache* 2011; **51**: 789–95.

[43] Kato K, Sullivan PF, Pedersen NL Latent class analysis of functional somatic symptoms in a population-based sample of twins. *J Psychosom Res* 2010; **68**: 447–53.

[44] Kronke K, Spitzer RL, Williams JBW, *et al.* Physical symptoms in primary care: predictors of psychiatric disorders and functional impairment. *Arch Fam Med* 1994; **3**: 774–9.

[45] Smith GR, Jr., Monson RA, Ray DC. Psychiatric consultation in somatization disorder. A randomized controlled study. *N Engl J Med* 1986; **314**: 1407–13.

[46] Creed F, Barsky A. A systematic review of the epidemiology of somatization disorder and hypochondriasis. *J Psychosom Res* 2004; **56**: 391–408.

[47] Greeven A, van Balkom AJ, Visser S, *et al.* Cognitive behavior therapy and paroxetine in the treatment of hypochondriasis: arandomized controlled trial. *The Am J Psychiatry* 2007; **164**: 91–9.

[48] Walker J, Vincent N, Furer P, Cox B, Kjernisted K Treatment preference in hypochondriasis. *J Behav Ther Expe Psychiatry* 1999; **30**: 251–8.

[49] Thomson AB, Page LA Psychotherapies for hypochondriasis. *Cochrane Database Syst Rev* 2007; **17**: CD006520.

[50] Kanaan RA, Wessely SC Factitious disorders in neurology: an analysis of reported cases *Psychosomatics* 2010; **51**: 47–54.

[51] Solomon S, Lipton RB Headaches and face pains as a manifestation of Munchausen syndrome *Headache* 1999; **39**: 45–50.

[52] Reich P, Gottfried LA. Factitious disorders in a teaching hospital. *Ann Intern Med* 1983; **99**: 240–7.

[53] Kwan P, Lynch S, Davy A. Munchausen's syndrome with concurrent neurological and psychiatric presentations *J Roy Soc Med* 1997; **90**: 83–5.

[54] Yassa R. Munchausen's syndrome: a successfully treated case. *Psychosomatics* 1978; **19**: 242–3.

[55] Rogers R Development of a new classificatory model of malingering *Bull Am Acade Psychiatry Law* 1990; **18**: 323–33.

[56] Berry TR, Nelson NW DSM V and malingering : a modest proposal. *Psychol Injury Law* 2010; **3**, 295–303.

[57] Fishbain DA, Cutler R, Rosomoff HL, Rosomoff RS Chronic pain disability exaggeration/malingering and submaximal effort research. *Clin J Pain* 1999; **15**: 244–74.

[58] Greve KW, Ord JS, Bianchini KJ, Curtis KL Prevalence of malingering in patients with chronic pain referred for psychologic evaluation in a medico-legal context *Arch Phys Med Rehab* 2009; **90**: 1117–26.

[59] Maizels M, Smitherman TA, Penzien DB. A review of screening tools for psychiatric comorbidity in headache patients *Headache* 2006; **46** :S98–109.

[60] Goldberg D, Gask L, O'Dowd T. The treatment of somatization: teaching techniques of reattribution. *J Psychosom Res* 1989; **33**: 689–95.

[61] Sumathipala A. What is the evidence for the efficacy of treatments for somatoform disorders? A critical review of previous intervention studies. *Psychosom Med* 2007; **69**: 889–900.

Index